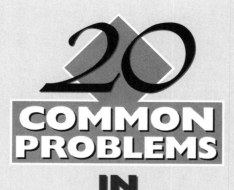

20 COMMON PROBLEMS

IN

Gastroenterology

EDITOR

STEVEN A. EDMUNDOWICZ, M.D.

Associate Professor of Medicine
Chief of Endoscopy
Director of Interventional Endoscopy
Division of Gastroenterology
Washington University School of Medicine
St. Louis, Missouri

SERIES EDITOR

BARRY D. WEISS, M.D.

Professor of Clinical Family and Community Medicine
University of Arizona College of Medicine
Tucson, Arizona

McGraw-Hill

Medical Publishing Division

New York   Chicago   San Francisco   Lisbon   London   Madrid   Mexico City
Milan   New Delhi   San Juan   Seoul   Singapore   Sydney   Toronto

McGraw-Hill

*A Division of The **McGraw·Hill** Companies*

ISBN 0-07-022055-7

This book was set in Garamond by V&M Graphics, Inc.
The editors were Susan R. Noujaim, Andrea Seils, and Regina Brown.
The production supervisor was Catherine Saggese.
The cover was designed by Marsha Cohen/Parallelogram.
The index was prepared by Jerry Ralya.
R.R. Donnelly & Sons was the printer and binder.

Library of Congress Cataloging-in-Publication Data

20 common problems in gastroenterology / editor, Steven Edmundowicz.
    p. ; cm.
  Includes bibliographical references and index.
  ISBN 0-07-022055-7
  1. Gastrointestinal system—Diseases. 2. Primary care (Medicine) I. Title:
Twenty common problems in gastroenterology. II. Edmundowicz, Steven.
  [DNLM: 1. Gastrointestinal Diseases—diagnosis. 2. Gastrointestinal
Diseases—therapy. WI 143 Z999 2002]
RC801.A12 2002
616.3′3—dc21   2001030900

To my wife, Annemarie, who constantly provides love, encouragement, humor and guidance for me and our four children, Bobby, Cara, Ryan and Brent. Without her presence and support this project and many others would never come to fruition and our family's journey in life could never be as interesting or pleasurable.

*—**Steven A. Edmundowicz**—*

Contents

Contributors

ABNORMAL LIVER FUNCTION TESTS (CHAPTER 19)

Minhhuyen T. Nguyen, MD
Clinical Assistant Professor of Medicine
MCP Hahneman University
Division of Gastroenterology
Graduate Hospital
Philadelphia, PA

ACUTE ABDOMINAL PAIN (CHAPTER 7)

Mohan Charan, MD, MRCP (UK)
Felllow in Gastroenterology
Graduate Hospital
Philadelphia, PA

Steven A. Edmundowicz, MD
Assistant Professor of Medicine
Chief of Endoscopy
Director of Interventional Endoscopy
Division of Gastroenterology
Washington University School of Medicine
St. Louis, MO

ACUTE DIARRHEA IN ADULTS (CHAPTER 12)

David D. K. Rolston, MD, FACP
Clinical Assistant Professor of Medicine
Co-Program Director Internal Medicine Residency Program
MCP Hahneman University
Graduate Hospital
Philadelphia, PA

ACUTE LOWER GASTROINTESTINAL BLEEDING (CHAPTER 9)

Chandra Prakash, MD, MRCP (UK)
Assistant Professor of Medicine
Division of Gastroenterology
Washington University School of Medicine
St. Louis, MO

ACUTE UPPER GASTROINTESTINAL BLEEDING (CHAPTER 8)

Mary F. Chan, MD
Assistant Professor of Medicine
Division of Gastroenterology
Washington University School of Medicine
St. Louis, MO

ANAL PAIN (CHAPTER 15)

James Fleshman, MD
Professor of Surgery
Director of Colorectal Surgery
Washington University School of Medicine
St. Louis, MO

BILIARY OBSTRUCTION (CHAPTER 20)

Marc Bernstein, MD
Digestive Disease Medical Consultants PC
Missouri Baptist Hospital
St. Lukes Hospital
St Louis, MO

CHRONIC ADDOMINAL PAIN: THE FUNCTIONAL GASTROINTESTINAL DISORDERS (CHAPTER 6)

Pradip Cheran, MD, MRCP (UK)
Attending Physician
Doylestown Hospital
Doylestown, PA

Susan Gordon, M.D.
Professor of Medicine
MCP Hahneman University
Division of Gastroenterology
Graduate Hospital
Philadelphia, PA

COLORECTAL CANCER SCREENING (CHAPTER 14)

David S. Weinberg, MD, MSc
Associate Professor of Medicine
Temple University School of Medicine
Director of Gastroenterology
Fox Chase Cancer Center
Philadelphia, PA

Christine Laine, MD, MPH
Clinical Associate Professor of Medicine
Jefferson Medical College
Thomas Jefferson University
Philadelphia, PA

CONSTIPATION (CHAPTER 13)

Dordaneh Maleki, MD, FACP
Atlantic Gastroenterology Associates PA
Egg Harbor Township, NJ

DYSPEPSIA (CHAPTER 5)

Alan M. Adelman, MD, MS
Professor Department of Family and Community Medicine
Penn State University College of Medicine
Hershey, PA

DYSPHAGIA (CHAPTER 3)

Richard Lynn, MD
Associate Professor of Medicine
Division of Gastroenterology and Hepatology
Jefferson Medical College
Thomas Jefferson University
Philadelphia, PA

FLATULENCE (CHAPTER 11)

Anita C. Lee, MD
Clinical Assistant Professor of Medicine
MCP Hahneman University
Graduate Hospital
Philadelphia, PA

HEARTBURN (CHAPTER 1)

Philip O. Katz, MD
Kimbel Professor and Chairman
Department of Medicine
Chief, Division of Gastroenterology
Graduate Hospital
Philadelphia, PA

LIVER MASSES (CHAPTER 18)

Yogesh K. Govil, MD, MRCP (UK)
Fellow in Gastroenterology
Graduate Hospital
Philadelphia, PA

Minhhuyen T. Nguyen, MD
Clinical Assistant Professor of Medicine
MCP Hahneman University
Division of Gastroenterology
Graduate Hospital
Philadelphia, PA

NAUSEA AND VOMITING (CHAPTER 2)

Debra Feldman, MD
Clinical Associate Professor of Medicine
MCP Hahneman University
Division Chief
General Internal Medicine
Graduate Hospital
Philadelphia, PA

OCCULT BLEEDING AND IRON DEFICIENCY ANEMIA (CHAPTER 10)

Sreenivasa S. Jonnalagadda, MD
Assistant Professor of Medicine
Division of Gastroenterology
Washington University School of Medicine
St. Louis, MO

RIGHT UPPER QUADRANT PAIN: GALLBLADDER DISEASE AND ITS COMPLICATIONS (CHAPTER 17)
Cheryl A. Cox, MD
Fellow in Gastroenterology
University of Virginia Health Sciences Center
Charlottesville, VA

Stephen J. Bickston, MD
Assistant Professor of Medicine
Division of Gastroenterology
University of Virginia Health Sciences Center
Charlottesville, VA

VIRAL HEPATITIS (CHAPTER 16)
Saeed Zamani, MD
Fellow in Gastroenterology
Jefferson Medical College
Philadelphia, PA

Steven K. Herrine, MD
Clinical Associate Professor of Medicine
Division of Gastroenterology and Hepatology
Thomas Jefferson University
Philadelphia, PA

WEIGHT LOSS (CHAPTER 4)
Arun Khazanchi, MD
Fellow in Gastroenterology
Graduate Hospital
Philadelphia, PA

Steven A. Edmundowicz, MD
Associate Professor of Medicine
Chief of Endoscopy
Director of Interventional Endoscopy
Division of Gastroenterology
Washington University School of Medicine
St. Louis, MO.

Preface

As medical information continues to expand, the task of managing and applying this information in particular clinical settings becomes more challenging. 20 Common Problems in Gastroenterology is another key text in the McGraw-Hill's *20 Common Problems* series that provides concise, practical information for health care professionals. This text focuses on the most common gastroenterologic problems encountered in a primary practice setting and represents a selection of 20 clinical issues that every practitioner of primary care and general Gastroenterology will encounter on a regular basis. The chapters of the text are organized to allow rapid access to the information necessary to evaluate and treat most patients with these problems.

The text is organized into three sections: general Gastroenterology, gastrointestinal bleeding, and hepatic & biliary problems. Each chapter is based on a problem or typical patient presentation in Gastroenterology. The chapters are intended to follow the same general headings for each problem. Familiarity with this structure allows the reader to quickly find similar information regarding different problems. The chapter outline provides a quick reference guide to direct the reader to specific headings

of interest. In addition to the text, most chapters contain a diagnostic and treatment algorithm to provide a general approach to the typical patient presentation. Each chapter contains selected references to guide the interested reader to more detailed information.

The algorithm and treatment recommendations in this book are provided by authors who are clinically active and use this information in their practice of medicine. By design, algorithms are generalized approaches to specific problems and will not necessarily always provide the most direct or ideal evaluation for a particular patient's condition. However, they are useful guides for evaluating common problems, which is in line with the major goal of this text. One should also be cautioned that practice guidelines and algorithms should be, and in fact are, heavily influenced by evidence-based medicine. This implies that guidelines could change rapidly and dramatically if well-designed studies are suddenly available. The most recent advances in clinical Gastroenterology have been incorporated into this text; in the future, additional progress will undoubtedly change the approach to some of the 20 problems discussed.

Acknowledgements

While this is a work of many, I owe a special thanks to those key individuals who made this text a reality. Dr. Barry Weiss initiated this entire series and personally reviewed each contribution to this text. His enthusiasm and energy for this series has been an inspiration to all involved. I must also thank the many authors and their secretarial staffs who generously contributed their work to this project. Without their time and effort (much of which came from "free nights and weekends") this text would never have materialized. Special thanks to Susan Noujaim and the McGraw-Hill editorial staff who kept us all on target despite our many moves and missed deadlines. Finally, special recognition to Karen Miklosey, Dianne Oliver, and most importantly, Julie Wood who have provided outstanding secretarial support to me and my office during this entire process.

Steven A. Edmundowicz, M.D.

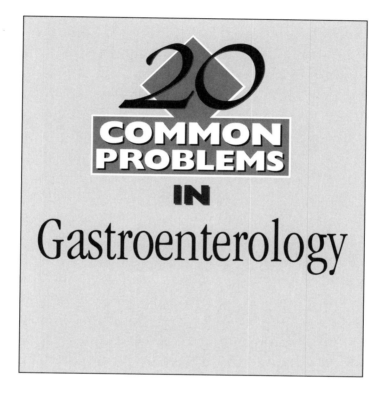

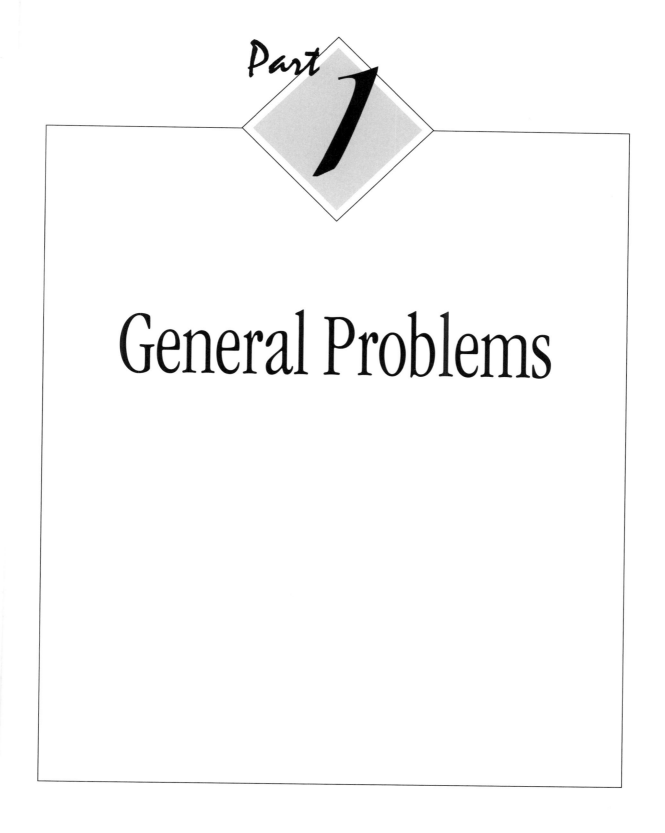

Part 1

General Problems

Philip O. Katz, M.D.

Heartburn

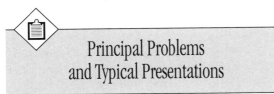

How Common Is Heartburn?

Heartburn and acid indigestion affect at least 95 million Americans monthly. Over $1 billion of over-the-counter therapies are consumed in the United States yearly. Many would agree this is the most common symptom seen in clinical practice. Close to 1 million cardiac catheterizations are performed in the United States yearly. Of these, 10 to 30 percent are normal, making unexplained or noncardiac chest pain a common diagnosis. Both are common symptoms of gastroesophageal reflux disease (GERD). The gastrointestinal causes of chest pain, with a focus on GERD, will be presented in this chapter.

Principal Problems and Typical Presentations

Gastroesophageal Reflux Disease

Heartburn is the primary symptom of GERD, occurring daily in 7 to 10 percent of the U.S. population. Of these, 25 to 50 percent will have intermittent heartburn at least monthly. Heartburn occurs in 33 percent of pregnant women. The recent explosion in the over-the-counter H_2-receptor antagonist (H_2RA) market underscores the importance of this symptom in the lives of our patients. Close to 80 percent of the over-the-counter antacid usage in the United States is for heartburn and/or acid regurgitation.

The patient with heartburn will describe a burning sensation under the breastbone with radiation up toward the throat or mouth, which occurs shortly after meals, with heavy lifting, or upon bending over. Large meals, spicy foods, citrus products, high-fat meals, colas, coffee, teas, and beer have an acidic pH and will exacerbate symptoms. Meals close to bedtime or alcohol with meals may increase nighttime symptoms. Symptoms may be relieved with an over-the-counter antacid preparation, H_2RA, and often by drinking water. Regurgitation—the spontaneous feeling of acid or a bitter taste in the chest or mouth—may accompany heartburn and is a distinct symptom. GERD may present with nonspecific upper gastrointestinal symptoms, such as nausea, dyspepsia, bloating, belching, or indigestion. These symptoms lack specificity for GERD in the absence of predominant heartburn or acid regurgitation. Waterbrash—the sudden filling of the mouth with a clear, salty fluid—is not heartburn. Waterbrash reflects the increase in salivary secretion seen as a reflex response to reflux or regurgitation of gastric acid into an inflamed distal esophagus.

Heartburn is often described in patients with achalasia. Fermentation of undigested food resulting in an acidic pH coupled with esophageal inflammation causes a heartburn-like sensation in the absence of true GERD. With this major exception, if heartburn is the only presenting esophageal symptom, GERD is the diagnosis.

The clinician must be aware that neither the frequency nor severity of heartburn correlates with the severity of GERD. Severe disease, including Barrett's esophagus and peptic strictures, may present with infrequent or absent complaints of heartburn, while many patients with daily heartburn have no endoscopic abnormalities. Patients with extraesophageal manifestations of GERD (chronic cough, asthma, hoarseness, etc.) often have minimal to no heartburn. It has been reported that patients commonly do not understand the term *heartburn*; in one series only 70 percent of patients who complained of heartburn were thought to have classic heartburn after questioning. In the same series, 23 percent of patients who initially denied heartburn were believed to have symptoms consistent with true heartburn on further interview.

Regurgitation is defined as the effortless return of gastric contents into the esophagus and, more frequently, into the mouth. It is often associated with heartburn and GERD. If the two symptoms present together, the diagnosis of GERD is likely.

Regurgitation without heartburn should raise suspicion of Barrett's esophagus (because of reduced acid sensitivity), achalasia, or anatomic obstruction. Regurgitation is a prominent symptom, in patients with extraesophageal manifestations of GERD, particularly pulmonary symptoms, and is an important prognostic factor for predicting outcome of therapy. Patients with regurgitation are more likely to respond to proton-pump inhibitors (PPI). Regurgitation is not vomiting. The absence of nausea is the major distinguishing feature between these two symptoms.

There are many so-called extraesophageal or atypical presentations of GERD. Up to 75 percent of asthmatics will have associated GERD, independent of bronchodilator use. Suspicion should be highest in patients with adult-onset asthma and nocturnal asthma, those wheezing after a large meal or an alcohol binge, or in patients with unresponsive or nonallergic asthma. The third most common cause of chronic cough with a normal chest x-ray is GERD. A large number of patients with chronic laryngitis, posterior pharyngitis, or sore throat may also have GERD. Apthous ulcers, erosion of dental enamel, and chronic nausea have been associated with GERD. Heartburn and regurgitation are infrequent and may even be absent. Patients presenting with essential or non-ulcer dyspepsia may also have GERD. A high index of suspicion is required.

Myocardial Ischemia or Infarction

Recurrent substernal chest pain indistinguishable from cardiac angina may be due to an esophageal etiology. A key point is that the medical history itself cannot be used to exclude cardiac disease or rule in an esophageal cause for recurring substernal chest pain. A cardiac etiology of the presentation must be considered and excluded before considering esophageal disease. The presence of heartburn and/or dysphagia increases the likelihood of an esophageal etiology. Pain occurring with or after meals, in the supine position, lasting greater than 1 h, and/or awakening the patient

from sleep suggests esophageal pain. Further specific cardiac diagnostic testing is indicated if there is any suggestion of a cardiac etiology of the chest pain. While up to 50 percent of patients with non-cardiac recurrent chest pain will have GERD, all of the esophageal etiologies of chest pain should be considered after cardiac etiologies have been excluded.

Esophageal Motility Disorders and Hypersensitivity

Esophageal motility abnormalities can be seen in patients with chest pain who do not have GERD or angina. These include nutcracker esophagus, diffuse esophageal spasm, hypertensive lower esophageal sphincter, and ineffective esophageal motility. There are many patients with chest pain who have neither a definable motility disorder nor a documented GERD in whom chest pain can be provoked with either intraesophageal balloon distension or by the injection of edrophonium (Tensilon), a cholinesterase inhibitor that augments esophageal contraction amplitude and duration. These patients are suspected to have a "hypersensitive" or "irritable" esophagus.

Other Causes of Chest Pain

The differential diagnosis of chest pain is quite broad and encompasses many other areas of medicine that are beyond the scope of this chapter. However, several life-threatening diagnoses should be mentioned and promptly excluded in those patients who present with the appropriate clinical symptoms. While pulmonary diseases including pulmonary embolus, pneumothorax, and malignancies typically present with shortness of breath, this can be absent initially. Vascular disorders including aortic dissection should also be considered and excluded. Rarely pericarditis or myocarditis may present with chest pain as the initial manifestation.

Occasionally, other gastrointestinal disorders can lead to symptoms of chest pain. Gallbladder disease and acute cholecystitis may present with vague chest discomfort. Rarely, acute pancreatitis and complications of chronic pancreatitis may also lead to chest symptoms. Finally, individuals with rare disorders of the esophagus, including those with spontaneous perforation, infectious esophagitis, Crohn's disease, or even malignancy, will have chest pain.

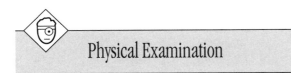

Physical Examination

The physical examination in patients with heartburn, unexplained chest pain, and GERD is usually normal unless there is coexisting systemic disease. Patients with extraesophageal symptoms will exhibit abnormalities in the organ of presenting symptoms. For example, patients with asthma will have pulmonary findings typical of someone with asthma. Patients with otolaryngologic symptoms will have vocal cord edema and erythema. Physical examination of patients with throat and voice complaints must be comprehensive. A thorough head and neck examination is always included, with attention to the ears and hearing, nasal patency, oral cavity and temporomandibular joints, signs of allergy, larynx, and neck. At least a limited general physical examination is included to look for signs of systemic dysfunction that may present as throat or voice complaints.

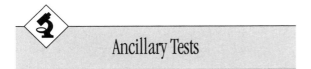

Ancillary Tests

Endoscopy

Endoscopy is performed in the evaluation of patients with heartburn, GERD, and chest pain for the following reasons: to exclude other diseases or complications when symptoms are not clear cut or have alarms, such as signs of bleeding, dysphagia, or weight loss; to screen for Barrett's esophagus in patients with long-standing symptoms; to diagnose and grade the severity of esophagitis; and to attempt to direct therapy and predict chronicity. Endoscopy for the most part is diagnostic of GERD if erosive esophagitis or Barrett's esophagus is found, although confusion may arise in selected patients with erosive esophagitis resulting from infections or pill-induced injury. Endoscopy is often normal; only 30 to 40 percent of patients undergoing endoscopy for troublesome heartburn will have erosive esophagitis. It has been suggested that the presence of severe esophagitis can guide therapy and help predict the response to treatment, relapse rate, and chronicity. It is unusual to perform endoscopy for this reason. The main problem with grading esophagitis is the lack of an approved standardized classification system. It has been estimated that there are more than 30 endoscopic classification systems reported in the literature, none of which is universally accepted. Many gastroenterologists consider erythema, friability, and blurring of the squamocolumnar junction as criteria for the diagnosis of GERD. This approach increases the sensitivity of endoscopy at the expense of reduced specificity. Another area of controversy is the role of esophageal biopsy in diagnosing GERD. Even though pathologic changes suggestive of GERD have been noted for decades, the value of these abnormalities is limited and not helpful in the evaluation of patients with endoscopy-negative reflux disease. Current recommendations are that endoscopy should be performed in patients with alarm symptoms of dysphagia, weight loss, or bleeding and in patients with suboptimal response to empiric therapy. Patients with reflux symptoms for 5 or more years' duration should be considered for endoscopy to screen for Barrett's esophagus. At present, it is recommended that if Barrett's metaplasia is not seen, repeat endoscopy should not be necessary. When screening for Barrett's esophagus, it is recommended that patients be treated with a proton-pump inhibitor until asymptomatic to minimize the possible erosive or ulcerative changes that might otherwise mask the columnar epithelium and make it more difficult to guide biopsies.

Endoscopy has even lower yield in patients with chest pain. Less than 10 percent of patients with noncardiac chest pain will have abnormal endoscopy, making this test of little use in this population.

Prolonged pH Monitoring

Prolonged ambulatory esophageal pH monitoring has the ability to quantitate esophageal acid exposure and has contributed greatly to the understanding of GERD. The test is currently performed in an ambulatory setting with compact portable data loggers, miniature pH electrodes (<2 mm in diameter), and computerized data analysis. Patients should have unrestricted diets and activities during the monitoring period. Prolonged pH monitoring helps to identify patients with GERD by demonstrating a pathologic or abnormal degree of reflux and allows symptom correlation with reflux events. A pH monitoring of 24 h has been shown to offer a good discrimination between normal controls and patients with esophagitis.

Patients with heartburn rarely require prolonged pH monitoring to make a diagnosis of GERD; however, the procedure is quite useful in patients with this symptom and who appear refractory to antisecretory (or other medical) therapy. Ambulatory pH monitoring, while the patients continue medication, is helpful in determining if esophageal acid exposure continues and if symptoms are associated with GERD. Ambulatory pH monitoring is the diagnostic procedure of choice in patients with unexplained chest pain.

The correlation between reflux and symptoms is of particular use in these patients. Up to 60 percent of patients with unexplained chest pain have demonstrated abnormal esophageal acid exposure or a high-symptom correlation (greater than 50 percent correlation of symptom and reflux events) when studied with ambulatory pH monitoring. The presence of a high-symptom index is predictive of a good response of chest pain to PPIs.

Radiology

Barium esophagograms have been used for the evaluation of GERD and its complications. Barium studies are useful in the evaluation of GERD patients with dysphagia and have a high accuracy for the diagnosis of hiatal hernia, esophageal strictures, and esophageal rings. Barium studies can detect esophagitis with increasing sensitivity as the esophagitis worsens. Radiological studies may suggest Barrett's esophagus by demonstrating a reticular pattern of the mucosa; however, barium studies have a low sensitivity for the diagnosis of GERD when compared with pH monitoring. Therefore, barium studies are of limited use in the evaluation of patients with GERD who do not suffer from dysphagia.

Provocative Testing

Provocative tests attempt to provide proof that patients' symptoms are due to reflux. The Bernstein test involves the infusion of 0.1 N HCl into the esophagus with a saline infusion as placebo. A positive test result is defined as reproduction of patients' typical symptoms with acid perfusion but not with saline. The test is considered to be highly specific in implicating reflux as the cause of symptoms, but has a low sensitivity and is less useful than pH monitoring with symptom-reflux association in the evaluation of patients with unexplained chest pain. The Bernstein test should rarely be performed and is reserved for situations in which pH monitoring is not available or when patients have infrequent symptoms that were not reported during pH monitoring.

Esophageal Manometric Studies

Esophageal manometry has a limited role in the initial evaluation of suspected GERD. Manometry, however, can be useful in situations in which the diagnosis is unclear and can predict severe GERD if a hypotensive lower esophageal sphincter or peristaltic dysfunction is found. It is generally accepted that manometry is needed preoperatively in patients evaluated for fundoplication or endoluminal therapies to assess peristaltic function in the distal esophagus and to decide on the type of the fundoplication or endoscopic procedure to perform.

Therapeutic Trial for Diagnosis

A therapeutic trial is appealing in the evaluation of GERD because it answers one of the most important questions: Is the patient going to improve on therapy directed against GERD? This question is important because there is no true, highly reliable gold standard test for the diagnosis of GERD, and it is possible that patients with GERD are undiagnosed by the available tests. Even though the therapeutic trial has been used clinically for many years, it has not been assessed objectively until recently. The term *omeprazole test* was initially used in 1992 when the symptom response to a single dose of 80 mg of omeprazole compared favorably with the Bernstein test, endoscopy, and pH monitoring in 30 patients with unexplained chest pain. In 1995, a study was performed to assess the value of empiric acid reduction as a diagnostic test for GERD in 33 consecutive patients with GERD symptoms, normal endoscopy, and abnormal pH monitoring. The patients were treated for 1 week to 10 days with ranitidine, 150 mg twice a day, omeprazole, 40 mg daily, and omeprazole, 40 mg twice a day without a placebo arm. A positive test was defined as that which had a 75-percent reduction in symptoms. Omeprazole, 40 mg twice a day, had the best sensitivity (83.3 percent), and all patients on this regimen had reduction in mean acidity on pH monitoring.

Three other groups have reported experience with the omeprazole test in patients with symptoms suggestive of GERD. Another group studied 85 patients with grade 0 or 1 esophagitis and compared the results of pH monitoring with blinded response to either a placebo for 2 weeks or omeprazole, 40 mg daily, for 2 weeks. Response

to omeprazole had sensitivity and specificity similar to pH monitoring. A 1-week course of omeprazole, 20 mg twice a day, versus the placebo in patients with a diagnosis of GERD based on either abnormal pH monitoring or grade 2 or 3 esophagitis revealed treatment with omeprazole had a high sensitivity and a low specificity (75 percent and 55 percent, respectively). Several patients with normal pH monitoring in both studies had symptomatic improvement with omeprazole. Both studies did not include symptom-reflux association in their analysis, and therefore some of the omeprazole responders with normal pH monitoring might have had an acid-sensitive esophagus. Patients with unexplained chest pain have been tested in this manner. All patients underwent endoscopy and 24-h pH and were randomized to either the placebo or omeprazole (40 mg in the morning and 20 mg in the evening for 7 days). Patients were subsequently crossed over to the other arm. The investigators concluded that the omeprazole test had a sensitivity of 78 percent and specificity of 85.7 percent and that it results in cost savings primarily by decreased use of endoscopy. The patients studied, however, had a high incidence of reporting typical GERD symptoms, and approximately 40 percent reported dysphagia. Because endoscopy is not systematically required in the work-up of chest pain and because patients with dysphagia need further testing, the investigators' economic analysis may not be accurate.

There are several limitations for embarking on a therapeutic trial as a diagnostic test for GERD. Perhaps the biggest problem is in masking other diagnoses, such as peptic ulcer disease or a malignancy, by potent acid suppression. Another hazard is failing to diagnose possible Barrett's esophagus and associated dysplasia. These problems can be minimized by using upper endoscopy in suspicious cases and by careful follow-up of those treated with an empiric trial. Another problem is that the most cost-effective regimen and the optimal duration for a therapeutic trial are still unknown. This approach still has not been rigorously tested for patients with extraesophageal manifestations of GERD even though these patients pose a bigger diagnostic dilemma. Nonetheless, in the absence of alarm symptoms, an empiric trial with a PPI is a reasonable and appropriate initial diagnostic test for patients with suspected GERD.

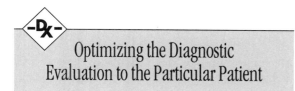

Optimizing the Diagnostic Evaluation to the Particular Patient

Patients presenting with classic symptoms of GERD rarely need confirmatory diagnostic tests. In most cases, a presumptive diagnosis can be established and therapy initiated. Additional testing should be reserved for instances in which a specific clinical question is asked. Table 1-1 summarizes the cost of various tests employed.

If the clinician wishes to know if the esophageal symptoms are due to GERD, ambulatory pH monitoring with reflux-symptom association is the diagnostic test of choice for patients' heartburn or chest pain provided that patients develop symptoms during the recording time. The option to use a diagnostic trial of high-dose omeprazole should be reserved for patients with frequent (more than three times per week) symptoms so rapid response can

Table 1-1

Cost Comparison

Test	Cost (U.S. $)*
Upper endoscopy	497.40
24-h pH	315.74
Esophageal manometry	342.25
Bernstein test	150.00
Barium esophagogram	225.00
Standard dose PPI (8 weeks)	203.28
High-dose PPI	406.56
(8 weeks; twice-daily dose)	

*Estimated from Medicare reimbursement data and typical pharmacy cost to patients. PPI, proton-pump inhibitor

be assessed. In this scenario, pH monitoring (while on therapy) is reserved for patients with poor or incomplete response to medication, and endoscopy is reserved for patients with alarm symptoms and for screening for Barrett's esophagus.

If patients with heartburn or chest pain fail to have symptom relief after a trial of antireflux therapy, the clinician must determine if the initial treatment has been ineffective or the symptoms may not be due to GERD. In this case, prolonged ambulatory pH monitoring is the diagnostic test of choice and should be performed while patients continue on therapy. It is well documented that PPIs given twice daily can fail to suppress gastric acid secretion. Endoscopy may be useful in evaluating patients with a poor response to empiric therapy because finding severe esophagitis justifies using a more intensive treatment.

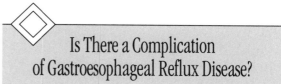

Is There a Complication of Gastroesophageal Reflux Disease?

Endoscopy is the procedure of choice for the identification of GERD complications, such as erosive esophagitis, esophageal ulcer, and Barrett's esophagus and associated dyplasia and adenocarcinoma. Patients with suspected Barrett's esophagus should undergo a systemic biopsy assessment for confirmation of the diagnosis of intestinal metaplasia and dysplasia. An endoscopic surveillance program consisting of endoscopy and biopsy every 2 to 5 years (debate exists as to the precise interval) should be undertaken. Barium studies are helpful in the evaluation of patients with dysphagia.

Summary

Patients with typical symptoms of heartburn or regurgitation require no diagnostic evaluation prior to initiation of the treatment. Endoscopy is indicated in patients suspected of having complicated GERD and in patients with long-standing

symptoms, severe symptoms, and frequent re-
lapses. Barium studies are indicated in patients
with dysphagia. Ambulatory pH monitoring is the
procedure of choice in patients with unexplained
chest pain, pulmonary and otolaryngologic symptoms, and poor response to medical therapy.
Symptom-reflux correlation and dual-probe use
increase the usefulness of pH monitoring. Esophageal manometry is of limited use except under
select circumstances. Given all of the diagnostic
options, a trial of acid suppression with a PPI is

likely the initial test in most patients with heartburn or chest pain and a high suspicion for GERD.

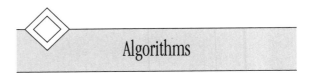

Algorithms

Algorithms for the diagnosis and treatment of
heartburn are depicted in Figures 1-1 and 1-2.

Figure 1-1

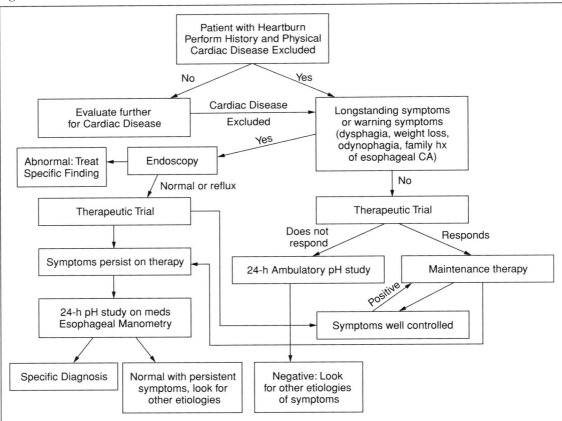

Diagnostic algorithm for patients with heartburn

Figure 1-2

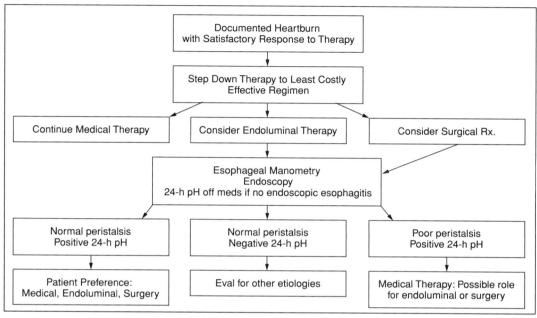

Treatment algorithm for patients with heartburn

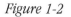

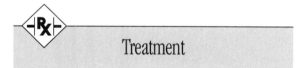

Treatment

Medical Therapy

Treatment should be based on four goals: elimination of symptoms, healing of esophagitis, management and/or prevention of complications, and maintenance of symptomatic relief over time. These goals can be accomplished with an individualized systematic approach to each patient using appropriate lifestyle changes, pharmacology, and antireflux surgery where appropriate.

Nonpharmacologic (Lifestyle) Therapy

Studies have indicated that elevation of the head of the bed, decreased fat intake, cessation of smoking, and avoidance of recumbency for 3 h postprandially all decrease distal esophageal acid exposure. Foods such as chocolate, alcohol, peppermint, and perhaps onions and garlic cause increased esophageal reflux. Coffee, whether caffeinated or not, also tends to promote reflux. Several medications decrease lower esophageal sphincter pressure, but no objective data are available to support improvement in symptoms or esophagitis after discontinuing these medications. Drugs that have been implicated in worsening GERD include, but are not limited to, theophylline, certain prostaglandins, anticholinergics, dopamine, nitrates, meperidine, diazepam, morphine, nitrates, and calcium-channel blockers. Avoiding late meals, following a prudent but not overly restrictive diet, and elevating the head of the bed should be emphasized. Patients should sleep on their left side if possible as this produces less esophageal acid exposure than when sleeping on the right.

These lifestyle modifications may not relieve symptoms in many patients; however, they are of low cost and pose no risk. It is for patients to judge how valuable these changes are in decreasing symptoms.

Patient-Directed Therapy (Over-the-Counter)

A wide variety of heartburn therapies are available without a prescription including simple antacids, antirefluxants, and reduced doses of H_2RAs. Proton-pump inhibitors (PPI) will most likely follow in the next few years.

Antacids and alginic acid are useful for relief of mild heartburn and indigestion, both shown to be more effective than a placebo in the relief of symptoms induced by a heartburn-promoting meal. Combined antacid and alginic acid therapy may be superior to antacids alone in reducing heartburn. These agents do not effectively treat chest pain due to GERD and are not useful as chronic continuous therapy. The comparison of several commonly used antacids is presented in Table 1-2.

The H_2RAs are available over the counter at a dose that is one-half of the standard prescription dose (Table 1-3). They appear to be equivalent clinically despite differences in potency, duration, and rapidity of action. These agents are particularly useful when taken before an activity that may cause heartburn (heavy meal or exercise).

Patients can often predict when they are going to have heartburn and can premedicate. All four agents have an excellent safety profile, although

Table 1-2

Commonly Used Antacids and Antirefluxants

MEDICATION	ACTIVE INGREDIENT	DOSAGE
Alternagel	Aluminum hydroxide (600 mg/5 ml)	5–10 ml (max. 90 ml/day)
Amphojel	Aluminum hydroxide (320 mg/5ml)	10 ml (max. 60 ml/day)
Gaviscon tablets	Aluminum hydroxide (80 mg) Magnesium trisilicate (20 mg) Alginic acid	2–4 chewed tablets up to 4 times daily
Gaviscon Extra Strength tablets	Aluminum hydroxide (160 mg) Magnesium carbonate (105 mg) Alginic acid	2–4 chewed tablets up to 4 times daily
Maalox	Aluminum hydroxide (225 mg/5 ml) Magnesium hydroxide (200 mg/5 ml)	10–20 ml up to 4 times daily
Maalox Plus tablets	Aluminum hydroxide (350 mg) Magnesium hydroxide (350 mg) Simethicone (25 mg)	1–3 chewed tablets up to 4 times daily
Mylanta	Aluminum hydroxide (200 mg/5 ml) Magnesium hydroxide (200 mg/5 ml) Simethicone (20 mg/5 ml)	10–20 ml up to 4 times daily
Mylanta Gelcaps	Calcium carbonate (311 mg) Magnesium carbonate (232 mg)	2–4 capsules up to 4 times daily
Mylanta Gas	Simethicone (40, 80, or 125 mg) Capsules	40–125 mg chewed up to 4 times daily
Tums	Calcium carbonate (500 mg)	No more than 16 per day
Tums E-X	Calcium carbonate (750 mg)	No more than 12 per day
Tums Anti-gas/antacid	Calcium carbonate (500 mg) Simethicone (20 mg)	No more than 16 per day

Table 1-3

Available Over-the-Counter H_2-Receptor Antagonists

MEDICATION	ACTIVE INGREDIENT	DOSAGE
Axid AR	Nizatidine (75 mg)	1 tablet once or twice daily
Mylanta AR	Famotidine (10 mg)	1 tablet once or twice daily
Pepcid AC	Famotidine (10 mg)	1 tablet once or twice daily
Tagamet HB	Cimetidine (200 mg)	1 tablet once or twice daily
Zantac 75	Ranitidine (75 mg)	1 tablet once or twice daily

cytochrome P-450 interactions may rarely occur with cimetidine. This interaction may become more important as the population ages and more elderly patients who are taking drugs such as theophylline, phenytoin, or warfarin concurrently take H_2RAs. The general public should be educated to the warning symptoms that may be associated with GERD and that may indicate a more serious underlying condition (dysphagia, weight loss, bleeding, or anemia).

There are little data comparing over-the-counter H_2RAs and antacids. It has been suggested that antacids provide a more rapid response, but gastric pH begins to rise less than 30 min after taking a dose of H_2RA, so that this does not seem to be a major factor. It is not appropriate for patients to self-medicate on a daily, long-term basis without consulting with their health care provider. If heartburn occurs more than twice a week, patients should be evaluated and therapy should be considered. In general, more severe symptoms often but not always break through the modest reflux control offered by nonprescription therapy; therefore, there is little concern that over-the-counter medications mask more serious conditions.

Antisecretory Therapy

Acid suppression remains the mainstay of the therapy for GERD; two major classes of agents currently available to suppress acid are full-prescription dosages of H_2RAs and PPIs. The four H_2RAs have been extensively studied (and used)

in the treatment of heartburn and GERD. Review of the literature reveals that when H_2RAs are used (equivalent of ranitidine, 150 mg twice daily doses), symptomatic relief can be expected in 32 to 82 percent of patients (with mean of 60 percent) and endoscopic resolution of documented esophagitis in 0 to 82 percent (mean 48 percent). To effectively treat patients who have anything more than trivial heartburn, twice-daily doses of these agents must be used. It is unusual to find a patient with GERD who hypersecretes acid, but even those who secrete normal amounts of gastric acid often need greater than normal amounts of H_2RA to control their disease. Higher and more frequent dosing of H_2RA appears to be more effective in the treatment of reflux symptoms and in healing of esophagitis in GERD. Famotidine, 40 mg twice daily, and ranitidine, 150 mg 4 times daily, result in higher healing rates than standard-dose H_2RA, but rates are still lower than those using PPIs. The cost of this regimen compared to PPIs (see later) precludes use in most circumstances. When equivalent dosages are studied, there is no clear difference between the four available agents. As a class, the H_2 blockers are among the safest drugs with a side-effect rate (most of which are minor and reversible) of about 4 percent. There have been some concerns about drug interactions with these agents. Serum concentrations of phenytoin, procainamide, theophylline, and warfarin have been altered after the administration of cimetidine and, to a lesser degree, ranitidine, whereas this interaction has not been reported with the other two H_2 blockers. The former concern that these agents might alter blood ethanol levels has been discounted.

The PPIs provide control of acid secretion and are the most effective agents in the therapy of GERD. The agents available in the United States (omeprazole, lansoprazole, pantoprazole, rabeprazole, and esomeprazole) provide an extensive and potent formulary for acid suppression (see Table 1-4). Doses of omeprazole as low as 20 mg daily have been shown to be more effective than is either the placebo or standard-dose H$_2$RA therapy. Symptomatic relief can be expected in 83 percent of cases (range, 71 to 96 percent). Omeprazole can be expected to heal esophagitis in 78 percent (range, 62 to 94 percent) over a 4- to 8-week period. The more severe the esophagitis, the lower the healing rate, leading to need for higher dosages in patients with more severe disease.

The PPIs provide the most rapid onset of control of both symptoms and endoscopic esophagitis, and PPI therapy also maintains control of heartburn in patients who have nonerosive GERD. The efficacy and side-effect potential of lansoprazole seems essentially identical to omeprazole.

Patients with chest pain due to GERD are best treated with PPIs; in many cases doses of 40 mg/day in divided doses (see later) will be necessary to control symptoms. A short course of omeprazole (40 mg in the morning and 20 mg in the evening for 1 week) was found to be 78 percent sensitive and 85 percent specific when compared to endoscopy and ambulatory pH study. The so-called omeprazole test may be considered a short-term, high-dose therapeutic trial in patients with frequent symptoms. As discussed earlier, the opti-mal therapeutic trial is not known; however, the most effective 24-h pH control can be achieved with a combination of a PPI twice daily (before breakfast and dinner) and an H$_2$RA at bedtime.

Therapy with PPIs does not result in gastric achlorhydria, and some patients with GERD continue to secrete gastric acid and have gastroesophageal reflux even on twice daily therapy. Increasing the PPI dose controls pH sufficiently in most, but not all, patients. When high doses of PPIs are used, they should be given in split doses and should always be given before meals. Patients usually take their morning dose before breakfast but tend to take their evening dose before bedtime, which results in a decrease in efficacy. Relief of symptoms, particularly in patients with Barrett's esophagus, does not guarantee control of GERD. The significance of this acid exposure in asymptomatic patients is unclear, but may effect proliferation of Barrett's epithelial cells.

Comparisons between the available agents are limited, but two large studies revealed lansoprazole, 30 mg/day, and omeprazole, 20 mg/day, are similar in healing and symptom relief. Rabeprazole, 20 mg once daily, and omeprazole, 20 mg once daily, were found to be equivalent in both the relief of reflux symptoms and in the healing of esophagitis. Esomeprazole, 40 mg daily, appears to be more effective than omeprazole and other PPIs for onset of symptom relief and healing by endoscopy.

The initial fears of complication with long-term PPI therapy have been largely eliminated. The modest increase in circulating gastrin levels seen in some patients on long-term PPI therapy is not felt to be clinically important. A relation between accelerated gastric atrophy and metaplasia in patients on PPI therapy who have *Helicobacter pylori* infection was suggested but has been refuted and should not be considered clinically important. Current guidelines do not support searching for and treating *H. pylori* in reflux patients on long-term PPI therapy. Some investigators believe that eradication of *H. pylori* in these patients may exacerbate GERD. Cobalamin absorption may be decreased while on long-term

Table 1-4

Available Proton-Pump Inhibitors

MEDICATION	EQUIVALENT DOSAGE
Omeprazole (Prilosec)	20 mg daily
Lansoprazole (Prevacid)	30 mg daily
Pantoprazole (Protonix)	20 mg daily
Rabeprazole (Aciphex)	20 mg daily
Esomeprazole (Nexium)	20 mg daily

PPI therapy, but no change in serum levels have been reported after 7 years of therapy. There has also been no evidence of bacterial overgrowth after long-term acid suppression and no effect on calcium or iron absorption.

In addition to providing the best initial healing of GERD, PPI therapy maintains symptom relief in the highest percentage of patients. High-dose ranitidine (300 mg twice a day) maintained remission in 32 percent of patients who were healed with a PPI, whereas lansoprazole or omeprazole is more effective. Similar effective maintenance should be expected with the new PPIs.

Side effects with any of the acid-suppressing agents have been only rarely reported (headache and diarrhea are most frequent) but do not differ from the placebo in randomized studies. When one of these rare side effects occurs, switching to a different agent may result in resolution of the symptom.

Promotility Therapy

The pathogenesis of reflux includes motility abnormalities including lower esophageal sphincter incompetence, poor esophageal clearance, and delayed gastric emptying. Ideal therapy for GERD would therefore correct these defects, making suppression of normal amounts of gastric acid unnecessary; however, the ideal agent is not currently available. Metoclopramide, a centrally acting dopamine antagonist, has been used in the therapy of GERD and appears equal in efficacy to H2RAs; however, the frequent central nervous system side effects of metoclopramide (e.g., drowsiness, irritability, and extrapyramidal effects) have decreased the regular use of this medication.

Cisapride is a benzamide compound that increases lower esophageal sphincter pressure in patients with a weak sphincter and accelerates gastric emptying. However, prolongation of the QT interval and reports of sudden and occasionally fatal arrhythmias in patients on this medication have led to the removal of cisapride from the U.S. market (1999). Although cisapride may have

been useful in certain patients with a combination of symptoms (nausea and constipation, among others), PPIs provide greater control of acid reflux, without the risk of cardiac rhythm disturbances. Several newer promotility agents under development may prove to be useful with less potential side effects.

Combination Therapy

A combination of a PPI and H2RA may be effective in some patients with refractory GERD. Healthy subjects were given omeprazole, 20 mg twice a day, and then an additional medication at bedtime. Superior control of gastric acidity (by pH testing) was obtained with either 150 or 300 mg of ranitidine, as compared with an additional 20 mg of omeprazole. This combination also reduced esophageal acid exposure when compared to therapy with PPIs twice daily on a small group of patients with refractory GERD. Omeprazole, 20 mg twice a day (before breakfast and dinner) is superior to omeprazole, 20 mg in the morning, with ranitidine, 150 mg at bedtime, in nocturnal acid control. This suggests that a nocturnal H2RA cannot replace a second PPI in patients with resistant disease (Table 1-5).

Table 1-5
Relative Potency of Antireflux Therapies

PPI twice daily* with H2RA at bedtime†	Most potent
PPI twice daily‡	
PPI in a.m., H2RA at bedtime	
PPI once daily	
High-dose H2RA (2–3 times a day)	
H2RA	
OTC H2RA/Antacid	Least potent

*PPI should always be given before a meal.
†Needed only when twice-daily PPI therapy fails.
‡Often needed for extraesophageal symptoms.
PPI, Proton-pump inhibitor; H2RA, H2 receptor antagonist; OTC, over the counter.

Maintenance Therapy

Modern medical therapy allows the control of reflux in most, if not all, patients and is needed in most patients with symptomatic GERD. After initial treatment with a PPI, recurrence rates of 75 to 92 percent can be expected if the drug is discontinued. Famotidine and ranitidine maintain healing that is superior to the placebo but are not as effective as PPIs. In studies of patients who healed with omeprazole, continuing omeprazole, 20 mg/day, was superior to returning to ranitidine, 150 mg twice a day. Lower than full-dose PPI therapy may be effective in some patients. Lansoprazole, either 15 or 30 mg/day, maintains remission superior to a placebo. In one study, however, 30 mg was superior to 15 mg of lansoprazole. For maintenance of remission, 20 mg of omeprazole is superior to 10 mg. Some patients will relapse despite full doses of PPIs.

Surgical Therapy

The surgical options for GERD involve either a transthoracic or transabdominal approach with either a full or partial Nissen fundoplication. All of these procedures can be carried out using minimally invasive techniques (laparoscopy). The disadvantage of the thoracic approach is that it has a high morbidity with a long hospital stay and long recovery period. Laparoscopy is the preferred approach in almost all situations, except when several attempts at an abdominal repair have failed, if there are multiple adhesions from previous surgery, or if a concomitant pulmonary problem needs to be surgically addressed.

There is evidence that a 360° Nissen fundoplication results in significant dysphagia in up to 40 percent of patients with ineffective esophageal motility. These patients have been found by most to have less dysphagia than previously after a partial fundoplication (see Figure 1-3).

SHORT-TERM OUTCOME

Many thousand laparoscopic fundoplications have been reported with excellent short-term results. The operative mortality is 0.1 percent and the morbidity is low. Operative complications are pneumothorax, bleeding, and splenic, hepatic, esophageal, or gastric injury. These are rarely encountered in experienced hands and can be easily managed if they are identified at the time of the surgery. Early postoperative symptoms include dysphagia in 15 to 100 percent of patients, abdominal bloating, early satiety, and chest pain. Most of these symptoms will spontaneously disappear, but 15 percent will require endoscopy and a dilatation or medication. After 1 to 2 years following laparoscopic fundoplication, persistent bloating is reported in up to 15 percent of patients and is probably due to the habit of aerophagy. Diarrhea is seen in 8 percent of patients and some dysphagia occurs in 5.5 percent of patients; it is mild in most patients and easily treated by esophageal dilatation, which is required in a further 3.5 percent of patients. Many of these symptoms

Figure 1-3

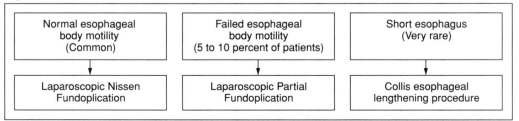

Surgical approach to patients with GERD confirmed by manometry.

were present before surgery, and it is not clear as to what the influence of surgery is in their genesis.

LONG-TERM OUTCOME

After 8 years, the long-term success rate of laparoscopic fundoplication is similar to the best-conducted long-term studies following open fundoplication. There is a 91 percent actuarially derived success rate in 100 patients followed up to 13 years (mean 45 months) and a 92 percent actuarially derived success rate in 160 patients followed up to 20 years (range 3 to 20 years; mean 136 months). The first laparoscopic fundoplications were performed in 1991, now allowing a 10-year follow-up. The results from the "best" surgeons indicate 88.3 percent are satisfied or very satisfied with the outcome, 8.2 percent find it acceptable, and 3.5 percent are not satisfied. Of interest is that some symptoms still persist, including bloating in 20.5 percent, occasional dysphagia in 27.5 percent, diarrhea in 12.2 percent, and heartburn in 5.9 percent. Of the total, 14 percent are found to be taking continuous antacid medications, but only 21 percent of these were on medications for clear GERD symptoms. Despite this, the patient satisfaction rate was high, with 93 percent reporting that they were satisfied with the decision to have surgery and an improvement in the quality of life score (1, worst, 10, best) from 2.2 before surgery to 8.8 after surgery.

New Endoluminal Therapies

New minimally invasive therapies have been described to treat GERD endoscopically or endoluminally. One treatment places sutures to create a gastroplication via a device attached to the tip of a standard flexible upper endoscope. The plication is made in the wall of the stomach just below the gastroesophageal junction to augment the lower esophageal sphincter zone. Another treatment uses radiofrequency energy to alter the region of the lower esophageal sphincter and reduce reflux. Many other approaches to nonsurgical treatment of patients with GERD are under development. There are currently no long-term data on the efficacy and safety of these new technologies.

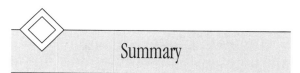

Summary

Chest pain is a common complaint in the practice of primary care. Once cardiac and other potentially life-threatening etiologies are excluded, a simple direct approach to the gastrointestinal etiologies can be completed. Most patients will have GERD. Once the diagnosis is confirmed, a number of treatment options can be instituted. Most patients will respond to medical therapy. Surgical and minimally invasive options are available for those patients not satisfied with medical therapy.

Bibliography

Dent J, Yeomans ND, Mackinnon M, et al: Omeprazole v ranitidine for prevention of relapse in reflux esophagitis. A controlled double blind trial of their efficacy and safety. *Gut* 35:590–598, 1994.

DeVault KR, Castell DO: Updated guidelines for the diagnosis and treatment of gastroesophageal reflux disease. *Am J Gastroenterol* 94 (6):1434–1442, 1999.

Euler AR, Murdock RH, Wilson TH, et al: Ranitidine is effective therapy for erosive esophagitis. *Am J Gastroenterol* 88:520–524, 1993.

Howden CW, Hunt RH: Guidelines for the management of *Helicobacter pylori* infection. *Am J Gastroenterol* 93:2330–2338, 1998.

Johnson LF, DeMeester TR: Evaluation of elevation of the head of the bed, bethanechol, and antacid foam tablets on gastroesophageal reflux. *Dig Dis Sci* 26: 673–680, 1981.

Katz PO, Dalton CB, Richter JE, et al: Esophageal testing of patients with noncardiac chest pain or dysphagia. Results of three years' experience with 1161 patients. *Ann Intern Med* 106:593–597, 1987.

Klinkenberg-Kriol EC, Festen HP, Jansen JB, et al: Long-term treatment with omeprazole for refractory reflux esophagitis: Efficacy and safety. *Ann Intern Med* 121:161–167, 1994.

Lieberman DA: Medical therapy for chronic reflux esophagitis. Long term follow-up. *Arch Intern Med* 147:717–720, 1987.

Marks RD, Richter JE, Rizzo J, et al: Omeprazole versus H2-receptor antagonists in treating patients with peptic stricture and esophagitis. *Gastroenterology* 106:907–915, 1994.

Mattox HE, Richter JE: Prolonged ambulatory esophageal pH monitoring in the evaluation of gastroesophageal reflux disease. *Am J Med* 89:345–356, 1990.

Ott DJ, Gelfand DW, Wu WC: Reflux esophagitis: Radiologic and endoscopic correlation. *Radiology* 103:583–588, 1979.

Sampliner RE: Practice guidelines on the diagnosis, surveillance and therapy of Barrett's esophagus. *Am J Gastroenterol* 93:1028–1032, 1998.

Sontag S, Robinson M, McCallum RW, et al: Ranitidine therapy for gastroesophageal reflux disease. Results of a large double-blind trial. *Arch Intern Med* 147:1485–1491, 1987.

Vigneri S, Termini R, Leandro G, et al: A comparison of five maintenance therapies for reflux esophagitis. *N Engl J Med* 333:1106–1110, 1995.

Wiener GJ, Koufman JA, Wu WC, et al: Chronic hoarseness secondary to gastroesophageal reflux disease: Documentation with 24-hr ambulatory pH monitoring. *Am J Gastroenterol* 84:1503–1508, 1989.

Debra Feldman

Nausea and Vomiting

The stomach starts to dance, the valves open,
and whoop, up it comes, a wild trumpet blast on
the unfortunate palate

　　　　　　　　　　　　　　　—Liam Farrell

Nausea and vomiting are common symptoms that herald a variety of medical conditions. A health survey from the U.S. Department of Health and Human Services lists vomiting as the eleventh most common reason for visits to emergency departments in 1997. In healthy persons, the symptoms of nausea and vomiting can be valuable responses that minimize the ill effects of toxins and contaminated food ingestion. Nausea and vomiting can also be stimulated by a wide variety of conditions that can be characterized as pathologic (e.g., bowel obstruction or pancreatitis), iatrogenic postsurgical and medication reactions (e.g., chemotherapy and radiation therapy), and reactive (e.g., overeating, pregnancy, or motion sickness).

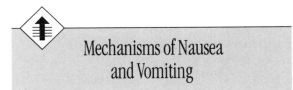

Mechanisms of Nausea and Vomiting

The word *nausea* originates from the Greek term for seasickness. Nausea is often described as an uncomfortable sensation, and it can occur independently of or prior to the onset of vomiting. Nausea is generally accompanied by decreased gastric tone and decreased or absent gastric peristalsis. Plasma vasopressin levels rise in nauseous humans, but the physiologic significance of this is unknown. Often, sweating, tachycardia, salivation, pupillary constriction, and skin vasoconstriction accompany nausea.

Vomiting occurs as the end result of several interrelated physiologic phenomena: The small intestine has retrograde contraction that returns its contents to the stomach, gastric tone decreases, the lower esophageal sphincter relaxes, the gastric

cardia rises, and, most importantly, the muscles of the diaphragm and abdomen forcefully contract. The net result is the expulsion of stomach contents. Hypersalivation, cardiac dysrhythmias, and the urge to defecate can accompany vomiting.

The physiologic mechanisms of vomiting are not clearly known, and many of the proposed mechanisms are based on animal experiments. A brief description of these mechanisms is helpful in understanding how so many varied conditions present with this symptom and in understanding medical therapy. The sensory components of the vagus nerve and sympathetic nerves are important in detecting luminal distension and in responding to chemical irritants and toxins. The area postrema, in the medulla, lies outside the blood-brain barrier and acts as the chemoreceptor trigger zone. Drugs and toxins in the bloodstream cause vomiting by stimulating this zone. The nucleus tractus solitarii and the medullary vomiting center respond to afferent input and initiate the motor activities that result in vomiting. Input from the vestibular system, the heart, the pharynx, the peritoneum, and the frontal cortex stimulate the vomiting reflex. Several receptors are involved in activating the vomiting reflex: muscarine, dopamine, histamine, serotonin, and neurokinin. Many medications used to treat vomiting block one or more these receptors.

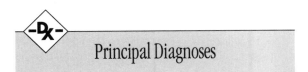

Principal Diagnoses

Disorders of almost every physiologic system can cause nausea and/or vomiting. Historical information, associated symptoms, and physical examination findings are essential for uncovering the root cause of nausea and vomiting. Table 2-1 provides a list of many causes of nausea and vomiting. A review of all causes of nausea and vomiting is beyond the scope of this chapter, so focus will be on the more common gastroenterologic causes. Common nongastrointestinal causes will be men-

Table 2-1

Possible Causes of Nausea and Vomiting

Pregnancy	Peptic ulcer disease
Motion sickness	Gastrointestinal infections
Migraine headaches	Acute or chronic pancreatitis
Alcohol and other substance abuse	Gallstone disease
Labyrinthine disorders	Gastric outlet obstruction
Chemotherapy	Gastrointestinal dysmotility
Radiation therapy	Toxin ingestion
Medications	Renal failure
Poorly controlled pain	Psychogenic causes
Postoperative causes	Endocrine disorders
Electrolyte disorders	Overeating

Table 2-2

Possible Gastrointestinal Causes of an Acute Abdomen

Acute appendicitis
Perforation of duodenal or gastric ulcer
Perforation of intestine
Acute peritonitis
Acute cholecystitis
Mesenteric ischemia
Acute pancreatitis
Large-bowel obstruction
Small-bowel obstruction
Perforated diverticulum
Ruptured abdominal abscess
Ruptured esophagus
Incarcerated hernia
Intussusception

tioned to aid in the approach to patients with nausea and vomiting. The principal diagnoses can be most usefully divided into acute and chronic presentations.

Acute Causes of Nausea and Vomiting

ACUTE ABDOMINAL EMERGENCIES

Any cause of an acute abdomen can present with the sudden onset of nausea and vomiting. The mechanism of nausea and vomiting may be mechanical obstruction, peritoneal inflammation, or severe pain. Causes of acute abdomen vary with age, with appendicitis being more common in children and young adults. While appendicitis remains an important diagnosis in middle-aged people and the elderly, bowel obstruction, bowel ischemia, perforation, and cholecystitis become more common. Malignancies of the gastrointestinal tract and metastatic cancers from other sites can cause bowel obstruction and perforation (Table 2-2). Nonabdominal emergencies can pre-

sent with acute abdominal pain, nausea, and vomiting. Myocardial infarction, aortic dissection or rupture, ectopic pregnancy, and pelvic inflammatory disease are important diagnoses to consider (Table 2-3).

GASTROINTESTINAL INFECTIONS

Nausea and vomiting are common features of gastrointestinal infections. Other common symptoms include abdominal pain, cramping, fever, diarrhea, and anorexia. Dehydration may occur in any age group, but is more common and more likely to be severe in infants, young children, and elderly and immunocompromised persons.

GASTROENTERITIS

Viral infections are the most common cause of episodic gastroenteritis. Rotavirus is the most common viral agent of gastroenteritis in children. Norwalk-like viruses (also known as small round structured viruses) are food-borne viral pathogens that commonly cause nausea and vomiting in adults.

Epidemic outbreaks can be caused by food-borne pathogens. Common bacterial pathogens

Table 2-3
Key History and Physical Features of Emergent Conditions That Can Present with Nausea and Vomiting

CAUSE	KEY HISTORY	KEY PHYSICAL
Toxin ingestion	Drugs or medications, including over-the-counter medications; suicidal ideation; consumption of unusual or spoiled foods, e.g., mushrooms, shellfish	Dehydration; constriction or dilatation of pupils; cardiac dysrhythmias; orthostatic hypotension; hyperthermia; anhidrosis; hyperhidrosis; alterations in consciousness
Gastrointestinal causes	Presence, nature, or timing of bowel gas, predisposing medical conditions, such as hypertension, atherosclerotic disease, or gallstones	Fever, decreased or absent bowel sounds, abdominal distension, peritoneal signs, abdominal pain
Myocardial infarction	Characteristic chest pain, epigastric pain, risk factors for atherosclerotic disease, symptoms of congestive heart failure	Hyper- or hypotension, tachycardia, diaphoresis, findings of congestive heart failure
Aortic dissection or rupture	Severe pain, often radiating to back; history of aneurysm or hypertension	Unable to sit still, hypertensive or hypotensive, tachycardia, pulsatile mass, loss of distal pulses
Ectopic pregnancy	Menstrual history, sexual history, history of tubal ligation or pelvic inflammatory disease	Pelvic or abdominal pain, fever, pelvic mass
Increased intracranial pressure	Headache, change in mental status, neurologic symptoms, cancer or head trauma	Papilledema, altered consciousness, neurologic findings, severe hypertension

include *Salmonella* spp., *Helicobacter* spp., *Clostridium botulinum*, *Escherichia coli* 0157:H7, *Shigella* spp, and *Staphylococcus aureus*. Episodic gastroenteritis can occur unrelated to contaminated food ingestion and often occurs in institutionalized settings. Most episodes of gastroenteritis are self-limited, lasting between 1 and 3 days. Abdominal pain is usually diffuse and crampy. If pain is severe and accompanied by fever, an invasive bacterial pathogen is more likely. Parasitic infections usually present with lower gastrointestinal tract symptoms.

INFECTIOUS HEPATITIS

The most common causes of infectious hepatitis are viral. Though there are seven types of viral

hepatitis identified, over 90 percent are caused by hepatitis A, B, and C virus. Hepatitis A and B often present with nausea and vomiting. Other clinical symptoms include anorexia, fatigue, malaise, and abdominal pain. Hepatitis A, responsible for about 35 percent of cases of acute hepatitis in the United States, is spread through contaminated food or water and from person to person. Hepatitis B is transmitted through blood products, sexual contact, and perinatal transmission. While both hepatitis A and B can present with fatigue and anorexia, hepatitis A is a self-limited disease. Hepatitis B can be a more prolonged illness, which is accompanied by jaundice, and may progress to acute liver failure in a few patients. Hepatitis B may also develop into a chronic infection that will cause chronic liver disease in a percentage of patients.

NONINFECTIOUS HEPATITIS

Drugs and toxins may cause noninfectious hepatitis. Acetaminophen toxicity can cause acute hepatitis with liver failure if not recognized and treated. Autoimmune hepatitis is a chronic hepatitis that usually does not present with acute nausea and vomiting.

GALLSTONE DISEASE

Most patients with gallstones never develop any symptoms. Those patients who do develop symptoms will often experience pain. The pain associated with biliary colic is in the right upper quadrant or epigastric area of the abdomen and can radiate to the right scapula, shoulder, or chest. The pain is not intense and usually peaks in late evening. The relation of the pain to fatty meals is not specific. The most common symptomatic presentations are from intermittent obstruction of the cystic duct, choledocholithiasis (intermittent common bile duct obstruction), acute cholecystitis (cystic duct obstruction), and cholangitis (common bile duct obstruction with bacterial infection). Nausea is a common accompaniment to biliary colic, acute cholecystitis, and choledocholithiasis. Vomiting often occurs in acute cholecystitis.

ACUTE AND CHRONIC PANCREATITIS

Epigastric abdominal pain radiating to the back is the most vivid presenting symptom of pancreatitis. Nausea and vomiting are frequent presenting symptoms.

Patients with chronic pancreatitis often have bouts of acute abdominal pain, nausea, and vomiting. Chronic pancreatitis results in permanent damage to pancreatic tissue. Causes of chronic pancreatitis include ethanol, hereditary causes, obstruction, hyperparathyroidism, and trauma.

Common bile duct gallstones and ethanol toxicity are responsible for 80 percent of cases of acute pancreatitis. Other causes include drugs, hyperlipidemia, and hypercalcemia. Acute pancreatitis can develop into necrotizing pancreatitis, which is a surgical emergency.

TOXIN INGESTION, PHARMACEUTICAL AGENTS, AND SUBSTANCE ABUSE

Almost any toxin can cause nausea and vomiting. Toxins can be food borne, such as those occurring from botulin, poison mushroom ingestion, or certain rare shellfish. Recreational or prescription drugs can cause nausea and vomiting, especially if taken in excessive dosages. Prescription drugs that cause vomiting include ipecac, chemotherapeutic agents, cardiac glycosides, levodopa, bromocriptine, ergot alkaloids, muscarinic receptor agonists, nicotinic receptor agonists, opiates, methylxanthines, aminoglycosides, high doses of estrogen, and progesterone compounds. Substances of abuse, such as ethanol and stimulant drugs, cause nausea and vomiting, both acutely and chronically. Withdrawal syndromes from opiates and alcohol may be accompanied by these symptoms.

Gastrointestinal Causes of Chronic Nausea and Vomiting

GASTRIC ULCERS AND DUODENAL ULCERS

Gastric and duodenal ulcers are usually benign, caused by *Helicobacter pylori* infection and/or acid breakdown of the stomach lining. Nonsteroidal anti-inflammatory drugs (NSAIDs) also cause ulcers. A small percentage of gastric ulcers are malignant. Nausea occurs in 40 to 70 percent of patients with gastric and duodenal ulcers. Vomiting is more likely to occur with gastric ulcers, but a significant proportion of patients with duodenal ulcers will also have vomiting. Severe pain and epigastric pain are associated with ulcer disease. The timing of pain in relation to meals is variable and cannot be used to diagnose peptic ulcer disease. Bloating is a common feature of both conditions.

Patients with ulcer disease usually give a history of chronic or subacute symptoms, but can also have acute nausea and vomiting.

GASTROINTESTINAL MOTILITY DISORDERS AND FUNCTIONAL GASTROINTESTINAL DISORDERS

Stomach and small-intestine motility disorders will present with symptoms of nausea, vomiting, early satiety, and bloating. Vomitus will often have a foul smell, indicating that stomach contents have been stagnant for several hours.

Gastroparesis occurs in those with diabetes, as well as in patients with progressive systemic sclerosis, and in patients who have had stomach surgery. Neurologic conditions, such as multiple sclerosis, amyloidosis, and brainstem infarctions, can also cause gastroparesis, as can anticholinergic drugs.

The small intestine may also have disordered motility, with inadequate contractions. Intestinal pseudo-obstruction is a motility disorder that can be difficult to distinguish acutely from mechanical obstruction.

Biliary dyskinesia occurs spontaneously or after cholecystectomy. Symptoms of biliary dyskinesia mimic obstruction of the biliary tract and include nausea, vomiting, and pain.

There is overlap between gastric motility disorders and what have been termed *functional gastrointestinal disorders*. Functional disorders include dyspepsia, irritable bowel syndrome, and biliary dyskinesia.

The Rome diagnostic criteria for functional dyspepsia define dysmotility-like dyspepsia as presenting with early satiety; postprandial fullness; nausea, recurrent retching, or vomiting; bloating of the upper abdomen; and upper abdominal discomfort aggravated by food. Motility abnormalities and increased sensitivity to sensory stimuli have been described for many of the functional disorders.

GASTRIC OUTLET OBSTRUCTION

Over half of patients with gastric outlet obstruction will have malignancies, either intrinsic or extrinsic to the gastrointestinal tract. Occasionally, peptic ulcer disease can cause the gastric outlet to be blocked. As with gastroparesis, patients vomit food that has been ingested several hours earlier. Abdominal pain, weight loss, and early satiety are other hallmarks of gastric outlet obstruction. Nausea develops in a large minority of patients.

Nongastrointestinal Causes of Nausea and Vomiting

Because of the many sensory inputs to the vomiting mechanism, many conditions result in nausea and vomiting. Table 2-1 lists many of the nongastrointestinal causes of nausea and vomiting.

Elevated intracranial pressure is an emergent diagnosis that can present with nausea and vomiting. Brain tumors, head trauma, ruptured aneurysms, strokes, bleeding, and infection of the central nervous system are among the conditions that cause elevations of intracranial pressure. In one survey, 9 of 10 patients with migraine headaches experience nausea, and 7 of 10 patients experience vomiting in association with headaches. Nausea and vomiting are presenting symptoms in motion sickness and other vestibular disorders such as Meniere's disease and acute labyrinthitis.

Chemotherapy and radiation therapy can cause disabling nausea and vomiting. Chemotherapy-associated vomiting can be immediate (occurring shortly after administration), delayed (occurring several hours later), or anticipatory (occurring prior to receiving treatment). Vomiting from radiation therapy is postulated to be secondary to the release of intracellular substances on cell death and is more likely to occur with abdominal or whole body irradiation.

One half of pregnant women will experience some degree of morning sickness. About 2 percent of these women will experience hyperemesis gravidarum, a potentially life-threatening refractory vomiting syndrome.

Psychogenic vomiting has been described as a manifestation of many psychiatric diseases. Bulimia is characterized by binge eating and purging methods, including self-induced vomiting. Extreme emotional distress may also be associated with nausea and vomiting, usually of limited duration. Vomiting is also a common postoperative complication and may be secondary to anesthetic agents, the surgery itself, or pain.

Severe pain of any type may be associated with nausea and vomiting. Renal colic is an example of a painful disorder that can present with nausea and vomiting. Medications used to treat pain, such as narcotic agents and NSAIDs, also cause nausea and vomiting.

Endocrine and metabolic diseases may present with a range of gastrointestinal symptoms, including nausea and vomiting. Adrenal insufficiency, pheochromocytoma, diabetic ketoacidosis, renal failure, hypercalcemia, and electrolyte disorders should be considered in the diagnosis of acute or episodic nausea and vomiting

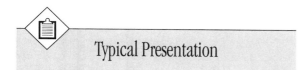

Typical Presentation

Acute nausea and vomiting are extremely uncomfortable symptoms that disrupt the ability of patients to function. Because so many conditions cause these symptoms, presentations will vary. Patients with severe or protracted nausea and vomiting may be dehydrated or have other complications of varying severity (Table 2-4). Patients who have had chronic nausea and vomiting may not volunteer these symptoms unless the primary care provider specifically asks about them. Their primary concern may be focused on another aspect of the illness causing the nausea and vomiting, such as abdominal pain or weight loss.

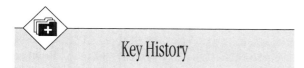

Key History

Nausea and vomiting are such ubiquitous symptoms that it is not possible to hone the key history to a few major points. No current research is available to guide the history-taking process of these two symptoms. Patients may have several conditions that can result in nausea and vomiting, so it may be difficult to distinguish which condition is

Table 2-4

Complications of Vomiting

Dehydration	Malnutrition
Metabolic alkalosis	Aspiration
Hypokalemia	Cardiac dysrhythmias
Esophageal tears or ruptures	Esophagitis

responsible. A complete history will be necessary to uncover the likely causes. Nonetheless, a few historical points are worth emphasizing.

Information regarding the frequency, onset, severity, and alleviating and exacerbating factors should be sought. Patients should describe the appearance and volume of the vomitus. Sometimes, patients may describe the production of respiratory secretions rather than the gastric contents.

Because nausea and vomiting can be symptoms of serious or life-threatening conditions, the initial history should be aimed at determining whether such conditions exist (Table 2-3). Most gastrointestinal causes of acute nausea and vomiting are associated with abdominal pain of some type and severity. The nature, timing, and location of the pain can be used to help differentiate such conditions as acute pancreatitis, gallbladder disease, and hepatitis (see principal diagnoses). When patients have a gastrointestinal infection, they can often identify a contact with similar symptoms or contaminated food ingestion. Associated symptoms will help narrow down the differential diagnosis.

Patients with chronic nausea and vomiting should be questioned about conditions that would predispose to motility disorders. Symptoms that suggest underlying malignancy, such as weight loss and anorexia, should be documented. A careful medication, substance abuse, and psychiatric history should be taken.

In both acute and chronic vomiting, symptoms of dizziness, decreased urine output, and weakness may indicate dehydration. In patients who are elderly, debilitated, or with altered sensorium, symptoms of shortness of breath could indicate aspiration.

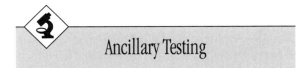

Physical Examination

A complete physical examination should be performed. The patient's general appearance will often provide information on the seriousness of the underlying cause. Some features associated with serious causes of nausea and vomiting are outlined in Table 2-3. Documented weight loss is a helpful clue to chronic serious illness. Health care providers should look for signs of dehydration, including orthostatic hypotension, tachycardia, dry mucous membranes, and anhidrosis. Fever suggests an infectious cause or a complication such as aspiration pneumonia. An abdominal examination may help localize the pain. Fecal occult blood testing may be helpful in diagnosing benign or malignant ulcer disease, bowel ischemia, or complications of vomiting.

Ancillary Testing

The history and physical examination should guide appropriate testing for the work-up. If acute infectious gastroenteritis is likely, and there is no evidence of significant dehydration, fever, or severe abdominal pain, no further testing is warranted. If invasive bacterial infection is suspected, stool samples should be sent, along with fecal leukocytes and fecal occult blood testing. An electrocardiogram should be performed if cardiac disease is suspected, either as the cause of nausea and vomiting, or as a complication. A chest x-ray should be done if an esophageal tear or aspiration is suspected. (Tables 2-5 and 2-6 list tests to consider in assessing the cause and in detecting spe-

Table 2-5

Laboratory Tests to Consider in the Evaluation of Nausea and Vomiting

Complete blood count (CBC)
Serum electrolytes
Blood urea nitrogen and creatinine
Calcium (Ca++)
Liver function tests (LFTs)
Amylase
Lipase
Hepatitis serology
Thyroid function tests
Toxicology screen
Urine or serum pregnancy test

cific gastrointestinal conditions of patients with acute nausea and vomiting.)

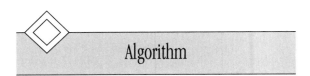

Algorithm

The algorithm depicted here is designed to guide the primary care provider through initial decisions in the assessment of acutely nauseous and/or vomiting patients (Figure 2-1). The first step is to determine whether these symptoms represent a serious or life-threatening condition. If so, appropriate referral to an emergency department or hospital admission with emergent evaluation is indicated. Pregnancy in women of childbearing age should be considered early in the evaluation.

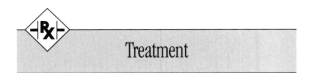

Treatment

The treatment of nausea and vomiting should be multidimensional, managing the underlying cause and providing symptomatic relief if the nausea and

Figure 2-1

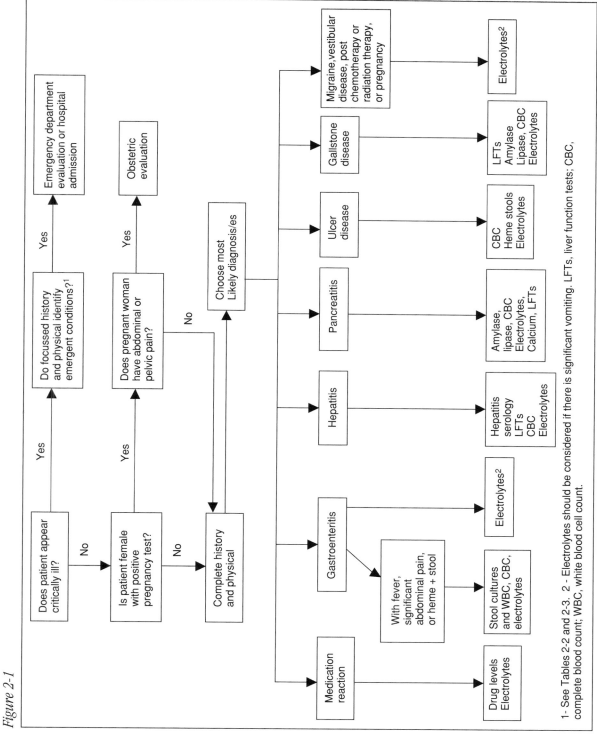

1 - See Tables 2-2 and 2-3. 2 - Electrolytes should be considered if there is significant vomiting. LFTs, liver function tests; CBC, complete blood count; WBC, white blood cell count.

Table 2-6

Diagnostic Tests to Consider for the Diagnosis of Gastrointestinal Causes of Nausea and Vomiting

TEST	CONDITIONS
Upper endoscopy	Gastric or duodenal ulcers, gastric malignancy
Upper gastrointestinal series	Gastric outlet syndrome, gastric or duodenal ulcer disease, gastric malignancy
Obstruction series	Bowel obstruction, small intestine pseudo-obstruction
Computed tomography scan of abdomen	Perforated diverticuli, abdominal abscess, ectopic pregnancy, gallstone disease
Gastric emptying study	Gastric motility disorder
Ultrasound of the abdomen	Gallstone disease
Gastrointestinal motility studies (manometry)	Gastric dysmotility, intestinal dysmotility, biliary dyskinesia

SOURCE: Modified from Kuczmarski et al

vomiting are severe or protracted. In some circumstances, vomiting may be protective, that is, if patients have ingested toxins or overdose. Clinicians will need to assess when the risks of nausea and vomiting become significant enough to warrant symptomatic treatment. Severe vomiting, especially in patients with altered mental status, may need to be managed initially in a hospital setting, where intravenous hydration and gastric decompression can be administered.

Table 2-7 summarizes considerations in choosing antiemetic medication. Much of the study of antiemetic treatments has been conducted in attempts to reduce chemotherapy-induced vomiting. The physiologic pathways of chemotherapy-induced vomiting are the same as the mechanisms described earlier; much of the information can be generalized to other conditions.

The mechanism of vomiting involves several neuronal pathways and a variety of neuroreceptors. Many antiemetics work by blocking one or more specific receptor sites and are presented by category of major receptor blockade.

PHENOTHIAZINES

The antiemetic effects of phenothiazines (e.g., prochlorperazine, chlorpromazine, and promethazine) intensify with increasing doses. Dosages are limited by significant side effects, including extrapyramidal reactions, hypotension, and dyskinesia. These medications are inexpensive and are used commonly to control symptoms related to acute benign conditions. Phenothiazines can be administered orally, rectally, or parenterally.

BUTYROPHENONES

Butyrophenones (e.g., haloperidol, droperidol, and domperidone) are often used to control postoperative vomiting and are modestly effective for chemotherapy-induced vomiting. Haloperidol and droperidol can cause extrapyramidal side effects. Domperidone is unique in that it does not cross the blood-brain barrier and so is unlikely to cause extrapyramidal side effects. It is used to treat vomiting induced by drugs for Parkinsonism and for chemotherapy.

SUBSTITUTED BENZAMIDES

Substituted benzamides (e.g., metoclopramide) are prokinetic agents. At high doses, metoclopramide can also block serotonin receptors. Drugs in this class can cause all the side effects associated with dopaminergic blockade, especially at

Table-2-7

Guide to Choosing Antiemetic Agents for Symptom Relief

SYMPTOM COMPLEX	DRUG OPTIONS	TYPICAL AGENTS	COST	COMMENTS	CAVEATS AND CAUTIONS
Mild symptoms: nausea without vomiting or occasional vomiting	None	None	None		
Moderate symptoms associated with a transient cause	Phenothiazines, benzamides	Prochlorperazine, chlorpromazine, promethazine, metoclopramide	Inexpensive		Extrapyramidal, reactions, dyskinesia
Motion sickness	Antihistamines, anticholinergic agents	Diphenhydramine, meclizine, doxylamine	Inexpensive, except transdermal formulations	Some antihistamine agents are non-prescription	Cautious use in elderly
Postoperative nausea and vomiting	Corticosteroids Benzamides, butyrophenones Serotonin receptor antagonists Nonpharmaceutical treatments	Dexamethasone Reglan Domperidol Odansetron Acupuncture	Inexpensive Inexpensive Inexpensive Expensive Variable	Combinations may be more effective	
Chemotherapy-induced nausea and vomiting	All listed classes, anxiolytics, acupuncture, hypnosis		Variable to expensive	Serotonin receptor antagonists and combination regimens effective with fewer side effects, antihistamines and corticosteroids used as adjunctive agents	
Motility disorders	Benzamides	Reglan	Inexpensive		Extrapyramidal effects

29

high doses. Metoclopramide is used widely to treat postoperative vomiting, chemotherapy- and radiation-induced vomiting, acute and chronic vomiting, and hyperemesis gravidarum. Metoclopramide can be used in the management of gastroparesis and other motility disorders, but is not used in motion sickness.

ANTICHOLINERGIC AGENTS

Anticholinergic agents (e.g., scopolamine= hyoscine, atropine, trihexyphenidyl=benzhexol, and benzatropine) act by blocking receptors in the afferent limb of the vomiting reflex. Side effects of dry mouth, orthostatic hypotension, blurred vision, urinary retention, and delirium can occur, particularly in the elderly and debilitated. Scopolamine has been used in motion sickness and is available in a transdermal patch. These agents have also been used perioperatively and are useful for drying secretions. Most anticholinergic agents are inexpensive, but the scopolamine transdermal patch is costly.

SEROTONIN RECEPTOR ANTAGONISTS

Serotonin receptor antagonists (e.g., odansetron, granisetron, dolasetron, and tropisetron), which block the 5-HT (sub 3) receptor, are effective in blocking emesis, especially triggered by chemotherapeutic regimens containing cisplatin. Though other antiemetics may be as effective, this group of medicines causes few and transient side effects. These side effects include headache, sedation, dry mouth, constipation, or diarrhea. Currently, their use is generally confined to vomiting resulting from chemotherapy, radiation therapy, and surgery. The cost of these medications is high, prohibiting their use for routine benign conditions.

Antihistamines

Antihistamines (e.g., diphenhydramine, meclizine, chlorphenylamine, dimenhydrinate, doxylamine, cyclizine, chlorcyclizine, and cinnarizine) reduce nausea and vomiting, but are generally not potent enough to be used as single agents in chemotherapy-induced vomiting. They are used in combination with antidopaminergic agents to reduce extrapyramidal side effects. Antihistamines, most of which are inexpensive, are also used for vestibular causes of nausea and vomiting.

Antiemetic Agents with Unknown Mechanism of Action

CORTICOSTEROIDS

The antiemetic mechanism of corticosteroids (e.g., hydrocortisone, dexamethasone, solumedrol) is unknown. They are mild antiemetics, usually used in combination with other agents. Side effects of corticosteroids are well known, and they should be used with caution in patients with diabetes mellitus. One of these agents, dexamethasone, is used for increased intracranial pressure.

CANNABINOIDS

Tetrahydrocannabinol, derived from marijuana plants, and synthetic cannabinoids (e.g., dronabinol and nabilone) are mildly effective in chemotherapy-induced vomiting. The mechanism of action is uncertain. These medications also stimulate weight gain and are most often used by patients with human immunodeficiency virus. Smoked marijuana is felt to be more effective by some patients, but has other side effects and cannot be dispensed legally.

Nonprescription Medications

Meclizine and dimenhydrinate are antihistamines that are available over the counter in several preparations. They are marketed to treat nausea, vomiting, and motion sickness. Phosphorylated carbohydrate solutions that coat the stomach lining are available to treat symptoms associated with gastrointestinal viruses and overeating. Bismuth salicylate is indicated for treatment of nausea and upset stomach.

Patient Education

Patients should be aware that nausea and vomiting are often the presenting symptoms of serious illnesses. Healthy patients with the acute onset of symptoms usually have self-limited conditions. However, they should report these symptoms to a health care provider if they do not resolve in several hours, if the nausea and vomiting are severe or progressive, or if there are accompanying symptoms of abdominal pain and/or fever. Elderly patients, patients with chronic medical illnesses, immunocompromised patients, and patients taking medications should report their symptoms to their health care provider and seek evaluation.

Nausea and vomiting associated with chronic benign conditions such as migraine headaches, motion sickness, vestibular disorders, and intestinal motility disorders can be managed with appropriate medical regimens. Patients should work with their primary care providers to establish treatment regimens that they can implement early in the development of symptoms.

Patients may seek information about digestive conditions from the National Digestive Disease Information Clearinghouse (NIDDK; *http://www. niddk.nih.gov/health/digest/pubs.htm*). A useful web site for many diseases, especially infectious diseases, is posted by the Centers for Disease Control and Prevention at *http:// www.cdc.gov.*

including herbal remedies and over-the-counter medications, should be considered as potential causes of nausea and vomiting. If patients are taking herbal remedies unfamiliar to the primary care provider, further information concerning these substances should be sought. Even properly prescribed and administered medications can cause toxicity. Elderly and debilitated patients may become toxic without taking overdoses. The possibility of systemic disease should always be sought, given the wide variety of conditions that cause nausea and vomiting. Again, elderly and debilitated patients should be given special consideration. The typical manifestations of serious disease, such as fever and tachycardia, may be absent in these populations, so a higher index of suspicion must be maintained in these groups.

Chronic nausea and vomiting may be symptoms of a variety of psychogenic disorders. Patients with eating disorders may hide these conditions from their health care provider. Similarly, patients who abuse alcohol or drugs may hide or deny their conditions. Providers should remain vigilant for the possible complications of nausea and vomiting. When deciding whether to treat symptoms, the primary care provider should consider that many antiemetic agents have extrapyramidal and anticholinergic side effects. For benign conditions, these side effects may be more problematic than are the symptoms. Severe vomiting should be controlled, beginning with the lowest doses of antiemetic medication available. Combinations of two low-dose antiemetics may be safer than increasing the dose of one medication.

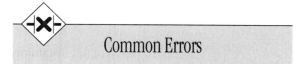

Common Errors

Significant errors in the diagnosis and management of nausea and vomiting arise when important historical clues are overlooked. Primary care providers should always consider pregnancy, especially ectopic pregnancy, early in the evaluation of women of childbearing age. Medication,

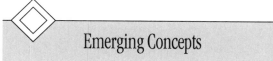

Emerging Concepts

As more information about the enteric nervous system is obtained, diagnostic testing may become more useful. Gastric and intestinal motility disorders can be detected via manometry, but the utility of these diagnostic tests in routine clinical practice is still being evaluated.

New treatment options are emerging that may reduce the nausea and vomiting that occur with radiation and chemotherapy treatments. Clinical trials indicate that substance P, a neurokinin neurotransmitter for sensory afferent neurons, will be effective against nausea and vomiting. Experimental agents targeted against neurokinin receptors are being developed. In 1998, a conference on acupuncture at the National Institutes of Health Consensus concluded that there is clear evidence that acupuncture is useful in the prevention of nausea and vomiting associated with chemotherapy and surgery.

Hypnosis and behavioral modification are now used to prevent anticipatory vomiting in chemotherapy patients. How to best combine nonpharmaceutical treatment with medication remains to be elucidated.

Bibliography

Abell TL, Werkman RF: Gastrointestinal motility disorders. *Am Fam Physician* 53:895–902, 1996.

American Gastroenterological Association: Medical position statement on nausea and vomiting. *Gastroenterology* 120:261–263, 2001.

Andrews PLR: Physiology of nausea and vomiting. *Br J Anaesth* 69(suppl 1):2S–19S, 1992.

Batal H, Johnson M, Lehman D, et al: Bulimia: A primary care approach. *J Womens Health* 7:211–220, 1998.

Chevalier A: *The Encyclopedia of Medicinal Plants*. New York, DK Publishing, 1996.

Drossman DA: Diagnosing and treating patients with refractory functional gastrointestinal disorders. *Ann Intern Med* 123:688–697, 1995.

Farrell L: ...a joy forever. *Br Med J* 318:1297, 1999.

Feldman M, Scharschmidt B, Sleisenger M, eds: *Sleisenger and Fordtrans's Gastrointestinal and Liver Disease: Pathophysiology, Diagnosis, and Management*, 6th ed. Philadelphia, W.B. Saunders Company, 1997.

Goyal RJ, Hirano I: Mechanisms of disease: The enteric nervous system. *N Engl J Med* 334:1110–1115, 1996.

Grunberg SM, Hesketh PJ: Drug therapy: Control of chemotherapy-induced emesis. *N Engl J Med* 329:1790–1796, 1993.

Hanson JS, McCallum RW: The diagnosis of nausea and management of nausea and vomiting: A review. *Am J Gastroenterol* 80:210–218,1985.

Heffernan AM, Rowbotham DJ: Postoperative nausea and vomiting—time for balanced antiemesis? *Br J Anaesth* 85:675–677, 2000.

Kapikian AZ: Overview of viral gastroenteritis. *Arch Virol* 12(S):7–19, 1996.

Khullar SK, DiSario JA: Gastric outlet obstruction. *Gastrointest Endosc Clin N Am* 6:585–603, 1996.

Koch KL: Dyspepsia of unknown origin: Pathophysiology, diagnosis and treatment. *Dig Dis* 15:316–329, 1997.

Lee A, Done ML: The use of nonpharmacologic techniques to prevent postoperative nausea and vomiting: A meta-analysis. *Anesth Analg* 88:1200–1202, 1999.

Marmor JB: Medical marijuana. *West J Med* 168:540–543, 1998.

Mergener K, Baillie J: Chronic pancreatitis. *Lancet* 350:1379–1385, 1997.

Mergener K, Baillie J: Fortnightly review: Acute pancreatitis. *Br Med J* 316:44–48, 1998.

Mitchelson F: Pharmacological agents affecting emesis: A review (part I). *Drugs* 43:295–315, 1992.

Mitchelson F: Pharmacological agents affecting emesis: A review (part II). *Drugs* 43:443–463, 1992.

NIH Consensus Conference. Acupuncture. *JAMA* 280:1518–1524, 1998.

Nourjah P: *Advance Data: National Hospital Ambulatory Medical Care Survey: 1997 Emergency Department Summary*. From Vital and Health Statistics of the Centers for Disease Control and Prevention/National Health Center for Statistics no 304, May 6, 1999.

Reasner CA, Isley WL: Endocrine emergencies: Recognizing clues to classic problems. *Postgrad Med* 101:231–242, 1997.

Silberstein S: Migraine symptoms: Results of a survey of self-reported migraineurs. *Headache* 35:387–396, 1995.

Soll AH: Medical treatment of peptic ulcer disease: Practice guidelines. *JAMA* 275:622–629,1996.

Traverso WL: Overview: Clinical manifestations and impact of gallstone disease. *Am J Surg* 165:405–409, 1993.

Wadibia EC: Antiemetics. *South Med J* 92:162–165, 1992.

Richard B. Lynn

Dysphagia

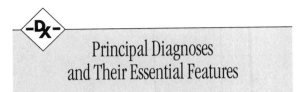

Definitions and Background

Dysphagia is defined as difficulty swallowing, most often described by patients as "the food gets stuck." This should be distinguished from odynophagia, which is pain with swallowing. Dysphagia generally is not painful. Globus (the sensation of a lump in the throat) and xerostomia (dry mouth) are separate disorders that a careful history should distinguish from dysphagia.

Dysphagia may be oropharyngeal or esophageal depending on the site of problem. Oropharyngeal and esophageal dysphagia have different presentations, etiologies, diagnostic evaluations, and treatments and will be treated separately in this chapter. A careful history is usually adequate to distinguish oropharyngeal from esophageal dysphagia. Oropharyngeal dysphagia is characterized by symptoms such as difficulty transferring food to the back of the throat in preparation for swallowing, difficulty initiating a swallow, nasal regurgitation, or aspiration when swallowing. Choking or coughing with swallowing are the hallmarks of oropharyngeal dysphagia. In contrast, patients with esophageal dysphagia report swallowing without choking or coughing, but then the food "gets stuck on the way down."

Epidemiologic data are scant, but the prevalence of dysphagia in the population over age 50 years is estimated in the range of 16 to 22 percent. Dysphagia affects about 12 percent of patients in acute care hospitals and 60 percent of nursing home occupants. The majority of the latter group have problems with oropharyngeal dysphagia.

The most important point to remember is that the symptoms of dysphagia always require a diagnostic evaluation to determine the etiology. The clinician should never attribute the symptoms to a "functional" disorder or empirically treat patients for some common disorder such as gastroesophageal reflux disease (GERD) without first completing an appropriate diagnostic evaluation. Dysphagia is caused either by obstruction or weakness of the muscles needed for propulsion of the bolus. The obstruction may be due to neoplastic, inflammatory, stricturing disorders or motility disorders that result in functional obstructions due to uncoordinated (nonpropulsive or spastic) contractions or failure of relaxation of a sphincter.

Principal Diagnoses and Their Essential Features

Oropharyngeal Dysphagia

Oropharyngeal dysphagia may be caused by a great variety of neuromuscular, head and neck, and gastrointestinal (GI) disorders (see Table 3-1). Typically, the underlying disorder is already apparent such as in the case of cerebrovascular accident (CVA) or advanced tumors of the head and neck. In these situations, patients are generally under the care of the appropriate specialist and the issues surrounding the dysphagia focus on management. However, sometimes oropharyngeal dysphagia is the presenting symptom and the primary care clinician must consider neuromuscular, head and neck, and GI etiologies. An appropriate history, physical examination, and initial diagnostic testing should allow for the identification of the likely etiology and for the direct referral to the appropriate specialist.

CEREBROVASCULAR ACCIDENT

Cerebrovascular accident is often complicated by oropharyngeal dysphagia. This complication is serious, as it is often accompanied by aspiration pneumonia. Oropharyngeal dysphagia can result from catastrophic CVAs, such as those involving a cerebral hemisphere or the brainstem, or from more minor CVAs and even lacunar infarcts. Patients with CVAs and oropharyngeal dysphagia are generally followed by a speech pathologist with special training and knowledge of swallowing disorders.

Table 3-1

Representative Causes of Oropharyngeal Dysphagia

Neurologic disorders
  Cerebral vascular accident
  Parkinson's disease
  Head trauma
  Amyotrophic lateral sclerosis
  Brainstem tumors
  Multiple sclerosis
  Central nervous system syphilis
  Polio and postpolio syndrome
  Myasthenia gravis
  Cerebral palsy

Muscle disorders
  Muscular dystrophies
  Polymyositis
  Dermatomyositis
  Metabolic myopathies (steroid,
    thyrotoxicosis, and myxedema)
  Amyloidosis
  Connective tissue diseases
  Sarcoidosis
  Paraneoplastic syndromes

Head and neck disorders
  Tumors
  Infectious (pharyngitis, abscess, and
    tuberculosis)
  Cervical webs
  Zenker's diverticulum
  Thyromegaly
  Osteophytes and cervical spine hyperostosis
  Surgical resections

Esophageal disorders
  Incomplete relaxation of the upper
    esophageal sphincter (cricopharyngeal
    achalasia and cricopharyngeal bar)
  Strictures
  Radiation inflammation or stricture
  Delayed relaxation of upper esophageal
    sphincter

Patients at risk of aspiration should take nothing by way of the mouth and be fed with a nasogastric feeding tube. In patients with more severe CVAs, it may be apparent within a matter of days that they will not recover adequately to take oral nutrition and a percutaneous endoscopic gastrostomy (PEG) should be placed to permit feeding.

In patients with milder neurologic damage, serial diagnostic evaluations either at the bedside or with videofluoroscopic studies should be performed until it is determined that they can swallow safely without undue risk of aspiration. Often patients will regain their ability to swallow adequately, but this recovery may take days, weeks, or months. However, in patients who have not recovered their ability to swallow safely by 3 months for hemispheric CVAs and 12 months for brainstem CVAs, it is unlikely that significant further recovery will occur. A PEG can be placed early in this process and can be removed easily when and if adequate ability to swallow is recovered.

AMYOTROPHIC LATERAL SCLEROSIS

Amyotrophic lateral sclerosis (ALS), or "Lou Gehrig's" disease, is a progressive neurologic disorder of the spinal cord. It can present with oropharyngeal dysphagia due to involvement of the bulbar spinal cord. The diagnosis is made by the characteristic findings on electromyography (EMG). This disorder inevitably requires placement of a PEG tube for enteral nutrition.

MYASTHENIA GRAVIS

Myasthenia gravis is an uncommon but important cause of oropharyngeal dysphagia. Myasthenia is a disorder characterized by weakness and fatigability of skeletal muscles. The disorder is due to loss of acetylcholine receptors at the neuromuscular junction. Difficulty swallowing is commonly encountered in myasthenia due to weakness of the muscles of swallowing, which are all skeletal muscles. The diagnosis is suggested by the physical examination demonstrating fatigability of muscles and confirmed with the anticholinesterase (edrophonium) test. These patients often do well with appropriate therapy. For this reason, myasthenia is an important cause of oropharyngeal dysphagia that should be considered in the differential diagnosis and tested for when appropriate. A reversible form of myasthenia can be caused by penicillamine, procainamide, large doses of aminoglycosides, and botulinum toxin.

PARKINSON'S DISEASE

Parkinson's disease is relatively common, particularly in the elderly population. This slowly progressive neurologic disorder is often complicated by either oropharyngeal or esophageal dysphagia. As with skeletal muscles elsewhere in the body, the swallowing muscles become rigid. While symptoms are usually mild, they can become moderate and even severe. The mild-to-moderate symptoms are often amenable to swallowing therapy (see patient education, later), but some patients with severe dysphagia may require treatment with nonoral feeding. The oropharyngeal dysphagia is often unresponsive to anti-Parkinsonian drug therapy; however, some patients do respond.

MYOPATHY

Any cause of skeletal muscle myopathy can cause oropharyngeal dysphagia (see Table 3-1). Dysphagia occurs when the propulsive muscles of the oropharynx are too weak to push the bolus through the residual pressure of the upper esophageal sphincter even after it relaxes during swallowing. In polymyositis, in addition to weakness of the propulsive muscles, the upper esophageal sphincter muscle can become fibrotic and represent an obstruction (see cricopharyngeal myotomy, later). This complex presentation needs to be recognized with the appropriate diagnostic tests to allow correction of the sphincter disorder as well as treatment of the myositis.

INCOMPLETE RELAXATION OF THE UPPER ESOPHAGEAL SPHINCTER

Incomplete relaxation of the upper esophageal sphincter is also known as cricopharyngeal achalasia since the cricopharyngeus muscle is the major muscle forming the upper esophageal sphincter. The problem is more likely to become symptomatic if there is also weakness of the muscles used to push the bolus through the sphincter during swallowing. Cricopharyngeal achalasia can be idiopathic but also occurs as a complication of CVA, polymyositis, or infiltrative disorders such as sarcoidosis.

The diagnosis may be suggested by the finding of a cricopharyngeal bar, which is the profile of the nonrelaxing cricopharyngeus muscle seen on the lateral view of a barium study. Esophageal manometry of the upper esophageal sphincter is the test of choice to make this diagnosis. It is important to have the head in the proper (straight) position since extension of the neck can cause manometry to record incomplete relaxation of the upper esophageal sphincter even in healthy individuals. Fixation of the head in extension, such as when the head is placed in a halo for a neck fracture, can cause this abnormality and result in symptoms. Patients with neck fractures often have dysphagia, and it is important to appreciate that the symptoms and finding of incomplete relaxation of the upper esophageal sphincter may be due to the fixation of the neck in extension and should not be treated until the test can be repeated with the head no longer in extension.

Esophageal Dysphagia

Esophageal dysphagia is due to either obstructing disorders or motility disorders. A careful history can often permit identification of the correct diagnosis. However, an obstructing lesion always needs to be sought either by a radiological (barium swallow) or endoscopic test.

ESOPHAGEAL CANCER

Esophageal cancer may be squamous cell carcinoma with risk factors of cigarette smoking and alcohol use, or adenocarcinoma arising in Barrett's esophagus and, therefore, resulting from GERD. Squamous cell carcinoma has historically comprised the vast majority of cases of esophageal cancer, but there has been a marked increase in the incidence of adenocarcinoma of the esophagus. The two types of esophageal cancer have the same presentations. Patients complain of increasing dysphagia to solids. A barium study can identify or "rule out" cancer of the esophagus. Endoscopic evaluation with biopsy provides the tissue diagnosis.

PEPTIC STRICTURE

Dysphagia due to a peptic stricture is typically preceded by years of reflux symptoms. These reflux symptoms can diminish and even resolve due to the antireflux barrier provided by the stricture. Benign strictures have a typical appearance on barium swallow, but require endoscopic evaluation (usually with biopsy and/or brushing) to rule out malignancy.

SCHATZKI RING

Schatzki ring, a common problem, is due to a mucosal invagination in the distal esophagus. The problem presents as intermittent dysphagia to solids. Because of a propensity for victims to choke on food in restaurants, it has acquired the nickname "steakhouse" syndrome. The episodes tend to be sporadic, occurring months or years apart. Between episodes, the patients are usually asymptomatic. The diagnosis is best made by a barium study, although it can be difficult to demonstrate a subtle ring. Swallowing a barium-covered marshmallow can increase the yield and should be specifically requested when ordering a barium swallow in search of a Schatzki ring. At endoscopy, the air insufflation can cause a ring to be unapparent. Treatment is a single pass of a large-bore dilator, which usually, but not always, provides complete and permanent resolution of the problem.

ACHALASIA

Achalasia is the classic esophageal motility disorder, characterized by incomplete relaxation of the lower esophageal sphincter and aperistalsis of the esophageal body. The disorder is due to loss of the myenteric ganglion neurons that innervate the sphincter and cause relaxation. Symptoms of dysphagia to solid and liquid foods may be present for years prior to presentation. Patients with short duration of symptoms, onset in old age, and weight loss should have tests checking for cancer as a possible etiology (pseudoachalasia). These patients will require endoscopy and a computed tomography (CT) scan to rule out malignancy of the gastroesophageal junction, proximal stomach, or lung directly invading the esophagus. Rarely, endoscopic ultrasound may be warranted to exclude a tumor in the submucosa of the esophagus.

For patients with primary achalasia, the diagnosis is suggested by the unique symptoms of food and liquid building up in the esophagus and then (when the weight of the column pushes open the lower esophageal sphincter) emptying completely. If patients become supine before the esophagus empties, nocturnal symptoms of regurgitation, coughing, and choking are common and can result in aspiration-induced lung disease. The barium swallow demonstrates a characteristic lower esophageal sphincter appearance of a "bird's beak" and a dilated esophageal body. Diagnosis is confirmed by esophageal manometry with two required findings of incomplete relaxation of the lower esophageal sphincter and aperistalsis of the esophageal body.

DIFFUSE ESOPHAGEAL SPASM

Diffuse esophageal spasm is a motility disorder of the esophagus characterized by disordered or "simultaneous" contractions of the esophageal body. Instead of a peristaltic wave of contraction progressing down the esophagus, different levels of the esophageal body contract simultaneously. As a result, the food bolus gets hung up by these contractions, instead of being propelled along, and patients complain of dysphagia. Diffuse esophageal spasm can also cause chest pain. This diagnosis probably includes a variety of motility disorders with the same manifestation of simultaneous contractions as reflected in the heterogeneity of the manometric findings and patient complaints.

APERISTALSIS OF THE ESOPHAGEAL BODY

Aperistalsis results in dysphagia for the obvious reason that there are no contractions strong enough to propel the food bolus. The lower esophageal sphincter pressure can be normal but is often weak. The finding of aperistalsis on manometry is not as uncommon as one might think. Esophageal aperistalsis can occur in scleroderma, CREST syndrome, other connective tissue diseases, and diabetes mellitus and can be idiopathic. Up to 70 percent of patients with scleroderma have "scleroderma esophagus," characterized by aperistalsis of the esophageal body and weakness of the lower esophageal sphincter. In addition to dysphagia, patients with scleroderma esophagus are at increased risk of GERD, which can be asymptomatic and may cause severe complications. For this reason, all patients with scleroderma should be studied with esophageal manometry and, if they have scleroderma esophagus, then prophylaxis with long-term acid suppression should be recommended.

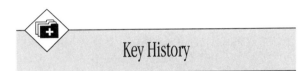

Key History

As discussed earlier, a careful history is important in distinguishing oropharyngeal from esophageal dysphagia. Oropharyngeal dysphagia is characterized by difficulty transferring food to the back of the throat in preparation for swallowing, difficulty initiating a swallow, nasal regurgitation, or aspiration when swallowing. Choking or coughing with swallowing are the hallmarks of oropharyngeal dysphagia. In contrast, patients with esophageal dysphagia report swallowing without choking or coughing.

Globus is the sensation of a lump or fullness in the throat. There is no difficulty swallowing or disruption of transport of the food bolus. Indeed, globus sensation is usually most apparent to patients between meals and improves or resolves completely while eating. The cause of globus is not known, but may be a motor, sensory, or psychological disorder. The diagnosis of globus is made by the typical history. A careful history, physical examination, and laryngoscopy should

be performed to rule out other diagnoses. Treatment for globus sensation consists of explanation and reassurance.

Xerostomia, or dry mouth, is due to inadequate saliva. These patients often complain of dysphagia, which is due to loss of the moistening and lubricating qualities of saliva. Xerostomia may be due to Sjögrens syndrome and may be associated with dry eyes, arthalgias, or arthritis. Medications with anticholinergic side effects are another important cause.

Oropharyngeal Dysphagia

The goal of both the history and physical examination is to determine if the problem is due to a neurologic, otolaryngological, or gastroenterological disorder so that patients can be evaluated appropriately. A thorough neurologic history is essential. Bulbar muscle dysfunction and other brainstem symptoms such as vertigo, nausea, vomiting, hiccups, tinnitus, diplopia, or syncope should be sought. Sudden onset of symptoms would suggest a CVA. Motor weakness or tiring of the facial muscles, such as that which occurs towards the end of a meal, might be an early symptom of myasthenia gravis. Weakness of the extremities associated with muscle pain or discomfort may be a clue in diagnosing inflammatory myositis. Patients should be questioned regarding any change in voice quality (dysphonia). Nasal speech can be indicative of soft palate dysfunction. Tremor or ataxia might suggest Parkinson's disease. A lack of other neurologic symptoms does not rule out neuromuscular disorders since dysphagia may be the first symptom present. Medications should be considered as a cause—particularly cholesterol-lowering HMG-CoA reductase inhibitors, which can cause toxic myopathy. Other medications that may contribute to oropharyngeal dysfunction include anticholinergics, phenothiazines, penicillamine, amiodarone, procainamide, or high doses of aminoglycosides. Finally, history and physical examination should seek evidence of such complications as aspiration pneumonia and weight loss.

Esophageal Dysphagia

History can be helpful in suggesting a likely diagnosis. However, history must not be considered definitive, and a proper diagnostic evaluation to define the disorder must be pursued as described later. A history of dysphagia that progressively worsens over months and is associated with weight loss is worrisome for esophageal cancer. A history of heartburn or other symptoms of GERD may suggest a benign peptic stricture, especially if these symptoms resolved as the dysphagia progressed. Dysphagia to only solids suggests an obstructive disorder, while dysphagia to both solids and liquids suggests a motility disorder. Patients with obstructive disorders often perceive the food sticking either at or above the level of the actual obstruction. Thus, it may be an inaccurate observation if patients report that the food sticks high substernally: Even distal esophageal cancers can present with that symptom. However, it is generally accurate if patients report food sticking in the distal esophagus. Finally, symptoms of systemic disorders such as scleroderma should be sought, including Raynaud's phenomenon and arthritic symptoms, especially in the hands.

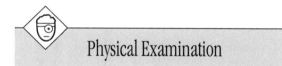

Physical Examination

In oropharyngeal dysphagia, the physical examination should include a complete neurologic exam with special attention to motor strength. Individual muscles of the head and neck such as the sternocleidomastoid or extraocular muscles should be tested for motor strength that fatigues against continued resistance; this is a specific finding suggestive of myasthenia gravis. The neck should be palpated for cervical masses, adenopathy, or thyromegaly. Careful inspection of the oropharynx is appropriate. Since an oropharyngeal exam will miss many important tumors of the pharynx and larynx, it is usually appropriate to further evaluate patients who

have dysphagia with nasolaryngoscopy. The presence or absence of the gag reflex is not helpful as it is absent in 20 to 40 percent of healthy adults.

The physical examination in esophageal dysphagia is not particularly helpful. A routine complete examination of the neck, chest, and abdomen should be performed for findings suggestive of a mass or metastatic disease. Findings suggestive of scleroderma or CREST syndrome should be sought, such as joint abnormalities, tight skin around the mouth and hands, or telangiectasias.

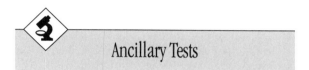

Ancillary Tests

Creatine phosphokinase is an important test for detecting inflammatory myopathies. Thyroid-stimulating hormone is also important as both hyper- and hypothyroidism can cause myopathy. The diagnosis of myasthenia gravis is suggested by the presence of AChR antibodies and a positive Tensilon (edrophonium) stimulation test. An EMG can be diagnostic of a variety of myopathies and neurologic disorders, including myasthenia gravis and ALS.

Videofluoroscopy (Cine Swallowing Study)

Videofluoroscopy involves swallowing liquid barium, barium paste, or barium-coated materials with continuous radiological filming. This is the most useful test to study the swallowing mechanism and to identify aspiration. It is of little value when evaluating esophageal dysphagia. Videofluoroscopy is best performed with a speech pathologist present. The speech pathologist can direct patients to perform certain maneuvers that may improve swallowing and decrease aspiration. With this approach, the videofluoroscopic study can be both diagnostic and therapeutic. This test can be repeated serially to assess improvement in patients' swallowing, such as after a CVA. Videofluoroscopy should always include a view of the entire esophagus (esophagram), as distal esophageal disease can be mistaken for oropharyngeal dysphagia.

Barium Swallow (Esophagram)

Barium swallow, a simple and commonly used test, is appropriate for the initial evaluation of esophageal dysphagia. When a barium swallow or esophagram is ordered, the radiologist usually examines the esophagus and lower esophageal sphincter only, while an upper GI series usually includes the entire esophagus, stomach, and duodenum. However, during the upper GI series the esophagus may receive less attention.

The barium swallow is sensitive in detecting obstructing lesions such as cancers and benign strictures, and a normal esophagram essentially rules out all these worrisome diagnoses. Certain motility disorders may have some characteristic findings such as a dilated esophagus with a "bird's beak" lower esophageal sphincter in achalasia or a "corkscrew" esophagus in severe diffuse esophageal spasm. However, diffuse esophageal spasm and other motility disorders often appear normal on barium swallow.

Endoscopy (Esophagoscopy)

Esophagoscopy is routinely performed as part of a complete esophagogastroduodenoscopy (EGD). Endoscopy can be performed as the initial evaluation of esophageal dysphagia. When endoscopy is performed to evaluate dysphagia without a previous barium swallow, the endoscopist should pass the scope under direct visualization to avoid complications such as entering and perforating a Zenker's diverticulum. A Zenker's diverticulum is an outpouching in the cervical esophagus that can present with dysphagia due to extrinsic pressure on the esophagus by a large diverticulum filled with fluid or food.

Endoscopy provides more accurate assessment of the mucosa than can the barium swallow and

allows biopsy. Many abnormalities identified by barium swallow require endoscopy to make a more definite diagnosis. Endoscopy is often needed for therapeutic interventions such as dilating strictures and stenting obstructing cancers and is increasingly used for treatment of motility disorders such as using pneumatic dilation or injection of botulinum toxin for achalasia.

Esophageal Manometry

Esophageal manometry is performed by placing a soft catheter nasally into the stomach. The catheter is then pulled back gradually and pressures are measured, both at rest and with a water swallow, of the lower esophageal sphincter, esophageal body (3 levels 5 cm apart), upper esophageal sphincter, and pharyngeal function. The procedure takes approximately 15 min and has an excellent safety record.

Esophageal manometry is useful in the evaluation of oropharyngeal dysphagia and is often used to complement the videofluoroscopic study to combine visual appearance and pressure recording to fully define the function of the swallowing mechanism. Manometry is useful for identifying weakness of the pharyngeal muscles, which might be the earliest clue to a myopathic disorder such as polymyositis.

Esophageal manometry is the test of choice for the diagnosis of motility disorders of the esophagus and is generally employed after the barium swallow or endoscopy have excluded significant obstructing pathology. Esophageal manometry is usually required for the diagnosis of achalasia, diffuse esophageal spasm, and scleroderma esophagus.

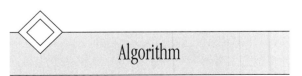

Algorithm

An algorithm for the evaluation of symptoms of dysphagia is depicted in Figure 3-1. Figure 3-2 is an algorithm for the management of dysphagia.

Figure 3-1

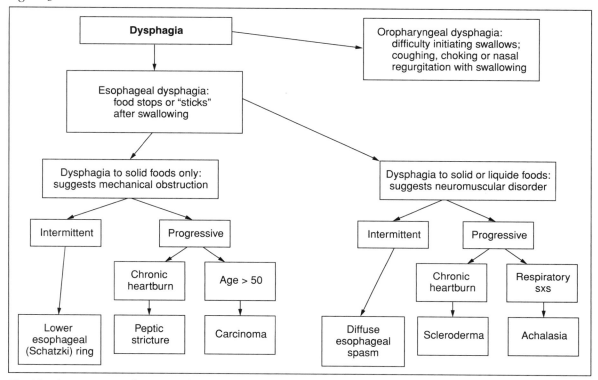

Algorithm for assessment of symptoms for patients with dysphagia. Confirmation of diagnosis with appropriate evaluation is necessary. Adapted with permission from Castell DO. Dysphagia: A general approach to the patient. In: Gelfand DW, Richter JE (eds): *Dysphagia Diagnosis and Treatment.* New York, Igaku-Shoin, 1989, page 4.

Figure 3-2

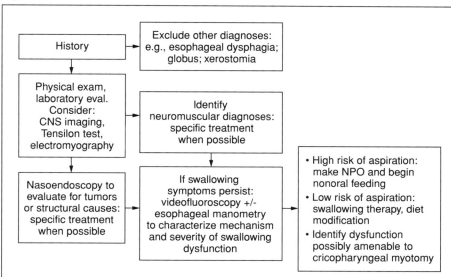

Algorithm of approach to diagnosis and management of oropharyngeal dysphagia.

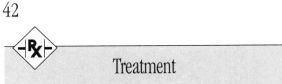

Treatment

Oropharyngeal Dysphagia

Whatever the cause of oropharyngeal dysphagia, the first issue to be addressed is the risk of aspiration and the safety of continuing oral feeding. Useful advice regarding this issue will be provided by speech pathologists who have special training and experience with swallowing disorders. These professionals are typically found in hospital-based rehabilitation departments, since patients hospitalized for acute CVAs are the most common patients needing their assistance. Patients with milder symptoms managed as outpatients can be taught techniques (see patient education) to decrease their symptoms such as a change in head position when swallowing or a change in food consistency. For patients at risk of aspiration, techniques such as a supraglottic swallow can reduce the risk of aspiration and pneumonias.

Patients who present with aspiration pneumonia or who, because of the severity of their neurologic or head and neck disorders are at high risk of aspiration, should be evaluated by a speech pathologist in combination with videofluoroscopy so that the risk of aspiration can be assessed. The speech pathologist can then teach the appropriate techniques and demonstrate that they are adequate in preventing aspiration.

If patients are found to be at high risk of aspiration, then nutrition should be provided by a nasogastric feeding tube for short-term management and a PEG for long-term management. The speech pathologist can reevaluate patients periodically to assess whether the risk of aspiration has been decreased and oral feeding can be restarted. Tube feeding does not completely eliminate the risk of aspiration pneumonia due to aspiration of feedings or oral secretions. There are a variety of surgical procedures that can eliminate these risks (e.g., glottic closure or tracheoesophageal diversion), but they are rarely employed.

Percutaneous Endoscopic Gastrostomy

Percutaneous endoscopic gastrostomy (PEG) will allow adequate enteral nutrition and avoid prolonged use of nasogastric tubes, which are a bit of a nuisance and may increase the risk of aspiration pneumonia. Alternatively, for the patients who do not want a PEG or are poor candidates for PEGs, prolonged use of the nasogastric feeding tube for enteral nutrition is acceptable.

The PEG is placed by a needle puncture through the abdominal wall directly into the stomach under endoscopic guidance. A wire is placed through the needle, grabbed via an endoscope passed into the stomach via the mouth, and withdrawn orally. The feeding tube is placed orally over the wire and passed out through the abdominal wall. When complete, the tube is maintained in the stomach by the intragastric anchor that is formed at the end of the tube.

The PEG placement may be complicated by infection of the skin around the PEG site, or infection in the abdominal wall that can dissect along tissue planes and allow abscess formation. In addition, leakage of gastric contents into the peritoneum can occur if the PEG is too loose. If the PEG is placed too tightly, pressure necrosis can occur. This can present with bleeding from a gastric ulcer at the PEG site. Once the gastric-cutaneous tract has matured (usually about 3 weeks), complications are uncommon. In fact, PEGs do not routinely need to be changed and can last many months. When it is no longer needed, the PEG can be easily removed by pulling on the catheter. The intragastric anchor is soft and malleable and will pop out. The tract will close within a couple of days. Removal of the PEG is best performed by the physician who placed it to ensure the nature of the anchoring mechanism is fully understood when attempting removal.

For patients who will receive radiation and/or chemotherapy for cancers of the head and neck or esophagus and are expected to develop severe dysphagia, the PEG can be placed prior to beginning the treatment. This way the PEG site will be mature by the time the consequences of radiation and/or chemotherapy set in and complications due to the PEG can be minimized and nutrition can be maintained without interruption.

Esophageal Dysphagia

Obstructing lesions and achalasia should be referred to a gastroenterologist or surgeon for appropriate treatment. Peptic strictures (due to GERD) should be treated with aggressive acid suppression with proton-pump inhibitors; this can improve the dysphagia and decrease the need for subsequent dilations. In some patients with mild narrowing of the distal esophagus, proton-pump inhibitors alone can improve the dysphagia adequately, thus avoiding the need for dilation. Once patients have peptic strictures, long-term treatment with proton-pump inhibitors will be needed to minimize the need for further dilations. Dilation can be performed with a variety of techniques, and three techniques are commonly used today. A Savory dilator is polyvinyl and passed over a guidewire that is endoscopically placed across the stricture and can be monitored fluoroscopically. A Maloney dilator is mercury-filled with a flexible tapered tip and is placed blindly through the mouth and across the stricture. Balloon dilators are passed through the endoscope and placed across the stricture under direct visualization. In general, dilation of esophageal strictures is done with serial dilations of increasing size performed during a single endoscopic examination, but it may need to be performed over multiple visits.

Achalasia is most often treated with pneumatic dilation, which employs a large-volume balloon to dilate the lower esophageal sphincter. Because of the size of the balloon, pneumatic dilation has a higher perforation rate than other types of dilation. Alternative therapies of achalasia include surgical myotomy, which can be done laparoscopically in selected cases and is typically performed after pneumatic dilation has failed or if there is a contraindication to dilation. A newer therapy for achalasia is injection of botulinum toxin (Botox) into the lower esophageal sphincter. This therapy is generally reserved for old or sick patients who are at high risk for surgery and, therefore, also poor candidates for pneumatic dilation as surgery may be needed in case of perforation. Botulinum toxin injection is a safe procedure and works well for achalasia, but the effect is transient, lasting from only months to as long as 1 to 2 years. The long-term safety of injection of botulinum toxin into the esophagus has not yet been determined. For this reason we generally reserve this therapy for elderly patients.

Hyperkinetic disorders of the esophagus such as diffuse esophageal spasm can be frustrating to treat. As chest pain is a common symptom in patients with this disorder, reassurance of the good prognosis of these disorders is important. Cardiac disease must be ruled out before initiating treatment of esophageal motility causes of chest pain. Chest pain of esophageal origin often mimics angina pectoris—a source of great anxiety to patients. It has been demonstrated that a major benefit of esophageal manometry can be to demonstrate a motility disorder of the esophagus, thereby providing further evidence to patients that the pain is not of cardiac origin. Treatment of chest pain related to diffuse esophageal spasm often begins with an empiric trial of gastric acid suppression, preferably with a proton-pump inhibitor, as GERD may be the underlying etiology of the motility disorder in a sizable fraction of these patients. Beyond this, a long-acting calcium channel blocker to decrease smooth muscle activity in the esophagus is usually tried but with variable success.

Patients with scleroderma esophagus (aperistalsis of the esophageal body and weak lower esophageal sphincter pressure) should be treated with acid-suppressing medications prophylactically because they are at risk of developing complications of GERD. If they are asymptomatic, an H_2-receptor antagonist is adequate. If they have any symptoms of GERD, then a proton-pump inhibitor is appropriate to control symptoms and prevent complications.

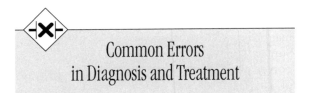

Patient Education

Dietary Modification and Swallowing Therapy

Altering the texture of liquids can improve swallowing. For example, thickened liquids are less likely to spill over the tongue base and can decrease aspiration in patients with disordered tongue function, impaired laryngeal closure, and aspiration that occurs before swallowing. Alternatively, thin liquids can help in patients with weak pharyngeal contraction or a narrowed cricopharyngeal opening.

Postural adjustments can compensate for focal muscle weaknesses. For example, patients with unilateral pharyngeal weakness after CVA can rotate the head toward the affected side forcing the bolus to travel down the unaffected side. Compensatory strategies and positions such as head rotation, head tilt, chin down, chin up, or lying down have been demonstrated to improve swallowing in 75 percent of patients and eliminate aspiration in 25 percent.

Swallowing therapy also offers active maneuvers that can decrease the risk of aspiration. For example, with the supraglottic swallow patients use breath holding, forceful expiration, and double swallowing to ensure closure of the vocal cords before and during swallowing. These types of swallowing therapies require adequate cognitive and neurologic function so that patients can understand and comply with the maneuvers. Dietary changes and postural adjustments can be instituted by caregivers even in the absence of normal cognitive function.

An important point is that the efficacy of each of these techniques in individual patients can be demonstrated during videofluoroscopy. This allows the speech pathologist to determine if the technique adequately protects the patient from aspiration, thereby providing some confidence that it is safe to proceed with oral feeding. Other techniques exist, but a detailed discussion of these

is beyond the scope of this review. One technique worthy of mentioning involves strengthening exercises for patients with pharyngeal weakness. As with other muscles in the body, response to exercise varies with the severity of the neurologic damage. While exercise of the swallowing muscles has not been demonstrated to be effective for most patients, in the individual patient it is certainly worth a try.

Esophageal Motility Disorders

Unlike patients with swallowing disorders, patients with esophageal dysphagia can do little to improve function. However, patients with poor peristalsis, such as in scleroderma esophagus or aperistalsis of the esophageal body, in whom an obstructing lesion or obstructing motility problem, such as incomplete relaxation of the lower esophageal sphincter in achalasia, has been ruled out can be reassured that the food passage is clear. When they feel food get stuck, they should remain calm, wait a few seconds, and then swallow again or take a sip of water to push a food bolus down and continue eating.

Common Errors in Diagnosis and Treatment

Empiric Treatment without Full Work-Up

Oropharyngeal and esophageal dysphagia are symptoms that require an appropriate diagnostic evaluation. In addition, the clinician should beware that when patients report that the food gets stuck in the throat or neck, this sensation may not be accurate. It is a common occurrence that more distal esophageal obstructions are mistakenly reported by the patient as occurring at more proximal locations. Therefore, the entire esophagus must be adequately evaluated on videofluoroscopic and barium studies performed for swallowing disorders.

Emergent Removal of Obstructing Food

When food gets stuck in the obstructed or partially obstructed esophagus, this represents an urgent situation that must be dealt with promptly. Food stuck in the esophagus can cause ischemia, infarction, and perforation of the esophageal wall, which can be a catastrophic problem requiring emergency resective surgery. If the food bolus is removed promptly, the damage to the esophagus is usually minimal. These patients often seek medical attention in the late evening after eating beef or chicken for dinner and complain accurately of food impaction. The inability for even saliva to pass the impaction may be apparent by frequent expectoration. Emergency endoscopy and removal of the impacted food is the treatment of choice and should be performed that night and not postponed until morning.

Cervical Osteophytes

Cervical osteophytes occur in 6 to 30 percent of elderly patients and, therefore, are a common incidental finding in patients with dysphagia due to other causes. Prominent osteophytes can cause dysphagia by compression of the posterior pharyngeal wall, perhaps in combination with inflammation induced by motion over the osteophytes. Surgical treatment, which involves removal of the bony spur, is controversial and has significant risk of complications. In light of these issues, cervical osteophytes are best treated conservatively and surgery should only be considered for patients with the most severe dysphagia.

Lateral Pharyngeal Diverticula

Small lateral pharyngeal diverticula are a commonly encountered incidental radiographic finding. Symptoms may be erroneously attributed to this disorder, which is usually asymptomatic. Lateral diverticula occur in the midpharynx and should not be confused with the posterior, hypopharyngeal diverticulum (Zenker's), which can cause symptoms. Lateral diverticula may be con-

genital or acquired, are frequently bilateral, and are more common in the elderly. Although there are sporadic case reports of surgical treatment alleviating dysphagia, in most cases these diverticula are asymptomatic and should not be treated.

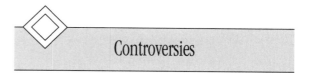

Controversies

Cricopharyngeal Myotomy

Surgical treatment of dysphagia with cricopharyngeal myotomy can be used to reduce the resting pressure of the upper esophageal sphincter. The controversy is in choosing appropriate patients for this treatment. Myotomy is most efficacious when used to treat patients with cricopharyngeal achalasia or structural disorders affecting the sphincter with preserved pharyngeal contractions such as postcricoid stenosis, cervical webs, and Zenker's diverticulum. In Zenker's diverticulum myotomy is essential for successful long-term relief of dysphagia. Treatment of Zenker's diverticulum with diverticulectomy or diverticulopexy combined with cricopharyngeal myotomy achieves good or excellent response in 80 to 100 percent of patients.

The role of cricopharyngeal myotomy in treatment of dysphagia due to neurologic disorders is much less clear. While the surgery seems to benefit some patients, it remains difficult to identify the population of patients in whom success can be predicted with acceptable confidence prior to recommending the surgery. Intuitively, patients with failure of relaxation of the upper esophageal sphincter with retention of adequate pharyngeal contraction would be expected to benefit from myotomy. Radiological criteria for incomplete relaxation of the sphincter are not reliable enough. Current solid-state manometric techniques are providing more reliable assessment of upper esophageal sphincter pressures and hopefully will be useful in predicting response to myotomy, although the data are not yet established. Parkinson's disease provides a good example of the problem. Incomplete relaxation of the upper esophageal sphincter is common in patients with Parkinson's disease; however, results with crico- pharyngeal myotomy are variable and more data are needed before this surgery should be recom- mended for patients with Parkinson's disease. For now, the role of cricopharyngeal myotomy in treatment of dysphagia due to neurologic disor- ders remains unsettled.

Botox for Esophageal Motility Disorders

Botulinum toxin (Botox) has been used for years to successfully treat spastic muscle disorders. Botox has been injected directly (via an endoscope) into the lower esophageal sphincter to treat achalasia with great success and apparent excellent safety. This treatment is generally reserved for the elderly or those too sick to tolerate standard therapy such as surgery or pneumatic dilation. Botox injection has been avoided in the young because of the unknown long-term safety profile.

Other hyperkinetic motility disorders of the esophagus such as diffuse esophageal spasm or hypertensive lower esophageal sphincter can cause severe symptoms without satisfactory med- ical or surgical treatments available. Currently, some gastroenterologists advocate injecting Botox into the lower esophageal sphincter to treat these disorders. Although preliminary data are encour- aging, efficacy has not yet been established. Addi- tionally, these disorders commonly affect young adults and, therefore, the unknown long-term risk of injecting Botox into the esophagus needs to be considered and discussed with the patient.

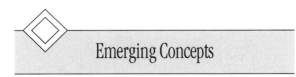

Emerging Concepts

Functional Oropharyngeal Dysphagia

Normal work-up including careful neurologic examination, direct laryngoscopy, cine swallowing study, and esophageal manometry is reassuring for ruling out significant pathology. However, many patients with mild symptoms have a negative work-up and the etiology of their symptoms is unclear. These patients are often dismissed with "symptoms are all in their head." A more appropri- ate explanation for some patients is that they have a subtle motor or sensory disorder of the orophar- ynx that is not detected by our rather crude testing. These patients can be categorized as having a func- tional disorder of swallowing. Of course, the pos- sibility of an early presentation of a significant neuromuscular or head and neck disorder must be considered and the patient followed carefully over time. Once it is apparent that the symptoms are not progressing then the diagnosis of a functional dis- order of swallowing is likely. Again, this diagnosis is best thought of as "a disorder of the motor or sensory function of the oropharynx that we are not yet able to diagnoses," and the patient should be reassured about the excellent prognosis.

Esophageal Dysphagia after Antireflux Surgery

Gastroesophageal reflux disease is increasingly being treated with surgical antireflux procedures such as the Nissan fundoplication. This surgery can be performed open or laparoscopically and essentially involves wrapping the fundus of the stomach around the distal esophagus, creating a new antireflux barrier. One problem with this approach is that the new antireflux barrier does not relax with swallowing to let the bolus pass, and some patients complain of dysphagia. Many patients have transient dysphagia after the surgery due to swelling. This dysphagia usually resolves by 3 months. On rare occasions, how- ever, the dysphagia can be permanent and require repeat surgery to undo the fundoplication. To decrease the risk of this problem, patients should undergo an esophageal manometry prior to surgery. Patients with weak contractions in the esophageal body (ineffective esophageal motility) are recommended to undergo a "loose" fundopli- cation, which generally entails a partial (270° or toupee) procedure. Patients with aperistalsis of the esophageal body (can be idiopathic or due to scleroderma) are at high risk of developing dysphagia, and antireflux surgery should be avoided in these patients.

Bibliography

American Gastroenterological Association: Medical position statement on treatment of patients with dysphagia caused by benign disorders of the distal esophagus. *Gastroenterology* 117:229, 1999.

Bastian RW: Contemporary diagnosis of the dysphagic patient. *Otolaryngol Clin North Am* 31:489, 1998.

Castell DO, ed: *The Esophagus*, 2nd ed. New York, Little, Brown and Company, 1995.

Cook IJ, Kahrilas PJ: American Gastroenterological Association: Medical position statement on management of oropharyngeal dysphagia. *Gastroenterology* 116:452, 1999.

Dray TG, Hillel AD, Miller RM: Dysphagia caused by neurologic deficits. *Otolaryngol Clin North Am* 31:507, 1998.

Ekberg O, Olsson R: Dynamic radiology of swallowing disorders. *Endoscopy* 29:439, 1997.

Gelfand DW, Richter JE, eds: *Dysphagia Diagnosis and Treatment*. New York, Igaku-Shoin, 1989.

Mujica AR, Conklin F: When it's hard to swallow. What to look for in patients with dysphagia. *Postgrad Med* 105:131, 1999.

Plant RL: Anatomy and physiology of swallowing in adults and geriatrics. *Otolaryngol Clin North Am* 31:477, 1998.

Poertner LC, Coleman RF: Swallowing therapy in adults. *Otolaryngol Clin North Am* 31:561, 1998.

Rothstein RD: A systematic approach to the patient with dysphagia *Hosp Pract* 15:169, 1997.

Sallout H, Mayoral W, Benjamin SB: The aging esophagus. *Clin Geriatr Med* 15:439, 1999.

Schechter GL: Systemic causes of dysphagia in adults. *Otolaryngol Clin North Am* 31:525, 1998.

Spechler SJ: AGA technical review on treatment of patients with dysphagia caused by benign disorders of the distal esophagus. *Gastroenterology* 117:233, 1999.

Wisdom G, Blitzer A: Surgical therapy for swallowing disorders. *Otolaryngol Clin North Am* 31:537, 1998.

Arun Khazanchi
Steven Edmundowicz

Chapter

4

Weight Loss

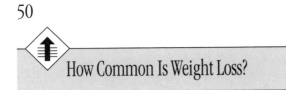

How Common Is Weight Loss?

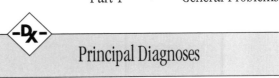

Principal Diagnoses

Patients' weight loss is a common complaint that often challenges the primary care physician. Fluctuations in weight over a period of time can often be attributed to diet, exercise, or intrinsic body rhythms; yet involuntary weight loss is of significant concern. Body weight is stable over long periods of time because food intake is matched to energy expenditure by neural activity in the hypothalamus that provides signals for "feeding" and "satiety." In fact, body weight may fluctuate as much as 1.5 percent from day to day in order to compensate for the metabolic demands. In some studies, mortality rates have been lower for individuals whose body weight fluctuates near the normal mean than they were for those whose weight fluctuates up or down considerably. Moreover, the incidence of cardiovascular and biliary tract disease is lower than it is for increased weight changes. However, an unexplained loss of more than 5 percent of the normal body weight within the past 6 months should warrant a thorough investigation and explanation.

The best way to document weight loss is to compare the current weight to previously recorded values over a period of time. In some instances patients may claim a significant weight loss that cannot be documented. In a survey of 1200 patients by Marton et al., only 50 percent of those who reported a loss of more than 5 lb in the past 6 months were actually verified. Therefore, proper documentation is necessary. In the absence of recorded documentation, a history of weight loss may be obtained from the patients' recollection of previous measured weights in the past year or changes in clothing sizes. Friends and relatives might be helpful in corroborating the changes in weight. If it is not possible to verify a weight loss, patients should be followed at regular intervals with repeat examinations since occult illness causing weight loss may not manifest itself for a period of time.

There are three basic mechanisms of weight loss that may occur alone or in combination in a given patient: increased metabolic rate, increased loss of energy, and decreased intake. The causes of unintentional weight loss in three large series are listed in Table 4-1.

Decreased food intake is by far the most common mechanism and is usually due to loss of appetite but may be attributed to physical factors such as obstruction in the esophagus or stomach secondary to stricture, compressive mass, or infiltrating malignancy causing early satiety (Table 4-2). Unpleasant symptoms associated with eating (impaired sense of taste and smell or painful mouth), dietary idiosyncrasies, and psychiatric conditions such as depression and anorexia nervosa may also play a pivotal role. Some common causes of *increased metabolism* or energy expenditure (Table 4-3) are hyperthyroidism, pheochromocytoma, inflammation, burns, bone fractures, cancer, and major exercise programs. *Increased loss of energy* generally is due to either diabetes mellitus with glycosuria or intestinal malabsorption with steatorrhea. Chronic pancreatitis in alcoholics is the most common cause of steatorrhea, but malabsorption can occur with intestinal lymphoma, celiac sprue, islet cell tumors (such as somatostatinomas or gastrinomas), radiation injury, biliary tract obstruction, inflammatory bowel disease, and a variety of other disorders (Table 4-4). If the weight loss occurs with a history of increased food intake and appetite, another diagnosis such as diabetes mellitus (polyuria and polydipsia), hyperthyroidism (stare, fine tremor, warmly moist skin, and tachycardia), or malabsorption syndrome (fatty and malodorous stools) is more likely. Occasionally leukemias and lymphomas, carcinoid tumors, and infection by intestinal parasites may present with weight loss in the absence of anorexia or even with increased food intake.

Table 4-1

Causes of Unintentional Weight Loss

DIAGNOSIS	CALIFORNIA STUDY MARTIN ET AL.* (%)	ISRAEL STUDY RABINOWITZ ET AL.† (%)	GEORGIA STUDY THOMPSON AND MORRIS‡ (%)
Unknown	26	23	2
Malignancy	19	36	16
Gastrointestinal disorders	14	17	11
Psychiatric	9	10	20
Cardiovascular	9	0	0
Alcohol	8	0	0
Pulmonary	6	0	0
Endocrine or metabolic	4	4	9
Infectious	3	4	2
Inflammatory	2	1	0
Renal	0	4	0
Neurologic	0	0	7
Medication	0	0	9
Miscellaneous	4	1	5

*Marton KI et al: Involuntary weight loss: Diagnostic and prognostic significance. *Ann Intern Med* 95:568–574, 1986.
†Rabinowitz M et al: Unintentional weight loss. A retrospective analysis of 154 cases. *Arch Intern Med* 146:186–187, 1986.
‡Thompson MP, Morris LK: Unexplained weight loss in the ambulatory elderly. *J Am Geriatr Soc* 39:393, 1991.
Adapted from Drossman DM: Approach to the patient with unexplained weight loss. In Yamada T, ed. *Textbook of Gastroenterology*, 2nd ed. Philadelphia. JB Lippincott Company, 1995, vol. 32; p 721.

Medications

Certain medications may be a cause of weight loss in an individual. Many drugs may cause nausea and thus decreased food intake. In particular, theophylline as well as many other drugs may cause nausea and loss of appetite. Laxative abuse in young men or women may be a surreptitious cause of weight loss. Therefore, a careful and complete record of all medications including herbal medications should be recorded.

Psychological Causes

Depression is the leading psychological cause for weight loss seen in the primary care office setting. The symptoms can be recognized by appetite and sleep disturbance, anhedonia (low energy, poor motivation, and decreased libido), feelings of sad-

ness, agitation or psychomotor retardation, and poor concentration or memory. A diagnosis of depression or other psychosocial problems does not, of course, rule out the simultaneous presence of a physical cause for weight loss, because both may be present independently or they may be related (depression appearing as an early manifestation of malignancy).

Anorexia nervosa most often occurs in adolescent women who lose weight as a result of decreased intake, frequently accompanied by self-induced vomiting, laxative abuse, or excessive physical activity. The disorder often first appears shortly after separation from previous social support (leaving home, divorce, separation, or death). The diagnosis should be considered in any young female who is losing weight. Diagnostic criteria outlined in the Diagnostic and Statistical Manual of Mental Disorders (DSM-IV) include intense fear of becoming obese (not diminished by progres-

Table 4-2

Causes of Decreased Food Intake

SYMPTOMS	POSSIBLE ETIOLOGIES
Abdominal pain with fear of eating (sitophobia)	Channel ulcer Partial intestinal or gastric obstruction Intestinal ischemia Pancreatitis Pancreatic cancer Cholecystitis Choledocholithiasis Gastric bezoar Psychiatric (e.g., conversion disorder) Irritable bowel syndrome
Abnormal taste (dysgeusia)	Hepatitis Medications Psychiatric (e.g., depression or psychosis) Zinc deficiency Vitamin B deficiency Sinusitis Malignancy
Loss of appetite with the thought, sight, or odor of food (anorexia)	Malignancy Medications Psychiatric (e.g., depression or psychosis) Alcohol or drug abuse AIDS Eating disorders Chronic renal disease
Mechanical pain with swallowing (dysphagia or odynophagia) or dyspnea limiting ingestion	Oral/dental disease Esophageal stricture or motor disorder Neurologic (bulbar) disturbance Severe cardiopulmonary disease
Lethargy, weakness	Severe malnutrition of any cause Neuromuscular disease Psychiatric (e.g., depression) Cancer chemotherapy
Poverty	

Adapted from Heizer WH: Weight loss. In Dombrand L, Fletcher R, Hoole A, Pickard G, eds. *Clinical Problems in Ambulatory Care Medicine*. Boston, Little, Brown, and Company 1992, p 15.

sive weight loss); disturbance of body image (claiming to feel fat even when very thin); refusal to maintain a body weight over a minimal normal weight for age and height; and absence of physical illnesses that would account for the weight loss. Failure to recognize the syndrome is likely to precipitate an inappropriately extensive medical evaluation. In contrast, few cases are so clearly

Table 4-3

Increased Metabolic Rate

POSSIBLE ETIOLOGIES
Autoimmune deficiency syndrome
Bone fractures
Burns
Chronic infections (tuberculosis, fungal infections, and endocarditis)
Chronic obstructive pulmonary disease
Congestive heart failure
Diabetes mellitus (uncontrolled)
Exercise programs
Hyperthyroidism
Malignancy (advanced)
Pheochromocytoma

Table 4-4

Causes of Malabsorption and Maldigestion

Bacterial overgrowth
Bile duct obstruction
Celiac sprue
Chronic pancreatitis
Congestive heart failure (advanced) with bowel edema
Crohn's disease
Enteroenteric fistula
Gastrinoma
Hypoalbuminemia (usually seen only with serum albumin <2.5 mg/dl)
Intestinal lymphoma
Lymphatic obstruction
Pancreatic duct obstruction
Parasitic infestation
Radiation injury
Scleroderma
Somatostatinoma

evident initially that all diagnostic testing can be avoided. Patients with inflammatory bowel disease and brain tumors have been mistakenly diagnosed as having anorexia nervosa.

Typical Presentation

In the majority of instances in which a physical cause for weight loss can be found, the cause will be obvious after the history, physical examination, and a minimal laboratory investigation are completed. For example, of 91 male veterans evaluated for involuntary weight loss, the cause was clinically evident on the initial evaluation in 55 of the 59 patients with identified physical causes. The likelihood of a physical cause was the increase in the presence of nausea or vomiting; recent change in cough; and a variety of physical findings such as cachexia, abdominal mass, adenopathy, or thyromegaly. Physical causes were less likely in patients who did not smoke heavily (<20 pack-years) or who maintained their usual activity level.

Large prospective studies of the causes of weight loss are not available, and the five retrospective studies published since 1981 involve relatively small numbers of patients. In young persons, the most likely diagnoses are diabetes mellitus, hyperthyroidism, anorexia nervosa, or infection, especially human immunodeficiency virus (HIV). In elderly persons, cancer is the most likely cause of significant weight loss, with psychiatric illness such as Alzheimer's disease and depression being a distant second.

Under most circumstances the diagnosis of the cause of weight loss is not difficult and is revealed by history, physical examination, and routine laboratory screening. The most common occult condition is cancer. Gastrointestinal, pancreatic, and hepatic malignancies are particularly prone to cause early weight loss. Infectious disease may occasionally be symptomatically silent. Weight loss may occur in HIV infection prior to autoimmune deficiency syndrome (AIDS) defining illness, and tuberculosis, fungal disease, bacterial endocarditis, or hepatitis may present as weight loss in the absence of defining symptoms. Eating disorders, early Alzheimer's disease, and depression may cause unexplained anorexia and weight loss. Uremia and hypercalcemia may be asymptomatic but are easily recognized through screening laboratory examination. Elevated calcium levels not only produce anorexia but sometimes induce nephrogenic diabetes insipidus, compounding the weight loss by volume depletion. Weight loss may or may not be a prominent feature of pheochromocytoma. Pernicious anemia may cause anorexia before hematologic changes occur, and early adrenal insufficiency can cause weight loss in the absence of electrolyte changes, nausea, vomiting, or hypotension. Other causes of anorexic weight loss are chronic obstructive pulmonary disease and emphysema, congestive heart failure, chronic liver disease, and neurologic diseases such as Parkinsonism. For those returning from foreign countries, parasitic disease must always be considered.

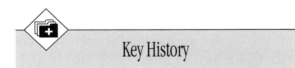

Key History

One should first attempt to determine the degree and rate of weight loss in patients. It is important to establish a rapport with patients before proceeding to more difficult issues including psychological causes of weight loss. The examiner must be aware that in some situations patients may be in denial and unaware of the degree of weight loss that has occurred. In attempting to determine how changes in food intake or physical activity may be contributing to weight loss, it is helpful to ask patients to describe a typical day: time of arising, meals, snacks, activities, time of going to bed, and amount of sleep.

A general review of systems should be useful in detecting any symptoms that may provide a clue to underlying medical conditions that could lead to weight loss. A detailed social history, including a travel history to consider infections or parasites, and a description of the social support system for patients are helpful. If the history suggests reduced oral intake, eliciting the circumstances contributing to decreased food intake may suggest a specific cause, as detailed in Table 4-2. A careful history from patients who have main-

tained or increased their oral intake should explore issues of increased physical activity, change in bowel habits (diarrhea with steatorrhea), and the causes of increased metabolic rate, as listed in Table 4-3.

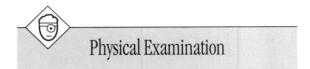

Physical Examination

The physical examination should assess nutritional status as well as identifying underlying causes of weight loss. General findings, such as wasting, fever, tachycardia, and apathetic appearance, should be noted. An effort to detect underlying causes to further direct the evaluation should include, but is not limited to, findings of glossitis; mouth lesions; poor dentition or loss of dental enamel; goiter; adenopathy; masses in the abdomen, rectum, or pelvis; organomegaly; or peripheral neuropathy. In appropriate patients, the examination should also include sampling the stool for occult blood, as well as a pelvic or prostate examination for occult malignancy detection.

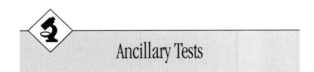

Ancillary Tests

Laboratory evaluation should be guided by the results of the history and physical examination. In patients without specific findings on the history or exam, an initial battery of tests might include a complete blood count with differential, urinalysis, serum chemistry profile with glucose, creatinine, albumin, liver function tests, and stool specimens for occult blood. Thyroid function tests should be performed for all elderly patients with weight loss because of the high incidence of thyroid dysfunction in this age group, and they should be considered for other patients in whom the history strongly suggests that food intake has not decreased.

Laboratory studies for malabsorption should be considered when food intake is normal and there is no evidence of causes of increased metabolic rate from diabetes, thyroid disease, or tumor. Screening tests for malabsorption should include a Sudan stain of the stool for fat and tests for serum carotene and folic acid. These tests are valid only when patients have been eating an adequate diet for several weeks. The definitive test for malabsorption is a quantitative determination of fat absorption by means of a 72-h stool collection with a dietician's assessment of fat intake during the collection.

If the cause of weight loss is not evident on history and physical examination or basic laboratory testing, then the best management might be watchful waiting, with further investigation primarily dictated by continuing weight loss or development of new symptoms. Follow-up visits should also be used to reevaluate any possible psychological causes of weight loss.

In appropriate patients with increased risk factors for malignancy or occult disease, radiographic imaging may be useful to secure a diagnosis. Chest radiography should be considered in smokers or those with a history of smoking exposure. Computed tomography is often overutilized in the evaluation of patients with unexplained weight loss; however, it is one of the only methods of detecting some occult malignancies or infections. In general, a more intensive imaging evaluation than that which is described here is usually unrewarding without specific symptoms or findings to evaluate.

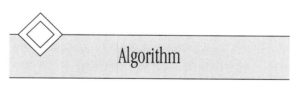

Figure 4-1 shows a diagnostic and treatment algorithm for weight loss.

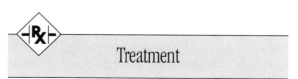

Management of patients with weight loss is directed toward diagnosing and treating the underlying medical problem. In the primary care setting, weight loss is often more important as an indica-

Figure 4-1

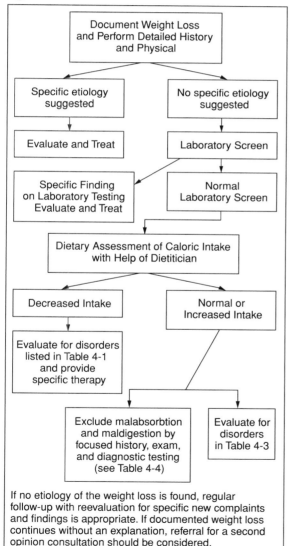

If no etiology of the weight loss is found, regular follow-up with reevaluation for specific new complaints and findings is appropriate. If documented weight loss continues without an explanation, referral for a second opinion consultation should be considered.

Diagnostic and Treatment Algorithm for Weight Loss

tion of the presence and severity of underlying disease than as a medical problem requiring treatment. The initial effort should include a thorough evaluation for a medical or psychological cause of the weight loss while supplying nutritional support. At some point, weight loss itself may become a significant medical problem. Many studies show that life expectancy is greatest for individuals with weights 5 to 20 percent below U.S. average, excluding cigarette smokers and people with pre-existing disease. Furthermore, a modest degree of weight loss is probably a beneficial adaptive response in some illnesses, including chronic obstructive pulmonary disease, congestive heart failure, and possibly some cancers.

Although data are limited, it is likely that at a loss of 10 to 20 percent of normal body weight, medically significant manifestations of malnutrition begin to appear. These include weakness, decreased stamina, depressed immune function, increased tendency for breakdown of the skin, increased susceptibility to infection, and emotional changes of apathy and irritability. An individual of average weight would be expected to lose approximately 15 percent of body weight in 3 weeks of total starvation, in 3 months of one-half normal food intake, and in 3 weeks of one-half the normal nutrient intake in the setting of significant trauma.

There are no measures of nutritional status suitable for clinical use that are both specific and sensitive. In addition to weight loss, measurements that may provide some quantitative assessment of the degree of protein-calorie malnutrition include skin-fold thickness, serum albumin and pre-albumin concentrations, total lymphocyte count, and delayed hypersensitivity by skin testing.

It is preferable to prevent rather than treat serious nutritional deficiency, and prevention should begin early. Most important is to discover and eliminate the cause of weight loss. In addition, attention should be directed toward increasing oral intake. This may include the following:

1. Frequent feeding of foods with high-calorie intake

2. Use of community resources such as senior center lunch programs and Meals-on-Wheels to provide calories for those who need social support
3. Arranging for properly fitting dentures
4. Avoiding restrictive diets of unproved benefit
5. Avoiding drugs that suppress appetite or hinder gastrointestinal function whenever possible (This usually means eliminating all drugs that are not required.)
6. Avoiding accidental or unnecessary restriction or intake in association with diagnostic procedures
7. Using commercial dietary supplements

Early consultation with a registered dietitian may be extremely helpful in the verification of caloric intake as well as directing nutritional support. In certain situations, reliance on patients' oral intake for nutrition will be inadequate and considerations for nutritional support options will include tube feeding or parenteral nutrition.

Enteral supplementation should be initiated early in the course of weight loss when the function of the gastrointestinal tract is not disrupted. If patients are unable or unwilling to consume adequate calories to maintain a reasonable nutritional status, then supplemental feedings by nasogastric, nasoenteric, or percutaneous tube feedings should be considered. Enteral feedings can be accomplished by these methods at home with minimal to no assistance depending on the patients' conditions and supports. The ethical issues surrounding the initiation of tube feedings in patients with terminal illness, refusal of oral intake, or psychiatric conditions are beyond the scope of this text.

Peripheral or central hyperalimentation can be used in those patients requiring nutritional support with a nonfunctional gastrointestinal tract. While more complex, expensive, and hazardous than enteral nutrition, both peripheral and central hyperalimentation provide an option for those patients who would benefit from supplemental or total nutritional support. Most home care nursing organizations have a home nutritional support team to facilitate this process from intravenous line placement to monitoring, patient and family education, and home visits. It is rare that this form of therapy would be necessary for patients without a defined underlying medical condition.

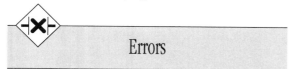

Errors

Two common errors are seen in the evaluation and management of patients with weight loss. The first is the failure to recognize and diagnose a serious underlying condition as the cause of unexplained weight loss in patients. This error is limited by pursuing a careful and thorough initial evaluation. If no explanation for weight loss is found, careful follow-up is necessary to be certain that patients have recovered and no underlying condition exists. The second common error is the failure to recognize eating disorders in young patients with weight loss. Often patients are unwilling to discuss the issues surrounding the condition and, unless a significant rapport can be established with them, recognition and therapy will be difficult.

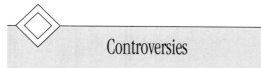

Controversies

A significant controversy persists regarding the use of feeding tubes in patients with weight loss and chronic medical conditions. The ethical issues regarding placement and removal of feeding tubes in patients with dementia and other irreversible conditions remain complex. These issues are best addressed with patients and family members long before the situation becomes critical.

Bibliography

Alpers DH, Rosenberg IH: Eating behavior and nutrient requirements. In Feldman M, Scharschmidt B, Sleisenger M, eds. *Sleisenger and Fordtrans's Gastrointestinal and Liver Disease: Pathophysiology,* *Diagnosis, and Management,* 6th ed. Philadelphia, W.B. Saunders Company, 1997.

Balaa MA, Drossman DA: Anorexia nervosa and bulimia: The eating disorders. *Dis Mon* 31(6):1–52, 1985.

Bonnisler BA, Harvard CW: Patients who lose weight (Editorial). *Br Med J* 286–289, 1993.

DeWys WD: Nutritional abnormalities in cancer. Weight loss in cancer patients: Prognostic and pathophysiologic considerations. In Kluthe R, Lohr GW, eds. *Nutrition and Metabolism in Cancer.* New York, Thieme-Stratton, 1981, p 8.

Drossman DA: Approach to the patient with unexplained weight loss. In Yamada T, ed. *Textbook of Gastroenterology,* 2nd ed. Philadelphia, JB Lippincott Company, 1995, pp 717–729.

Floch MH: Weight loss and nutritional assessment. In Floch MH, ed. *Nutrition and Diet Therapy in Gastrointestinal Disease.* New York, Plenum, 1981, p 101.

Forbes GB: Body composition: Influence of nutrition, disease, growth, and aging. In Shils ME, Young VR, eds. *Modern Nutrition in Health and Disease.* Philadelphia, Lea & Febiger, 1988, pp 533–556.

Foster DW: Gain and loss in weight. In Fauci AS, Braunwald E, Isselbacher KJ, et al, eds. *Harrison's Principles of Internal Medicine,* 14th ed. New York, McGraw-Hill, 1998, pp 244–246.

Garfinkel PE, et al: Differential diagnosis of emotional disorders that cause weight loss. *Can Med Assoc J* 129:939–945, 1983.

Grant JP, Custer PB, Thurlow J: Current techniques of nutritional assessment. *Surg Clin North Am* 61:437–463, 1981.

Grunfeld C: What causes wasting in AIDS? (Editorial.) *N Engl J Med* 333:123, 1995.

Halmi KA: Anorexia nervosa and bulimia. *Annm Rev Med* 38:373–380, 1987.

Haubrich WS: Weight loss. In Feldman M, Scharschmidt B, Sleisenger M, eds. *Sleisenger and Fordtrans's Gastrointestinal and Liver Disease: Pathophysiology, Diagnosis, and Management,* 6th ed. Philadelphia, W.B. Saunders Company, 1997.

Heizer WH: Weight loss. In Dornbrand L, Fletcher R, Hoole A, Pickard G, eds. *Clinical Problems in Ambulatory Care Medicine.* Boston, Little, Brown, and Company, 1992, p 15.

Iribarren C, et al: Association of weight loss and weight fluctuation with mortality among Japanese American men. *N Engl J Med* 333:686, 1995.

Marton KI, Sox HC Jr, Knupp Jr: Involuntary weight loss: Diagnostic and prognostic significance. *Ann Intern Med* 95:568–574, 1981.

Palenicek JP, et al: Weight loss prior to clinical AIDS as a predictor of survival. Multicenter AIDS Cohort Study Investigators. *J Acquir Immune Defic Syndr Hum Retrovirol* 10, 366, 1995.

Rabinowitz M, et al: Unintentional weight loss. A retrospective analysis of 154 cases. *Arch Intern Med* 146: 186–187, 1986.

Reife CM: Involuntary weight loss. *Med Clin North Am* 79:299, 1995.

Robbins LJ: Evaluation of weight loss in the elderly. *Geriatrics* 44:31–37, 1989.

Thompson MP, Morris LK: Unexplained weight loss in the ambulatory elderly. *J Am Geriatr Soc* 39:497, 1991.

Von Roenn JH, et al: Megestrol acetate in patients with AIDS-related cachexia. *Ann Intern Med* 121:393, 1994.

Alan M. Adelman

Chapter 5

Dyspepsia

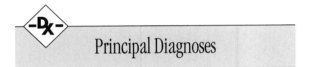

How Common Is Upper Abdominal Pain or Dyspepsia?

The complaint of upper abdominal pain or dyspepsia encompasses a wide variety of clinical presentations and diagnoses, ranging from mild gastrointestinal infections to such life-threatening conditions as perforated duodenal ulcer and pancreatic cancer. This can make it challenging to identify the specific cause of upper abdominal pain—even more so in primary care practice because the various conditions that cause abdominal pain do not always present with classic findings. With so many conditions resulting in dyspepsia, a review of all possible causes would require an entire textbook. This chapter will focus on the most common causes of dyspepsia seen in primary care practice.

Prevalence

According to the National Ambulatory Medical Care Survey, abdominal pain, classified as stomachache, cramps, or spasms, is one of the top 10 reasons why patients in the United States make office visits to physicians. The majority of these visits are to primary care clinicians. Over one-third of individuals with abdominal pain will localize their pain to the upper abdomen.

Virtually all individuals experience abdominal pain at some time in their lives, and between 14 and 27 percent report having had abdominal pain within the last 6 to 12 months. Of those who report abdominal pain, 20 to 38 percent seek medical care for their pain, with women more likely to seek care than do men.

Not surprisingly, individuals who have severe or frequent pain are more likely to seek medical attention than are others, averaging between one and three visits to a clinician for each episode of abdominal pain. Despite that only the more severe cases come to medical attention, almost 90 percent of patients who are evaluated by a clinician for abdominal pain will be pain-free within 2 to 3 weeks of the evaluation, even without any specific treatment. Only about 10 percent of patients seen in primary care practice for abdominal pain are referred to specialty clinicians for further evaluation. Fewer than 10 percent are admitted to a hospital.

Heartburn, the most common symptom of dyspepsia, is extraordinarily common. Over 6 million individuals in the United States experience heartburn every day, and nearly one-half of all U.S. adults have heartburn at least monthly. The problem is so common that 18 million Americans take antacids to relieve heartburn more than twice per week.

Principal Diagnoses

Dyspepsia describes a constellation of symptoms consisting predominantly of upper abdominal or epigastric discomfort. The major symptom of dyspepsia is upper abdominal or epigastric pain. Heartburn—the feeling of acid in the stomach—is also common. Other symptoms include bloating, nausea, vomiting, hiccuping, and/or belching.

About one-quarter of individuals with dyspepsia will consult a clinician. After evaluation by a clinician, the five diagnoses accounting for 80 to 90 percent of dyspepsia are nonulcer dyspepsia, gastroesophageal reflux disease, duodenal ulcer, gastritis, and gastric ulcer.

Nonulcer Dyspepsia

The most common cause of dyspeptic symptoms is "nonulcer dyspepsia," which refers to dyspepsia for which no specific cause can be identified. Thus, as with the general category of abdominal pain, the most common diagnostic outcome for patients with dyspepsia is to identify no specific cause for the symptoms.

The cause of nonulcer dyspepsia is unknown, though some experts believe it may represent a gastrointestinal motility disorder. Patients with non-ulcer dyspepsia have normal levels of gastric acid secretion, and the prevalence of *Helicobacter pylori* infection, the apparent cause of peptic ulcers, is no greater in persons with nonulcer dyspepsia than it is in the general population. In addition, treatment of *H. pylori* infection does not predictably lead to resolution of nonulcer dyspepsia.

The incidence of nonulcer dyspepsia decreases with advancing age. Thus, when young adults complain of dyspeptic symptoms, the likelihood that no specific pathology will be discovered (i.e., the diagnosis will be nonulcer dyspepsia) is relatively high. With increasing age, however, especially after age 50, the diagnosis of specific conditions such as gastritis, gastric cancer, peptic ulcer disease, or gastroesophageal reflux becomes more common.

Gastroesophageal Reflux Disease

The next most common cause of dyspeptic symptoms in primary care practice is gastroesophageal reflux disease (GERD). GERD involves reflux of stomach contents into the esophagus, which can cause injury to the esophagus [Fig. 5-1 (plate 1)]. Most symptoms of GERD are caused by reflux of acid, but pepsin, bile salts, and pancreatic enzymes may also contribute to symptoms and esophageal injury.

The principal pathophysiologic process that permits reflux to occur is weakness or incompetence of the lower esophageal sphincter. However, other processes also contribute, including abnormal esophageal motility, diminished resistance of the esophageal mucosa to refluxed gastric contents, and delayed postprandial emptying of the stomach.

Simple heartburn is the most common manifestation of GERD. However, gastric contents can damage esophageal mucosa, causing esophagitis—including erosive esophagitis [Fig. 5-2 (plate 2)]. Esophageal mucosa that is chronically exposed to gastric contents can also develop strictures. In addition, between 10 and 20 percent of patients who seek care for GERD will develop Barrett's esophagus (metaplasia of normal squamous esophageal

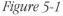
Figure 5-1

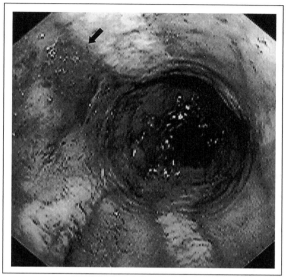

Esophagitis. Endoscopic view of the distal esophagus showing inflammation of the esophageal mucosa. The arrow indicates the most-inflamed area. *(Courtesy of Gregory Gambla, D.O., Milton Hershey Medical Centers, Penn State Geisinger Health System.) (See color plate 1).*

epithelium into columnar epithelium). Barrett's esophagus is of concern because the metaplastic epithelium can undergo further transformation to adenocarcinoma. Finally, in some patients, refluxed gastric contents can enter their airway, resulting in laryngitis, chronic cough, asthma-like wheezing, aspiration pneumonia, or chest pain.

Duodenal Ulcer

Duodenal ulcers are typically small (less than 1 cm) ulcerations of the proximal duodenal mucosa [Fig. 5-3 (plate 3)]. They occur at one time or another in about 10 percent of the U.S. population. Duodenal ulcers are thought to result from the action of gastric acid and digestive enzymes on a duodenal mucosa that is inadequately protected by mucus, bicarbonate, and prostaglandins. However, the gram-negative bacteria *H. pylori* also play a critical role, as the organism is present in nearly all individuals who develop duodenal ulcers. In addition, eradication of *H. pylori* with antibiotic therapy markedly reduces the risk of ulcer recurrence.

Duodenal ulcers are more common in persons who smoke cigarettes, and in individuals with chronic renal failure, alcoholic liver disease, and hyperparathyroidism. Persons with blood type O are also at increased risk, possibly because the O-antigen facilitates binding of *H. pylori* to duodenal mucosa.

Aside from the discomfort of dyspeptic symptoms, the major risk of duodenal ulcers is bleeding. Bleeding can be abrupt and of large volume, resulting in upper gastrointestinal hemorrhage. It can also be occult and manifest as chronic iron-deficiency anemia. Duodenal inflammation and edema associated with the ulcer can cause gastric outlet obstruction. Less commonly, duodenal ulcers can perforate the duodenal wall, spilling gastrointestinal contents into the peritoneal cavity or penetrating into adjacent structures such as the pancreas.

Figure 5-2

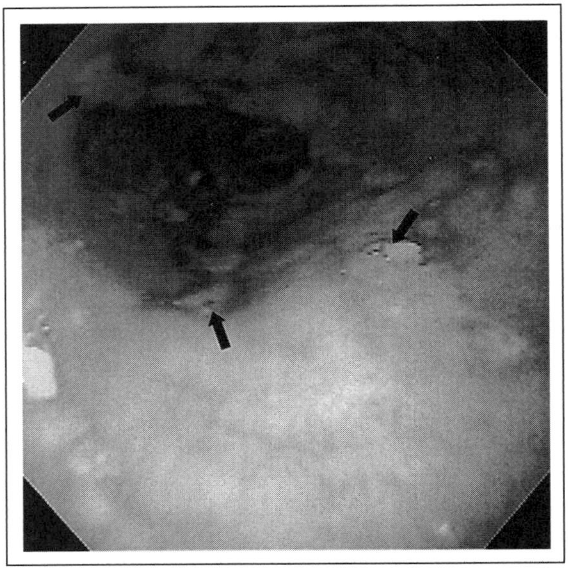

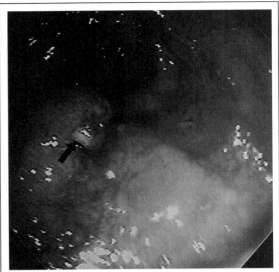

Figure 5-3

Duodenal ulcer. The ulcer is marked by the arrow. *(Courtesy of Gregory Gambla, D.O., Milton Hershey Medical Centers, Penn State Geisinger Health System.) (See color plate 3).*

Esophagitis with ulcerations. Endoscopic view of the distal esophagus demonstrating erythema and multiple erosions and ulcerations (examples marked with arrows). *(Courtesy of Gregory Gambla, D.O., Milton Hershey Medical Centers, Penn State Geisinger Health System.) (See color plate 2).*

Gastric Ulcer

Gastric ulcers are typically deep ulcerations through the mucosa of the stomach, often surrounded by areas of gastritis. They can be caused by ingestion of nonsteroidal anti-inflammatory drugs (NSAIDs), but they also occur in the absence of NSAID use. Gastric acid and pepsin are both involved in the pathogenesis of gastric ulcers but, as with duodenal ulcers, there is also strong evidence that *H. pylori* infection is of primary importance in gastric ulcers. In fact, *H. pylori* are present in the stomach of virtually all individuals who develop gastric ulcers. And, even in the 20 to 25 percent of gastric ulcers caused by NSAIDs, *H. pylori* is still thought to play an etiologic role in many individuals. The mechanism by which *H. pylori* causes gastric ulcers is not certain, but the organism secretes a variety of factors that may damage gastric mucosa and gastric mucus.

Gastric ulcers may be benign or malignant. Benign gastric ulcers are typically small and occur in the antrum of the stomach. They are almost always accompanied by antral gastritis due to *H. pylori* infection. Ulcers in the gastric fundus, in contrast, and larger ulcers, are more likely to be malignant. Endoscopy and biopsy are required to determine if a gastric ulcer is benign or malignant. Barium contrast radiological studies are unreliable, as they may be falsely negative in the presence of malignant gastric ulcers.

Gastric ulcers may also cause serious acute complications. These include hemorrhage, gastric outlet obstruction, and perforation of the stomach either into the abdominal cavity or posteriorly into the pancreas. Of note, duodenal ulcers are simultaneously present in about 10 percent of patients with benign gastric antral ulcers.

Gastritis

Gastritis (inflammation of the gastric mucosa) can result from a variety of causes, and it may be acute or chronic. In primary care practice, the most common causes of acute gastritis are *H. pylori* infection and NSAID ingestion. Acute gastritis may be mild and asymptomatic [Fig. 5-4 (plate 4)], or it may cause dyspeptic symptoms or gastrointestinal bleeding [Fig. 5-5 (plate 5)].

The common form of chronic gastritis seen in primary care practice is related to *H. pylori* infection. In young patients, the inflammation associated with *H. pylori* is typically in the gastric antrum (antral gastritis), whereas in old individuals, the entire stomach may be affected. Over time, the gastric mucosa involved in *H. pylori* gastritis may become atrophic, which increases the risk of gastric adenocarcinoma, though the mechanism by which *H. pylori* infection causes gastric cancer is not understood. It may be that the infection renders gastric mucosa more susceptible to dietary or environmental carcinogens, or it may be simply that the chronic inflammation leads to cell proliferation and subsequent development of cancer. Interestingly, chronic *H. pylori* gastritis is also associated with an increased risk of gastric lymphoma.

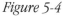

Figure 5-4

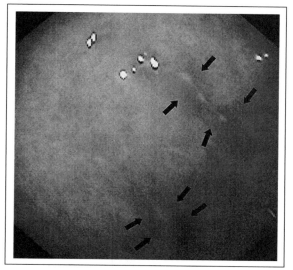

Gastritis. This patient has mild gastritis, manifest as areas of erythema on the gastric mucosa (arrows). *(Courtesy of Gregory Gambla, D.O., Milton Hershey Medical Centers, Penn State Geisinger Health System.) (See color plate 4).*

Figure 5-5

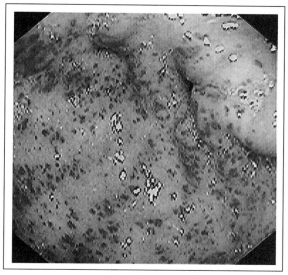

Gastritis. This patient has marked gastritis, with areas of intense erythema and numerous small mucosal hemorrhages. *(Courtesy of Gregory Gambla, D.O., Milton Hershey Medical Centers, Penn State Geisinger Health System.) (See color plate 5).*

Table 5-1
Causes of Dyspepsia

COMMON
Nonulcer Dyspepsia
Gastroesophageal Reflux Disease
Gastritis
Peptic Ulcer Disease (duodenal or gastric)
Cholelithiasis

UNCOMMON
Gastroparesis
Gastric Cancer
Pancreatic Cancer
Pancreatitis
Acute Myocardial Infarction
Perforated Duodenal Ulcer
Abdominal Aortic Aneurysm

Another, relatively uncommon, cause of gastritis is autoimmune gastritis. In this condition, antibodies develop against gastric parietal cells and intrinsic factor, resulting in malabsorption of vitamin B_{12} and subsequent pernicious anemia. There are also many other causes of gastritis that are almost never seen in primary care practice. These include sar-coidosis, Crohn's disease, and parasitic, mycobacterial, and fungal infections of the stomach.

Other Diagnoses to Consider

In addition to the common dyspepsia syndromes previously described, and some uncommon causes of abdominal pain listed in Table 5-1, there are also several serious or life-threatening conditions that should be considered in any patient who presents with abdominal pain. A discussion of these conditions is beyond the scope of this chapter, but a few of the more common conditions are listed in Table 5-2.

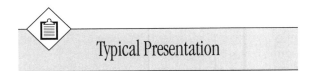

Typical Presentation

Most patients with dyspeptic syndromes, by definition, present with pain above the umbilicus. However, pain may not be a consistent presenting complaint. Other symptoms that may or may not be present include heartburn, bloating, nausea, vomiting, hiccuping, and/or belching.

Table 5-2
Serious or Life-Threatening Causes of Dyspepsia

CAUSE OF PAIN (EXAMPLES)	KEY HISTORY	KEY EXAM
• Gastric outlet obstruction	• Bloating, persistent emesis	• Tympanitic upper abdomen, succussion splash
• Cancer (gastric, pancreatic)	• Weight loss, anorexia, fatigue	• Jaundice, abdominal mass, rectal bleeding, anemia
• Abdominal aortic aneurysm	• Ripping or tearing pain, pain radiating or boring to the back, history of hypertension	• Loss of femoral pulses, pulsatile abdominal mass, hypotension
• Bowel perforation (duodenal ulcer)	• Pain, fever	• Absent bowel sounds, abdominal muscle rigidity
• Pancreatitis	• Epigastric pain, fever, emesis	• Distension, tachycardia
• Acute gastrointestinal bleeding	• Dizziness, weakness, hematemesis, melena, hemochezia	• Guiac-positive emesis or stool, tachycardia, hypotension

In primary care practice, patients' symptoms often do not fit classic patterns described in textbooks. This can make diagnosis difficult. The infrequency of classic patterns in primary care practice occurs for two main reasons.

First, patients often come to primary care clinicians early in the course of their disease. It is only with time that patients display the classic presentations of a particular condition. Dyspeptic syndromes such as duodenal ulcer may initially present with nonspecific complaints such as nausea or lack of appetite, and only later will the possibility of an ulcer become apparent.

The second reason why classic presentations are uncommon in primary care is that most patients simply do not have the classic conditions described in textbooks. Many patients with "classic" ulcer symptoms will have nonulcer dyspepsia. Many patients will have undifferentiated symptoms that are not easily labeled and are never diagnosed with an identifiable cause for their pain.

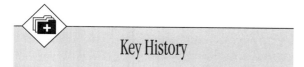

Key History

The history in patients with dyspepsia can be both helpful and confusing, because serious diagnoses occur infrequently, and many conditions have the same or overlapping symptoms. The combination of low prevalence of serious disease and overlapping symptoms makes the positive predictive value of most symptoms quite low.

For example, duodenal ulcer and nonulcer dyspepsia both can present with pain relieved by food or antacids. However, duodenal ulcer is fairly uncommon, whereas nonulcer dyspepsia is extremely common. The low frequency of duodenal ulcer means that even if patients have the classic ulcer symptom of pain relieved by food or antacids, the positive predictive value of these symptoms for duodenal ulcer is actually low. Furthermore, the presence of these symptoms is not a good discriminator between ulcers and nonulcer

dyspepsia. In such situations, in which the prevalence of serious disease is low, the challenge in taking a history is to identify those few patients with potentially serious problems from the majority who have no specific treatable problem or diagnosis.

Thus, the basic plan in taking a history from a patient with dyspepsia and/or abdominal pain is to first search for symptoms indicative of serious or life-threatening conditions. In addition, the patient should be asked about use of NSAIDs. Then, the clinician should seek symptom clusters that suggest or exclude one of the specific dyspepsia syndromes described earlier. If none are detected, the patient likely has nonulcer dyspepsia.

Symptoms Indicative of Serious Conditions

The first step in taking a history from patients with upper abdominal pain is to seek clues to the presence of serious or life-threatening disease such as gastric-outlet obstruction, bowel perforation, gastrointestinal bleeding, and cancer. Important clues to these diagnoses include severe pain or vomiting, weight loss, melena, hemochezia, hematemesis, and orthostatic dizziness. Table 5-2 shows key history items for a number of serious conditions that may be encountered in primary care. As mentioned earlier, the conditions in Table 5-2 are uncommon in everyday office practice, but clinicians should briefly consider them in any patient with abdominal pain.

Myocardial ischemia, in contrast, is somewhat more common in primary care practice. Therefore, clinicians must always consider the possibility of ischemia or infarction in patients with dyspeptic symptoms. The likelihood of a cardiac cause for dyspepsia is higher in elderly patients, particularly those with risk factors for atherosclerosis, recent onset of symptoms, or other symptoms associated with heart disease. If ischemia is considered a possible cause for a patient's symptoms, the patient should be evaluated with resting and stress electrocardiography if the symptoms are chronic, and hospital admission to exclude acute infarction or unstable angina if symptoms are acute.

Nonsteroidal Anti-Inflammatory Drugs

Patients with dyspeptic symptoms should always be questioned about the use of NSAIDs, both prescription and over-the-counter. These medications are the second-most common cause of peptic ulceration after *H. pylori* infection. NSAID gastropathy is also a common cause of gastrointestinal bleeding, especially in elderly individuals.

Dyspeptic Symptoms

Assuming that history does not suggest any of the serious conditions discussed earlier and the patient is not taking NSAIDs, the next step is to focus on symptoms of dyspepsia. Differentiating the symptoms of nonulcer dyspepsia from the specific dyspeptic syndromes (duodenal ulcer, gastric ulcer, gastritis, and GERD) can be difficult, as there is poor correlation between symptoms and endoscopic findings. In addition, in primary care practice the classic history items, such as the relation of pain to food, timing of pain, and severity of pain, are all poorly predictive of the patient's actual diagnosis.

SINGLE SYMPTOMS

Single symptoms in patients with dyspepsia are poor predictors of the final diagnosis, with one exception. The exception—heartburn with a sensation of reflux into the esophagus or mouth (pyrosis)—is highly suggestive of GERD. Other less common, but relatively typical symptoms of GERD include dysphagia (manifest as food boluses getting stuck in the esophagus) and/or chronic cough not explained by a respiratory tract problem.

SYMPTOM CLUSTERS

Experienced clinicians tend to rely on patterns and clusters of symptoms for clues to the diagnosis, rather than seeking any one specific symptom. Table 5-3 summarizes the operating characteristics of various symptom clusters in patients with dyspepsia.

SYMPTOMS SUGGESTING NONULCER DYSPEPSIA   The first symptom cluster in Table 5-3 (food or milk aggravates pain, pain less severe, no night pain, no vomiting, no weight loss, and age under 40) is highly suggestive of nonulcer dyspepsia. If this symptom cluster is present, there is a 90 percent chance that the patient has nonulcer dyspepsia, and it is almost 10 times more likely that the patient has nonulcer dyspepsia than not. Thus, the presence of this symptom cluster is useful in diagnosing nonulcer dyspepsia.

SYMPTOMS SUGGESTING AN ORGANIC CAUSE OF DYSPEPSIA   The presence of nocturnal pain and advanced age are common to all the clusters associated with organic (i.e., other than nonspecific) causes of dyspepsia. In addition, clusters 4 and 6 are moderately useful in diagnosing cholelithiasis and peptic ulcer, respectively.

SYMPTOMS EXCLUDING AN ORGANIC CAUSE OF DYSPEPSIA   The absence of cluster 3 in Table 5-3 is useful for excluding peptic ulcer disease, and the absence of cluster 5 tends to exclude all organic causes of dyspepsia. Lack of previous peptic disease and young age are common to all the clusters that tend to exclude organic dyspepsia.

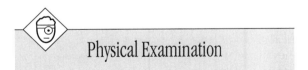

Physical Examination

In general, the physical examination is usually not helpful in the diagnosis of dyspepsia in primary care practice. While classic signs of peritonitis, gastric outlet obstruction, cholecystitis, or other serious conditions may sometimes be present, the more common situation is that the examination reveals few physical findings, most of which are nonspecific. The most common finding is usually mild mid-epigastric tenderness.

Table 5-3

Operating Characteristics of Symptom Clusters in Dyspepsia

SYMPTOM CLUSTERS	DISEASE	SENSITIVITY	SPECIFICITY	LR+	LF–	PV+	PV–
1. Food or milk aggravates pain, pain less severe, no night pain, no vomiting or weight loss, age under 40	Nonulcer dyspepsia	57	94	9.5	.46	90	67
2. Pain relieved by antacids, age above 40, previous ulcer disease, male gender, symptoms provoked by berries, night pain relieved by antacids or food	Organic dyspepsia	84	51	1.7	.31	41	88
3. Previous peptic ulcer, pain relieved with antacids, age above 40, smoking, pain relieved by food	Peptic ulcer	90	55	2.0	.18	27	93
4. Pain radiating to the back	Cholelithiasis	83	74	3.1	.23	36	96
5. Vomiting, smoking, previous peptic ulcer or hiatus hernia, high age, male gender	Organic dyspepsia	97	30	1.4	.10	34	97
6. Nocturnal pain, pain before meals or when hungry, absence of nausea, high age, male gender	Peptic ulcer	51	83	3.0	.59	49	84

ABBREVIATIONS: LR+ signifies the likelihood ratio that the disease is present if the symptom cluster is present, compared to if the symptom cluster were absent; LR– signifies likelihood ratio that the disease is absent if the symptom cluster is absent, compared to if the symptom cluster were absent; PV+ signifies positive predictive value for the disease of a symptom cluster; PV– signifies negative predictive value of a symptom cluster.

Adapted and reprinted by permission of Appleton & Lange, Inc., from: Muris JWM, Starmans R, Pop P, et al. Discriminant value of symptoms in patients with dyspepsia. *J Fam Pract* 38:139–143, 1994.

Nonetheless, an important purpose of the physical examination is to detect serious conditions, if they are present, and to seek findings suggestive of the specific dyspeptic syndromes. The absence of specific or classic signs, however, does not rule out any particular condition.

Detecting Serious Conditions

As with the history, initial attention during the physical examination should be focused on detecting signs of serious or systemic conditions. These include findings such as fever, significant weight loss, jaundice, abdominal rigidity, orthostatic hypotension, and blood in the stool. In addition, examination should include the lungs. Table 5-2 shows key examination findings for some of the serious conditions that can present with abdominal pain.

Identifying Dyspeptic Conditions

Most patients with dyspepsia have no examination findings or minimal epigastric tenderness. If present, however, findings that suggest complications of dyspeptic syndromes (i.e., perforated ulcer or bleeding from ulcers, gastritis, or GERD-related esophagitis) include orthostatic hypotension, blood in the stool, and peritoneal signs such as abdominal rigidity, distension, or absent bowel sounds.

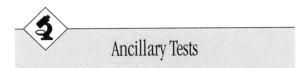

Ancillary Tests

As with the history and physical, ancillary tests in patients with dyspepsia are used to detect serious conditions or complications, and to diagnose and guide management of dyspeptic syndromes. There are no tests that should always be ordered in evaluating patients with dyspepsia, as such an approach to testing seldom leads to diagnoses not already suspected by the clinician. Instead, imaging and laboratory testing should be guided by findings of the history and physical.

The only exception to routine testing may be in elderly patients. In elderly individuals with dyspepsia, there is a high rate of serious abnormalities. The elderly frequently have atypical presentations and may not be able to communicate their symptoms to clinicians. Thus, while testing in geriatric-aged individuals should still be guided by the history and physical examination, clinicians should regularly consider obtaining complete blood counts, radiographic imaging or endoscopy, chemistry panels, and stool testing for patients in this age group who have dyspepsia. A similar approach is needed for immunocompromised patients, in whom symptoms and presentations are also frequently atypical and may represent serious disease.

Detecting Helicobacter Pylori

Methods for detection of *H. pylori* include blood testing, stool or saliva testing, breath analyses, and several tests that can be performed in conjunction with endoscopy.

BLOOD TESTS

Qualitative tests for anti-*H. pylori* antibodies in serum are widely available The serum tests are reasonably accurate (sensitivity 93 percent, specificity 90 percent, positive likelihood ratio of 9, and negative likelihood ratio of 0.08). However, not all individuals who test positive have ulcers or gastritis, and the test cannot be used to distinguish active from previously treated infection because serology remains positive even after treatment.

A quantitative enzyme-linked immunosorbent assay (ELISA) can also be used. It is even more accurate than a qualitative serology (sensitivity 95 percent, specificity 95 percent, positive likelihood ratio of 19, negative likelihood ratio of 0.05). More importantly, it can be used to document resolution of infection, because ELISA titers decrease after successful treatment of *H. pylori* infection. Repeat ELISA measurements can be performed following therapy (usually at 1, 3, and 6 months after treatment) to document eradication of the organism.

BREATH ANALYSIS

The ^{13}C-urea breath test is based on *H. pylori* being a urea-splitting organism. The test involves ingesting a gelatin-coated capsule that contains carbon-13-labeled urea. If *H. pylori* are present in a patient's stomach, the urea is split and releases radiolabeled CO_2 that can be detected in the patient's exhaled breath. The test is sensitive (96 percent), specific (98 percent), and has positive and negative likelihood ratios of 48 and 0.04, respectively. Breath analysis can be used for initial diagnosis of infection and to test for eradication of *H. pylori* after treatment.

STOOL TESTS

A stool antigen immunoassay was developed, but is not widely available. Its sensitivity is 96 percent and specificity is 93 percent. It can be used as an alternative to ^{13}C-urea breath testing.

ENDOSCOPIC TESTS

If endoscopy is performed, several methods can be used to detect *H. pylori* infection in biopsy specimens. The "gold standard" method is to culture the biopsy tissue specimen for *H. pylori*. In clinical practice, however, culture is used primarily when there is concern about antibiotic resistance.

Currently, the fastest and most frequently used method is the rapid urease test, also known as the *Campylobacter*-like organism (CLO) test, which tests a biopsy specimen of mucosa for bacterial urease. The CLO test detects the change in pH that occurs as a result of urease activity by changing the color of a phenol-red indicator. The CLO test has a sensitivity of about 95 percent and near-perfect specificity.

Histologic examination of the tissue specimen for the *H. pylori* organism can also be used. Special stains may be needed, however, and studies report variable sensitivity compared to culture, ranging from less than 90 percent to as high as 99 percent.

Finally, polymerase chain reaction testing of biopsy specimen has almost perfect sensitivity and specificity compared to culture. It is likely to become the test of choice in the future.

Other Testing

The tests most commonly used for diagnosing the specific cause of dyspepsia are endoscopic esophagogastroduodenoscopy and barium-contrast upper gastrointestinal (UGI) radiography. Esophageal pH monitoring is a useful adjunctive test for diagnosing GERD.

ENDOSCOPY

For most patients in whom examination of the upper gastrointestinal tract is needed, endoscopy is the preferred test. Endoscopy can reliably diagnose gastritis and is more sensitive and specific than is radiographic imaging for diagnosing ulcers and GERD. In fact, endoscopy is considered the gold standard for diagnosing ulcers, gastritis, and esophageal injury from GERD. In addition, the ability to obtain biopsies during endoscopic procedures permits identification of *H. pylori* infection.

Endoscopy should be performed if (a) there is no response to medical therapy, (b) signs of ulcer complications develop, (c) signs of systemic illness are present, or (d) symptoms recur after treatment. As will be discussed later, most experts now recommend that endoscopy be reserved for patients with persistent symptoms or if signs and symptoms of serious disease are present. Endoscopy is also recommended in patients with a long-standing history of untreated GERD, because such patients may have Barrett's metaplasia.

UPPER GASTROINTESTINAL RADIOGRAPHY

Upper gastrointestinal radiography x-rays are considerably less costly than is endoscopy (1996 Medicare reimbursement for physician and hospital costs of UGI was approximately $100, while the cost for endoscopy was over $400), and they can diagnose peptic ulcer, gastric ulcer, and GERD. Unfortunately, the false-negative rates are substantial. For peptic ulcers, the false-negative rate of UGI studies exceeds 18 percent, and it is much higher for GERD. In addition, UGI examinations are falsely positive for ulcers in up to one-third of examinations. For these reasons, UGI x-rays are not usually considered the test of choice for evaluating dyspeptic symptoms.

Upper gastrointestinal radiography series still has a role in diagnosis, however. In particular, UGI x-rays can be useful as an initial diagnostic test in patients with isolated dysphagia and in those for whom the sedation required for endoscopy would be excessively risky.

ESOPHAGEAL pH MONITORING AND MANOMETRY

Esophageal pH monitoring is useful for selected patients suspected of having GERD in whom endoscopy reveals no evidence of the condition. The procedure is performed by placing a probe through the nares into the distal esophagus to monitor esophageal pH. A fall in pH to <4 occurs when gastric contents reflux into the esophagus. Esophageal manometry can also be performed to measure the contractility of the lower esophageal sphincter, which is impaired in GERD. Manometry is not, however, a routine test in evaluation of patients with dyspepsia.

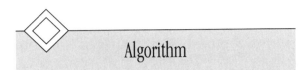

Algorithm

Many different recommendations have been made for how to approach dyspepsia. Figure 5-6 shows the diagnostic approach favored by many experts that can be used to evaluate patients with new symptoms of dyspepsia in the primary care setting. Note that this algorithm does not apply to patients with chronic or recurrent dyspepsia, in whom it is often appropriate to perform endoscopy at the onset of the evaluation.

For the individual with new-onset dyspepsia, the first step is to determine if the patient has any symptoms or signs of serious or life-threatening illness (Table 5-4). This should prompt an immediate evaluation to determine the cause of the

symptoms and signs. Age alone is a relative factor here. If an individual is ≥ 45 to 50 years and has no other danger symptoms and signs, they should be evaluated more aggressively than individuals ≤ 45 to 50.

Next, patterns or clusters of typical symptoms and signs should guide further evaluation and treatment. Heartburn and pyrosis typically indicate the presence of GERD. No further work-up is needed and symptomatic treatment may be initiated. The presence of crampy right upper quadrant to epigastric pain following a fatty meal and the pain radiating around to the back in a women over the age of 40 is typical for gallbladder disease. This patient should be evaluated appropriately to verify the presence of gallstones.

The next step is to determine whether the individual is taking a NSAID. If so, the NSAID should be discontinued. If dyspepsia persists after stopping the NSAID, the clinician should test for the presence of *H. pylori*. If positive, the patient should be empirically treated for *H. pylori*. If negative, endoscopy should be performed.

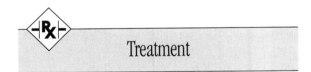

Treatment

Before seeking care from a clinician, many patients will have unsuccessfully self-treated themselves with nonprescription medications. The most commonly used medications are antacids and antisecretory histamine-2 (H2) receptor antagonists such as cimetidine, ranitidine, or famotidine. Because nonprescription H2 blockers and antacids are frequently taken in lower-than-the-recommended prescription dose, clinicians should ascertain the dose used before concluding that the patient's self-administered nonprescription treatment was truly unsuccessful. When symptoms are related to use of NSAIDs, these drugs should be stopped if at all possible.

In addition, some patients will have tried nontraditional self-treatments, including herbal reme-

Table 5-4

Symptoms/Signs of Serious or Life-Threatening Cause of Dyspepsia

SYMPTOMS AND SIGNS OF SERIOUS OR LIFE-THREATENING CAUSES
Persistent vomiting
Severe pain
Weight loss
Dysphagia
Gastrointestinal blood loss
Anemia
Abdominal mass
Abdominal lymphadenopathy

Figure 5-6

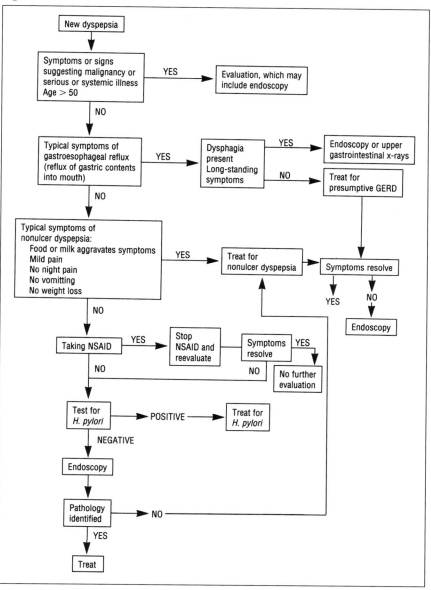

Algorithm for the diagnosis of new-onset dyspepsia in a primary care setting.

dies. One of the more widely used herbal reme-dies for dyspepsia is ginger, the underground stem of the *Zingiber officinale* plant. Several studies have shown some benefit from this treatment, and there are no reported side effects.

Treatment for Helicobacter Pylori *Infection*

If *H. pylori* infection is detected, eradicating infec-tion is the single most important intervention. While acid-reduction therapies are also used, they are of secondary importance. Failure to effectively treat and eliminate the infection is the major cause of recurrent ulcers and gastritis.

Several antibiotic regimens are effective for eradicating *H. pylori* infection, some of which combine antibiotics with acid-reduction therapy (Table 5-5). If the chosen antibiotic regimen does not include acid-reduction therapy, acid-reduction may be added as an adjunctive treatment, using the recommendations previously outlined.

Table 5-5

Several Drug Regimens for Eradication of *Helicobacter Pylori* Infection

MOC (87 to 91 percent effective):	cost, $200
Metronidazole*	500 mg bid × 14 days
Omeprazole	20 mg bid × 14 days
Clarithromycin	250 mg bid × 14 days
Helidac (77 to 90 percent effective)+	cost $45
Bismuth subsalicylate	2 tabs qid × 14 days
Metronidazole	250 mg qid × 14 days
Tetracycline	500 mg qid × 14 days
O + C (64 to 90 percent):	cost, $350
Omeprazole	40 mg qd × 14 days‡
Clarithromycin	500 mg tid × 14 days
BMTO (75 to 95 percent):	cost, $100
Bismuth	2 tabs qid × 10 days
Metronidazole	250 mg qid × 10 days
Tetracycline	500 mg QID × 10 days
Omeprazole	20 mg bid × 10 days
Tritec + clarithromycin (73 to 84 percent):§	cost, $200
Ranitidine/bismuth	400 mg bid × 2 weeks
Clarithromycin	500 mg tid × 2 weeks

*Substitute amoxicillin (1g bid) for metronidazole if metronidazole resistance is suspected.
+Helidac is nearly identical to classic triple therapy.
‡Continue omeprazole (20 mg qd) for 2 additional weeks if active ulcer is present.
§Continue ranitidine/bismuth (400 mg bid) for 2 additional weeks if active ulcer is present.

The most successful and widely used antibiotic regimen is the "triple therapy" combination of bismuth subsalicylate, metronidazole, and either amoxicillin or tetracycline. When combined with omeprazole, these regimens are effective at eradicating infection and healing ulcers in up to 90 percent of patients. However, the triple therapy regimen is somewhat cumbersome, in that patients must take pills 4 times per day, and side effects may occur including constipation, discoloration of the tongue and stool, and antibiotic-induced colitis. Therefore, alternative regimens are used with increased frequency. For example, the combination of clarithromycin and omeprazole, though considerably more expensive than triple therapy, is nearly as effective and much easier to administer (Table 5-5). In practice, the drugs available on the formulary of the health care organization in which a clinician practices frequently determine the choice of treatment regimen.

There are concerns about the developing problem of antibiotic-resistant *H. pylori*. Resistance is a particular problem with metronidazole, but may occur with all antibiotic regimens. If a patient has failed antibiotic therapy for *H. pylori*, then clinicians should strongly consider endoscopy in order to obtain culture and sensitivities.

Nonulcer Dyspepsia

For the treatment of nonulcer dyspepsia, no treatment has been shown to be consistently effective. Antacids and antisecretory agents (H_2 blocking agents) are often prescribed (see Table 5-6), but there is no convincing evidence that they alter the course of nonulcer dyspepsia. Similarly, as mentioned earlier, *H. pylori* infection is not thought to play a role in nonulcer dyspepsia, and treating the infection if present does not consistently improve symptoms. Thus, antibiotic treatment of *H. pylori* in patients with nonulcer dyspepsia is not considered appropriate therapy. Overall, despite the prevalence of nonulcer dyspepsia, clinical research provides clinicians with little guidance about how best to approach the treatment of this condition.

Table 5-6

Table 5-6

Medications Used in Treating Dyspepsia

STANDARD MEDICATION DOSES *	
H₂ Blockers blockers (antisecretory)	
• Cimetidine (Tagamet)	400 mg bid
• Famotidine (Pepcid)	20 mg bid
• Nizatidine (Axid)	150 mg bid
• Ranitidine (Zantac)	150 mg bid
Proton-pump inhibitors	
• Omeprazole (Prilosec)	20 mg qd
• Lansoprazole (Prevacid)	15 mg qd
• Rabeprazole (Aciphex)	20 mg qd
• Pantoprazole (Protonix)	40 mg qd
• Esomeprazole (Nexium)	20 mg qd
Protective coating agent	
• Sucralfate (Carafate)	1 gm qid
Antacids	
Aluminum hydroxide/magnesium hydroxide/simethicone antacids	
• Liquids	30 ml qid or prn
• Tablets	2 tablets qid
Prokinetic agents (for GERD)	
• Metoclopramide (Reglan)	10 mg qid

*NOTE: Some medications require dosing adjustments in renal or hepatic disease. Consult complete prescribing information before administering to patients.

Gastroesophageal Reflux Disease

Treatment of GERD involves lifestyle modifications, medications, and in some cases, surgery. In addition, an important part of managing GERD is surveillance for Barrett's metaplasia and esophageal adenocarcinoma.

LIFESTYLE MODIFICATIONS

Lifestyle modifications in GERD are aimed at decreasing exposure to substances that cause relaxation of the lower esophageal sphincter and avoiding physical and mechanical factors that predispose to reflux or esophageal irritation. Substances that decrease lower esophageal pressure include alcohol, caffeine, chocolate, and fatty foods. Physical and mechanical interventions include avoiding the supine position for several hours after eating, elevating the head of the bed during sleep, and avoiding large meals (which distend the stomach and predispose to reflux). Substances that directly irritate the esophageal mucosa include citrus, coffee, and spicy or tomato-based foods.

These lifestyle modifications are inexpensive and safe, but there is limited information about their benefit. The only study that examined long-term effectiveness of these treatments in primary care practice evaluated lifestyle modifications in combination with intermittent antacid therapy, rather than lifestyle modifications alone. Forty percent of patients in this study experienced relief of symptoms.

MEDICATIONS

Medications for treating GERD include antisecretory agents (H₂ blockers and proton-pump inhibitors) and prokinetic agents. Treatment, including presumptive treatment based on symptoms, typically begins with an H₂ blocker and/or a prokinetic drug. Proton-pump inhibitors are generally used for erosive esophagitis and for patients with GERD that has not responded to H₂ blockers.

H₂ RECEPTOR ANTAGONISTS H₂ blockers include cimetidine, famotidine, nizatidine, and ranitidine. All of the H₂ blockers inhibit about two-thirds of total daily gastric acid secretion, and they are more effective at decreasing nighttime acid production than postprandial acid secretion. None of the H₂ blockers has been shown to be superior to any of the others, though cimetidine interacts with the metabolism of many drugs, making it less desirable for some patients. The usual doses of H₂ blockers are shown in Table 5-6.

PROKINETICS Prokinetic drugs can be used as initial therapy, but they are more commonly used as adjuncts to H₂ blockers. Prokinetic drugs enhance esophageal peristalsis and gastric emptying, and they improve function of the lower esophageal sphincter. The only prokinetic drug approved in the United States for GERD is metoclopramide, a dopamine antagonist. Cisapride, a serotonin agonist that enhances release of acetylcholine from the esophageal myenteric plexus, was removed from the market in 2000 because of the risk of arrhthymias. Metoclopramide's extrapyramidal side effects limit its use, especially as a long-term therapy or in elderly patients. The usual dose of metoclopramide is shown in Table 5-6.

PROTON-PUMP INHIBITORS These drugs, which include omeprazole, lansoprazole, rabeprazole, pantoprazole, and esomeprazole, block the proton pump in gastric parietal cells that is responsible for acid secretion. Their effect on gastric acid secretion is far superior to that of H_2 blockers, decreasing acid production by over 90 percent. These drugs are the treatment of choice for patients with endoscopically documented erosive esophagitis. Resolution of esophagitis occurs in 80 to 90 percent of patients after 6 to 8 weeks of treatment. Proton-pump inhibitors are also indicated for documented GERD that has not responded to H_2 blocker treatment. In addition, patients who relapse after successful treatment with H_2 blockers may be candidates for therapy with proton-pump inhibitors. Finally, some patients will require long-term treatment to prevent relapse of GERD symptoms or esophagitis.

SURGERY

Antireflux surgery can be considered for patients who are refractory to medical treatment, develop recurrent esophagitis, or develop complications of esophagitis such as stricture or hemorrhage. Open surgical procedures for GERD have been available for years, but complication rates are relatively high and outcomes not optimal. Since the 1990s, laparoscopic surgical techniques have been used with success. The most common procedure is fundoplication, in which the gastric fundus is wrapped around the lower esophagus, increasing lower esophageal sphincter pressure. Success rates exceed 90 percent.

SURVEILLANCE FOR BARRETT'S METAPLASIA

About 10 percent of patients with GERD will develop Barrett's metaplasia, and these individuals have a risk of esophageal cancer up to 300 times higher than that of the general population. Thus, patients with esophagitis should be monitored for development of metaplasia and cancer. The ideal interval for monitoring is uncertain, but typical recommendations are that patients who have esophagitis without Barrett's changes should undergo an endoscopic examination every 3 to 5 years, while those with Barrett's metaplasia should be monitored endoscopically every 2 years unless dysplasia is found.

Gastritis, Duodenal Ulcers, Gastric Ulcers, and Nonsteroidal Anti-Inflammatory Drug Gastropathy

GENERAL CONSIDERATIONS

Patients with gastritis and peptic ulcers, including both duodenal and gastric ulcers, should avoid NSAIDs and alcohol (which irritate gastric and duodenal mucosa), discontinue or minimize nicotine and caffeine (both of which stimulate acid secretion), and avoid foods that aggravate symptoms. However, there is no evidence that any specific diets, such as "bland" diets or diets free of spices, are effective in relieving symptoms. Similarly, there is no evidence that "coating" the stomach with milk or cream is beneficial. In fact, milk and cream may actually be harmful because they stimulate gastric acid secretion; they also contribute to hyperlipidemia and atherosclerotic vascular disease.

For treatment of uncomplicated gastritis, duodenal ulcers, and gastric ulcers, the critical factor determining treatment is the presence or absence of *H. pylori*. If *H. pylori* are absent, then acid-reduction therapy with antisecretory drugs is indicated (Table 5-6). If *H. pylori* are present, antibiotics are prescribed, usually in combination with acid-reduction therapy (Table 5-5).

MEDICATIONS IF *HELICOBACTER PYLORI* INFECTION IS ABSENT

DUODENAL ULCER   For duodenal ulcers in the absence of *H. pylori* infection, treatment with H_2 blocking agents or proton-pump inhibitors is indicated. H_2 blocking agents are typically used as the first-choice treatment, but proton-pump inhibitors can also be used. Sucralfate, a complex salt of sucrose and aluminum that binds to ulcer craters, is also an acceptable first-line treatment. With sucralfate bound to the ulcer crater, the ulcer is protected from gastric acid, pepsins, and bile acid. Combination therapy (i.e., H_2 blockers plus proton-pump inhibitors or H_2 blockers plus antacids, etc.) has not been shown to be more effective than a single agent alone. Antacids are not appropriate for primary therapy of duodenal ulcer. Instead, they are used for breakthrough symptoms that occur while taking standard acid-reduction medications.

GASTRIC ULCER   For gastric ulcers in the absence of *H. pylori* infection, proton-pump inhibitors are the medications of choice because gastric ulcers heal faster with proton-pump inhibitors than they do with H_2 blockers. Benign gastric ulcers should heal within 2 to 3 months of beginning therapy. Failure to heal within that time interval suggests the possibility of malignancy and is an indication for endoscopy and biopsy.

GASTRITIS   Gastritis in the absence of *H. pylori* infection or NSAID use is not often encountered in primary care practice. Chronic gastritis can be due to an autoimmune process. Patients who do not have *H. pylori* typically have gastric mucosal atrophy and decreased acid secretion. Thus, acid-reduction therapy is not indicated. Treatments are directed at the underlying cause of the gastritis.

NONSTEROIDAL ANTI-INFLAMMATORY DRUG GASTROPATHY
When ulcers are related to use of NSAIDs, these drugs should be stopped if at all possible. Any approved therapy for ulcers can be used if the NSAID is discontinued. If it cannot be discontinued, the use of a proton-pump inhibitor is recommended. There are two types of NSAIDs: cyclooxygenase$_1$ (COX_1) inhibitors and the newer COX_2 inhibitors. The COX_2 inhibitors seem to have a low rate of gastrointestinal side effects. If the patient is taking a COX_1 inhibitor, the clinician can consider switching to a COX_2 inhibitor.

There are many options for the prevention of NSAID-induced ulcers. First, the clinician can avoid the use of NSAIDs. Factors that place patients at greatest risk for serious gastrointestinal complications from NSAIDs include a prior history of a gastrointestinal event (ulcer or bleeding), age greater than 60 years, high dosage of the NSAID, and concurrent use of corticosteroids or anticoagulants. Second, if an NSAID is necessary, the clinician can consider the use of a COX_2 inhibitor. And finally, misoprostol or a proton-pump inhibitor can be used in addition to the NSAID.

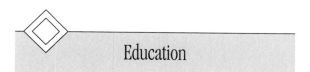

Education

The U.S. public has substantial misconceptions about the causes of dyspeptic syndromes. For example, most people believe that ulcers are caused by emotional stress and have no awareness that ulcers and gastritis are associated with an infection.

Thus, patients with peptic ulcers and gastritis should be provided with information about the cause of their condition and the lack of effect of dietary changes. Those with GERD should receive instruction regarding lifestyle interventions that may improve symptoms. Individuals with GERD and esophagitis should know about the importance of periodic surveillance for Barrett's metaplasia and cancer.

In the many patients for whom no specific diagnosis for dyspepsia is identified, clinicians should provide reassurance and emphasize that most dyspepsia resolves spontaneously. This is important because patients who seek medical attention for dyspepsia often are concerned about having cancer or heart disease. When possible, therefore, clinicians should explain the cause of symptoms to patients. If uncertainty about diagnosis exists, the uncertainty should also be explained.

Finally, it is important to inform patients about the need to seek medical attention if changes in symptoms indicate development of complications. Examples of such symptoms include increasing pain, hematemesis, melena, or orthostatic dizziness. Patients with GERD should seek attention for symptoms of dysphagia.

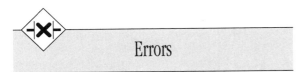

Errors

A variety of errors occur in the diagnosis and treatment of dyspepsia. The three most common errors are failure to consider important alternative diagnoses, inappropriate use of acid-reduction therapy, and inappropriate treatment of *H. pylori* infection.

Errors in Diagnosis

The most common serious error in diagnosis of dyspeptic symptoms is failure to consider and/or properly evaluate the possibility that symptoms are caused by myocardial ischemia. As noted earlier, inferior-wall myocardial ischemia frequently causes nausea, heartburn, and other symptoms typically associated with dyspeptic disorders. Failure to diagnose myocardial infarction is one of the 10 most common causes of malpractice allegations against family physicians in the United States and mistaking myocardial ischemia for dyspeptic symptoms is one of the common scenarios in which this failure occurs. Exclusion of a cardiac cause for dyspeptic symptoms should always take precedence over treatment of dyspepsia. If the diagnosis is uncertain, or if ischemia cannot be reliably excluded during an office encounter, clinicians should consider treadmill or other diagnostic testing, or hospital admission for cardiac monitoring and exclusion of ischemia and infarction.

Another error is disregarding signs or symptoms that indicate diagnoses other than the common dyspeptic syndromes. These missed diagnoses include the various conditions in Table 5-2. This error sometimes occurs because clinicians put too much weight on individual symptoms, signs, or laboratory tests; this can be avoided by knowing the operating characteristics of patients' symptoms (Table 5-3), signs, and test results. Errors in diagnosis also occur when clinicians fail to perform a systematic history and physical. For example, failure to perform a rectal examination for detection of fecal blood is a potentially serious error in evaluating patients with dyspepsia, because the therapy and follow-up can be substantially different in the presence of bleeding from gastritis, ulcers, or esophagitis.

A third diagnostic error is being unaware of the atypical presentation of dyspepsia in elderly or immunocompromised individuals. As discussed earlier, such individuals warrant more-intensive investigation because they frequently lack the expected signs and symptoms of serious intra-abdominal problems.

Inappropriate Use of Antisecretory Medications

While empiric treatment with antisecretory medications is acceptable, some clinicians prescribe these medications in inappropriate situations. For example, empiric antisecretory therapy is not appropriate for patients whose symptoms persist despite treatment, who have symptoms of dysphagia in association with reflux symptoms, or who have bleeding in their stool. Such individuals should undergo diagnostic tests (usually endoscopy) to accurately determine the cause of their symptoms.

Inappropriate Treatment of Helicobacter Pylori Infection

Similarly, acid-reduction therapy is not appropriate as sole treatment for ulcers or gastritis if *H. pylori* infection is present. Many clinicians make the error of prescribing H$_2$ blockers or proton-pump inhibitors without testing for *H. pylori*, perhaps because such tests are not readily available in the clinician's office. Failure to detect and treat *H. pylori* infection, however, markedly increases the rate of recurrence for ulcers and gastritis. Acid-reduction therapy should be considered an adjunct to antibiotic treatment of *H. pylori*-related ulcers and gastritis, not a principal treatment.

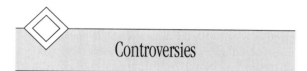

Controversies

There are two controversies surrounding the evaluation and management of dyspepsia. First, is the issue of how much diagnostic testing is necessary before treatment can be prescribed. That is, is it necessary to establish definitive diagnoses before beginning treatment, or is empiric treatment acceptable and appropriate? Because of the large number of individuals affected by these dyspeptic conditions, this controversy has substantial cost implications for society. Second, is the issue of treatment of *H. pylori* in the patient with the diagnosis of nonulcer dyspepsia.

Empiric Treatment

One proposed strategy involves empiric treatment. In this approach, patients are treated presumptively with either antisecretory agents or antibiotics, or both, based on symptoms indicative of gastritis or ulcers. The potential drawback of empiric antisecretory treatment is that malignant gastric ulcers will not be detected, nor will the presence of GERD-associated erosive esophagitis or Barrett's metaplasia be detected. The drawback to an empiric antibiotic is an increase in antibiotic-resistant *H. pylori*.

Treatment Based on Helicobacter Pylori Testing

Another strategy is to perform tests for *H. pylori* in patients who have symptoms suggesting ulcers or gastritis. At present, serologic testing is the most widely available. Individuals who test positive are treated with antibiotics, while those who test negative are treated empirically with antisecretory agents. This strategy is attractive because it eliminates the need for and cost of endoscopy. However, it will result in treatment of many persons who do not have demonstrable organic disease, because no diagnosis is established.

Routine Endoscopy Before Treatment

Another commonly proposed strategy is to perform endoscopy to make a definitive diagnosis in all patients with dyspepsia. If gastritis or ulcers are detected, testing for *H. pylori* is performed at the time of endoscopy. The cost of routine endoscopy would appear to make this approach expensive, but as subsequently noted, a controlled trial of various approaches to dyspepsia found it was more cost-effective to perform endoscopy early in the diagnostic evaluation than it would be to perform it later.

Resolving the Controversy

Over the past few years, several investigators have performed decision analyses to determine which of these or other strategies lead to the best outcomes at lowest cost. Unfortunately, there were differences between the specific strategies examined and each analysis reached different conclusions. Ebell, Warbasse, and Brenner examined seven different strategies and identified two that were most cost-effective: empiric *H. pylori* treatment and use of serologic tests to identify and treat patients with *H. pylori* infection. Ofman et al. examined patients who tested positive on serologic tests for *H. pylori* and found that the most cost-effective approach was to treat the infection without documenting an ulcer. Silverstein, Petterson, and Talley compared initial endoscopy and empiric therapy, with or without initial testing for *H. pylori*, and found that no strategy showed a clear advantage. Finally, the analysis of Fendrick et al. advocated initial empiric treatment of ulcers and *H. pylori* infection.

There is also a systematic review of the literature asking whether initial endoscopy improves patient outcomes. Ofman and Rabeneck found that initial endoscopy did not improve patient outcomes.

There are two randomized clinical trials that show conflicting results although the studies were not identical in their approach to the evaluation of dyspepsia. Bytzer, Hansen, and deMuckadell compared initial endoscopy before treatment to empiric treatment with antisecretory agents. The investigators found that it was more cost-effective to perform prompt endoscopy. Individuals treated in this fashion required less medication, lost fewer days from work, and used fewer health services than those treated empirically. A major limitation of this study, however, is that identification and treatment of *H. pylori* infection were not addressed. Heaney et al. compared empiric eradication of *H. pylori* with endoscopy-based management. They found that empiric eradication was better than initial endoscopy strategy for reducing dyspeptic symptoms and improving physical functioning.

Thus, while one study suggests that performing endoscopy before treatment may be the preferred approach to diagnosis and management of dyspeptic complaints, most experts tend to recommend testing for *H. pylori* and treating accordingly.

Treatment of Helicobacter Pylori *in Those with a Nonulcer Dyspepsia Diagnosis*

A meta-analysis concluded that there was an association between *H. pylori* and nonulcer dyspepsia and that eradication of *H. pylori* improved dyspeptic symptoms. However, there are two randomized

clinical trials that showed no improvement in symptoms. Talley et al. and Greenberg and Cello both showed that eradication of *H. pylori* does not improve dyspeptic symptoms in patients with nonulcer dyspepsia.

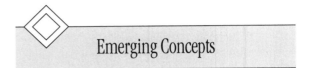

Emerging Concepts

Over the next few years, several emerging concepts should change our approach to dyspeptic abdominal pain syndromes. These include (a) development of new information on the diagnosis and management of dyspeptic syndromes, and (b) the possible relation between acid-reduction therapy and adenocarcinoma of the esophagus.

Diagnosis and Management of Dyspeptic Syndromes

As the influence of evidence-based medicine continues to grow, more information about the predictive values of symptoms, signs, and laboratory tests will emerge, permitting more accurate and rational diagnoses and treatment of dyspeptic disorders. Furthermore, controversies in the evaluation and management of dyspepsia, as outlined earlier, will likely be clarified. The possible development of office-based tests (e.g., breath analyses) for detecting *H. pylori* will further modify and facilitate the evaluation process.

Adenocarcinoma of the Esophagus

The incidence of adenocarcinoma among white men in the United States has increased substantially since 1970. Although controversial, some authors have proposed that the increase may be related to the increased use of H_2 blockers for treatment of GERD. The rationale for this hypothesis is that when used to treat GERD, antisecretory

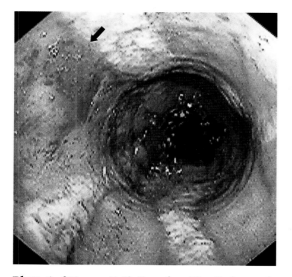

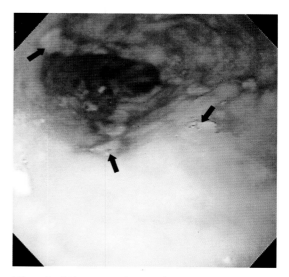

Plate 1 *(Figure 5-1)* **Esophagitis.** Endoscopic view of the distal esophagus showing inflammation of the esophageal mucosa. The arrow indicates the most-inflamed area. *(Courtesy of Gregory Gambla, DO, Milton Hershey Medical Centers, Penn State Geisinger Health System.)*

Plate 2 *(Figure 5-2)* **Esophagitis with Ulcerations.** Endoscopic view of the distal esophagus demonstrating erythema and multiple erosions and ulcerations (examples marked with arrows). *(Courtesy of Gregory Gambla, DO, Milton Hershey Medical Centers, Penn State Geisinger Health System.)*

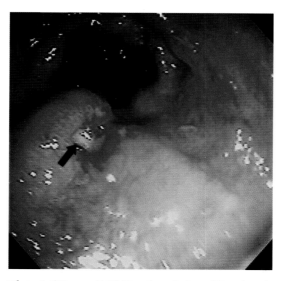

Plate 3 *(Figure 5-3)* **Duodenal ulcer.** The ulcer is marked by the arrow. *(Courtesy of Gregory Gambla, DO, Milton Hershey Medical Centers, Penn State Geisinger Health System.)*

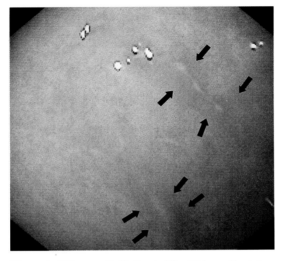

Plate 4 *(Figure 5-4)* **Gastritis.** This patient has mild gastritis, manifest as areas of erythema on the gastric mucosa (arrows). *(Courtesy of Gregory Gambla, DO, Milton Hershey Medical Centers, Penn State Geisinger Health System.)*

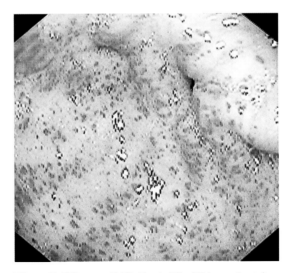

Plate 5 *(Figure 5-5)* **Gastritis.** This patient has marked gastritis, with areas of intense erythema and numerous small mucosal hemorrhages. *(Courtesy of Gregory Gambla, DO, Milton Hershey Medical Centers, Penn State Geisinger Health System.)*

agents only diminish acid production. While diminished acid production can eliminate the acid-related symptoms of reflux, antisecretory agents do not prevent reflux of pepsin and other gastric contents into the esophagus. Thus, patients' symptoms are relieved from antisecretory drugs, while reflux of pepsin and/or other gastric contents may continue to injure the esophagus and cause Barrett's metaplasia and adenocarcinoma. This concern has led some authorities to advocate increased use of laparoscopic fundoplication for treatment of GERD, as fundoplication decreases reflux of all gastric contents. However, some studies have demonstrated reversal of Barrett's metaplasia with proton-pump inhibitor therapy, suggesting that acid-reduction therapy is unrelated to the increased incidence of esophageal cancer. More research is needed to clarify these concerns.

Bibliography

American Gastroenterological Association: Medical position statement on evaluation of dyspepsia. *Gastroenterology* 114:579–581, 1998.

AGA Technical Review: Evaluation of dyspepsia. *Gastroenterology* 114:582–589, 1998.

Braden B, Teuber G, Dietrich CF, et al: Comparison of new faecal antigen test with ^{13}C-urea breath test for detecting *Helicobacter pylori* infection and monitoring eradication treatment: Prospective clinical evaluation. *Br Med J* 320:148, 2000.

Bytzer P, Hansen JO, deMuckadell OB: Empirical H-2 blocker therapy or prompt endoscopy in management of dyspepsia. *Lancet* 343:811–816, 1994.

Chang L: Gastroesophageal reflux disease: Pathophysiology, clinical symptoms, and diagnosis. *J Managed Care* 3, suppl:S6–11,1997.

Chow WH, Finkle WD, McLaughlin JK, et al: The relation of gastroesophageal reflux disease and its treatment of adenocarcinoma of the esophagus and gastric cardia. *JAMA* 274:474–477, 1995.

DeVault KR, Castell DO, and the Practice Parameters Committee of the American College of Gastroenterology: ACG Treatment Guideline: Updated guidelines for the diagnosis and treatment of gastro-esophageal reflux disease. *Am J Gastroenterol* 94: 1434–1442, 1999.

Ebell MH, Warbasse L, Brenner C: Evaluation of the dyspeptic patient: A cost-utility study. *J Fam Pract* 44: 545–555, 1997.

Fendrick AM, Chernew ME, Hirth RA, et al: Alternative management strategies for patients with suspected peptic ulcer disease. *Ann Intern Med* 123:260–268, 1995.

Foodborne and Diarrheal Disease Branch, Division of Bacterial and Mycotic Diseases, National Center for Infectious Diseases: Knowledge about causes of peptic ulcer disease—United States, March–April 1997. *MMWR* 46:985–987, 1997.

Fraser AG, Ali MR, McCullough S, et al. Diagnostic tests for *Helicobacter pylori*: Can they help select patients for endoscopy? *NZ Med J* 109:95–98, 1996.

Greenberg PD, Cello JP: Lack of effect of treatment for *Helicobacter pylori* on symptoms of nonulcer dyspepsia. *Arch Intern Med* 159:2283–2288, 1999.

Heaney A, Collins JS, Watson RG, et al: A prospective randomized trial of a "test and treat" policy versus endoscopy based management in young *Helicobacter pylori* positive patients with ulcer-like dyspepsia, referred to a hospital clinic. *Gut* 45:186–190, 1999.

Howden CW, Hunt RH, for and on behalf of the Ad Hoc Committee on Practice Parameters of the American College of Gastroenterology: Guidelines for the management of *Helicobacter pylori* infection. *Am J Gastroenterol* 93:2330–2338, 1998.

Jaakkimainen RL, Boyle E, Tudiver F: Is *Helicobacter pylori* associated with nonulcer dyspepsia and will eradication improve symptoms? A meta-analysis. *Br Med J* 319:1040–1044, 1999.

Johnsen R, Bernersen B, Straume B, et al: Prevalences of endoscopic and histological findings in subjects with and without dyspepsia. *Br Med J* 302:749–752, 1991.

Jones RH, Lydeard SE, Hobbs FDR, et al: Dyspepsia in England and Scotland. *Gut* 31:401–405, 1990.

Kuster E, Rose E, Toledo-Pimentel V, et al: Predictive factors of the long term outcome in gastroesophageal reflux disease: Six year follow up of 107 patients. *Gut.* 35:8–14, 1994.

Lanza FL and the Members of the Ad Hoc Committee on Practice Parameters of the American College of Gastroenterology: A guideline for the treatment and prevention of NSAID-induced ulcers. *Am J Gastroenterol* 93:2037, 1998.

Lehmann F, Drewe J, Terracciano L, et al: Comparison of stool immunoassay with standard methods for detecting *Helicobacter pylori* infection. *Br Med J* 319: 1409, 1999.

Mendall MA, Jazrawi RP, Marrero JM, et al. Serology for *Helicobacter pylori* compared with symptom questionnaires in screening before direct access endoscopy. *Gut* 36:330–333, 1995.

Muller JL, Clauson KA: Pharmaceutical consideration in common herbal medicine. *Am J Managed Care* 3: 1753–1770, 1997.

Muris JWM, Starmans R, Pop P, et al: Discriminant value of symptoms in patients with dyspepsia. *J Fam Pract* 38:139–143, 1994.

NIH Consensus Conference: *Helicobacter pylori* in peptic ulcer disease. NIH Consensus Development Panel on *Helicobacter pylori* in Peptic Ulcer Disease. *JAMA* 272:65–69, 1994.

Ofman JJ, Etchason J, Fullerton S, et al: Management strategies for *Helicobacter pylori*: Seropositive patients with dyspepsia: Clinical and economic consequences. *Ann Intern Med* 126:280–291, 1997.

Ofman JJ, Rabeneck L: The effectiveness of endoscopy in the management of dyspepsia: A qualitative systematic review. *Am J Med* 106:335–346, 1999.

Sampliner RE: Effect of up to 3 years of high-dose lansoprazole on Barrett's esophagus. *Am J Gastroenterol* 89:1844–1848, 1994.

Silverstein MD, Petterson T, Talley NJ: Initial endoscopy or empirical therapy with or without testing for *Helicobacter pylori* for dyspepsia: A decision analysis. *Gastroenterology* 110:72–83, 1996.

Soll AH, for the Practice Parameters Committee of the American College of Gastroenterology: Medical treatment of peptic ulcer disease: Practice guidelines. *JAMA* 275:622–629, 1996.

Talley NJ, Janssens J, Lauritsen K, et al: Eradication of *Helicobacter pylori* in functional dyspepsia: Randomized double blind placebo controlled trial with 12 months' follow up. *Br Med J* 318:833–837, 1999.

Yeomans ND, Tulassay ZT, Racz I, et al: A comparison of omeprazole with ranitidine for ulcers associated with nonsteroidal antiinflammatory drugs. *N Engl J Med* 338:719–726, 1998.

Wang HH, Hsieh CC, Antoniolo DA: Rising incidence rate of esophageal adenocarcinoma and use of pharmaceutical agents that relax the lower esophageal sphincter. *Cancer Causes Control* 5:573–578, 1994.

Pradip Cherian
Susan Gordon

Chronic Abdominal Pain: The Functional Gastrointestinal Disorders

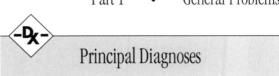

How Common Are Functional Gastrointestinal Disorders?

The term, *functional gastrointestinal disorders,* covers a variable combination of chronic, recurrent upper gastrointestinal disorders (dyspepsia) or lower gastrointestinal irritable bowel syndrome (IBS) symptoms, where an organic pathologic process or structural abnormality is absent. (The evaluations and treatment of patients who have dyspepsia due to identifiable etiologies are discussed in Chapter 5.) In contrast, the term, *functional bowel disorder,* usually refers to symptoms attributed to the lower gastrointestinal tract.

These disorders are among the more common gastrointestinal conditions diagnosed by both primary care physicians and gastroenterologists. Prevalence data for dyspepsia in the United States are sparse, but a study from Minnesota reported a 1-year prevalence of 26 percent. Prevalence of a single upper gastrointestinal symptom was more than 70 percent over a 1-year period. Several European countries have reported dyspeptic symptoms in 25 to 32 percent of the surveyed population in the year preceding the survey.

Symptoms of IBS account for 25 to 50 percent of consultations seen by gastroenterologists in the United States. A study from the United Kingdom reported that 22 percent of healthy volunteers had symptoms suggestive of IBS over a 1-year period. It must be noted that a significant proportion of patients meeting symptom criteria for dyspepsia also satisfy criteria for IBS, and in one study this figure was as high as 23 percent. Other studies have shown that more than 80 percent of patients with symptoms suggestive of IBS have concomitant dyspepsia. No formal analysis has been done to determine the costs of treating functional gastrointestinal disorders in the community. The health care expenditure in caring for patients with IBS is estimated at greater than $8 billion per year.

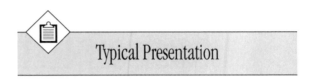

Principal Diagnoses

The evaluation of patients with dyspepsia of identifiable causes is discussed in Chapter 5. The currently used definitions (called the Rome criteria) for the commonly used terms in functional gastrointestinal disorders are given in Table 6-1.

Typical Presentation

Functional Dyspepsia

There is no typical presentation for patients who suffer from dyspepsia, because the term covers a broad range of symptoms. Patients may complain of upper abdominal pain, retrosternal pain, or discomfort accompanied by other symptoms referable to the upper gastrointestinal tract, such as nausea, vomiting, belching, bloating, or heartburn. There is no specific age group in which these symptoms are more common, and most studies have not shown specific gender predominance. Symptoms usually have been present for a few weeks and may suggest the presence of an ulcer, dysmotility, or reflux disease. Clinical evaluation and investigation, including endoscopy, reveal no definite cause for these symptoms.

Irritable Bowel Syndrome

The typical presenting features of patients with IBS are abdominal pain and a change in bowel habits. Symptoms seem to be more prevalent among women; but, in both sexes, symptoms seem to decrease with age. The classic study by Manning and coworkers identified several symptoms that were more common in patients with IBS than they were in the general population, and a

Table 6-1

Definition of Terms Used for Functional Gastrointestinal Disorders*

FUNCTIONAL DYSPEPSIA

1. Upper abdominal pain or discomfort centered in the upper abdomen.
2. No organic disease is likely to explain the symptoms.

Ulcer-like dyspepsia

Three or more of the following symptoms, but upper abdominal pain must be predominant:

        Epigastric pain

        Pain relieved by food

        Pain relieved by antacids or acid-reducing drugs

        Pain occurring before meals or when hungry

        Pain that at times awakens the patient from sleep

        Periodic pain with remission and relapses

Dysmotility-like dyspepsia

Pain is not a dominant symptom, but upper abdominal discomfort should be present and characterized by 3 or more of the following:

        Early satiety

        Postprandial fullness

        Nausea/retching and/or vomiting that is recurrent

        Bloating in the upper abdomen not accompanied by visible distension

        Upper abdominal discomfort often aggravated by food

Unspecified dyspepsia

        Dyspeptic symptoms that cannot be classified into the above 3 symptom profiles

IRRITABLE BOWEL SYNDROME

At least three months of continuous or recurrent symptoms of:

Abdominal pain or discomfort that is

        Relieved by defecation and/or

        Associated with a change in frequency of stool and/or

        Associated with a change in consistency of stool

        and

Two or more of the following, at least on one-fourth of occasion or days;

        Altered stool frequency

        Altered stool form

        Altered stool passage

        Passage of mucus

        Bloating or feeling of abdominal distension

*To be defined as a disorder the symptoms should have been continuous or recurrent for three contiguous months.

Table 6-2

Manning Criteria

Onset of pain associated with more frequent bowel movements than that which is normal for patient
Onset of pain associated with looser bowel movements than that which is normal for patient
Pain is relieved by bowel movements
Visible abdominal bloating is present
More than 1 in 4 bowel movements associated with a sense of incomplete evacuation
More than 1 in 4 bowel movements associated with mucus

set of six criteria were developed, later to be called "Manning criteria" (Table 6-2).

These criteria were modified by an international working team to establish the Rome criteria. Though two Manning criteria are needed to make a diagnosis, with a greater number of criteria present it is more likely that the patient has IBS.

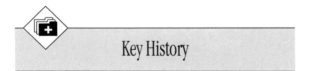

Key History

Functional Dyspepsia

Patients with functional dyspepsia could have a variety of symptoms, which seem to arise from the upper gastrointestinal tract and are not associated with defecation. These include epigastric discomfort or pain, epigastric or retrosternal burning, bloating or fullness, excessive belching, nausea, vomiting, or regurgitation. Nocturnal symptoms, such as burning, pain, and fullness, have also been described but are rare. It must be noted that most patients do not have one symptom alone but usually have two or more in combination.

There are some key points in the history that may suggest the presence of organic disease. First,

pain that is episodic (usually separated by weeks or months), severe, radiating to the back or scapula and accompanied by restlessness, sweating, or vomiting is strongly suggestive of biliary pain. Second, chronic recurrent heartburn, acid reflux or regurgitation, or difficulty in swallowing should suggest the possibility of gastroesophageal reflux disease (GERD), a condition that needs to be differentiated from dyspepsia. Third, medication history is important because several drugs may have side effects that can be mistaken for dyspeptic symptoms. Patients should be specifically asked about nonsteroidal anti-inflammatory drugs (NSAID) use and all over-the-counter medications. Finally, alarm symptoms such as weight loss, bleeding, anorexia, or dysphagia should immediately prompt an evaluation to exclude malignancy. (See Chapter 5 for further evaluation of dyspepsia due to organic causes.)

Irritable Bowel Syndrome

Lower or mid-abdominal pain is the classic symptom of patients with IBS, though descriptors of the pain vary from patient to patient. Some patients describe spasm or colic, which may vary in site and intensity, while others talk of pain that can last from minutes to several hours. The site of pain may vary from day to day. Pain is often related to changes in bowel habit. In some patients defecation relieves pain; while in others there is a change in stool frequency or consistency with pain. The stool appearance may change, with some patients describing "ribbon-like" stool while others describe "pellet-like" stool. A large fraction of patients with IBS complain of a feeling of incomplete evacuation, bloating, and abdominal distension, and have significant discomfort during these episodes, with passage of mucus in the stool. Again, key points in the history that suggest the presence of organic disease are the sudden appearance of symptoms for the first time in patients, age over 40 years, progressively worsening symptoms, new symptoms after a long period, nocturnal symptoms, fever, weight loss, or rectal bleeding.

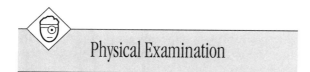

Physical Examination

Functional Dyspepsia

The physical examination may not contribute much toward the diagnosis of functional dyspepsia, but it is important to perform a thorough examination to exclude other disease processes. Occasionally, epigastric tenderness may be elicited, but this is a nonspecific finding. Any suggestion of ascites, palpable abdominal masses, visceromegaly, or fecal occult blood requires further diagnostic testing.

Irrritable Bowel Syndrome

Most people with IBS will have a normal physical exam. However, there may be some physical findings that are suggestive of the diagnosis of IBS. Patients may appear anxious or tense; the abdomen may appear slightly bloated; and there may be mild discomfort when the abdomen is palpated, especially in the region of the sigmoid colon. Any evidence of weight loss, fever, palpable abdominal masses, ascites, rectal bleeding, or fecal occult blood should suggest organic disease and prompt further investigation or testing.

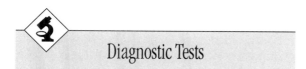

Diagnostic Tests

Functional Dyspepsia

There are no specific diagnostic tests to make the diagnosis of functional dyspepsia. This is essentially a diagnosis of exclusion after "reasonable" evaluation fails to reveal a cause for the symptoms. There is continued debate about how exhaustive an investigation is required to be considered reasonable. Some investigators have specified that there must be no cause identified on "the basis of clinical, biochemical, endoscopic, or radiological investigation." All patients should have a complete blood cell count and differential to look for anemia or inflammation, as well as a stool hemoccult test to detect occult GI bleeding. Based on consensus statements by the American Gastroenterology Association and the European *Helicobacter pylori* Study Group, some authors have recommended the following primary care options as a basis for diagnostic testing:

1. Patients <45 to 50 years old without alarm symptoms (weight loss, bleeding, anorexia, or dysphagia): Reassurance and lifestyle changes, including stress management, decrease of alcohol intake, discontinuance of NSAIDs, and if needed the trial of a course of H_2 antagonists or a prokinetic for 6 to 8 weeks. If there is no response, a referral for further investigation is advised.

OR

Noninvasive test for *H. pylori*; if positive, eradication therapy is given. If there is no response, referral for further investigation.

2. Patients >45 to 50 years old or if any "alarm" symptom present. Referral for further investigation at presentation.

Irritable Bowel Syndrome

As with functional dyspepsia, IBS is a diagnosis of exclusion and while some tests are recommended for all patients in a primary care setting, further testing may be required based on clinical history and examination. All patients should have a complete blood cell count, erythrocyte sedimentation rate, and differential to look for evidence of anemia or inflammation. A stool hemoccult test should also be done to detect evidence of gastrointestinal bleeding. Flexible sigmoidoscopy should be considered part of the initial work-up in most patients. At sigmoidoscopy, the mucosa should be free of ulcers, friability, bleeding, or any lesions or growths. Any significant finding in any of these tests should be an indication for further evaluation or referral to a gastroenterologist. Recurrent severe abdominal pain, long-standing diarrhea, severe constipation, or persistent dyspepsia are also indications for referral to a gastroenterologist.

Figure 6-1

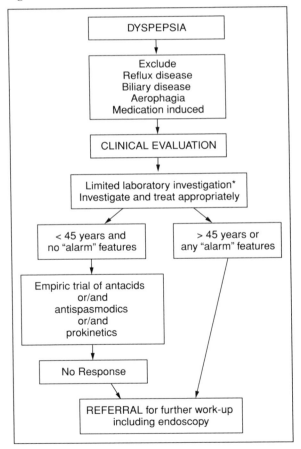

Algorithm: Evaluation of Dyspepsia. *See text and Chapter 5.

Additional Diagnostic Testing

Persistent dyspeptic symptoms, despite empiric treatment or the presence of alarm symptoms, are an indication for endoscopy. Reflux esophagitis, ulcers, and malignancy are quickly diagnosed by endoscopy. A normal endoscopy is also valuable because it reinforces the diagnosis of dyspepsia and has a reassuring effect on patients. Patients with suspected IBS, especially those with chronic diarrhea, may need extensive stool tests, large-bowel evaluation with colonoscopy or barium enema, and small-bowel evaluation with follow-through x-rays. Lactose tolerance tests should also be considered in patients with predominant diarrhea. If intractable constipation is the presenting feature, tests of colonic transit and anorectal and pelvic floor function may be useful.

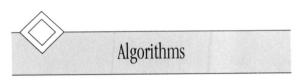

Algorithms for the evaluation and treatment of functional Dyspepsia and IBS are depicted in Figures 6-1 and 6-2.

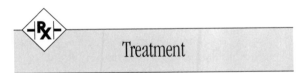

The most effective form of treatment begins with the establishment of a firm diagnosis after reasonable investigation. Unnecessary and repeated tests may undermine the confidence of patients in the diagnosis, and this must be avoided. Patients must be told that the diagnosis is benign and with no significant effect on life expectancy. Patients must also be told of the possibility of continuing and recurrent symptoms, but that the disease can be well controlled with patience, lifestyle and dietary changes, and the judicious use of medication.

Figure 6-2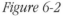

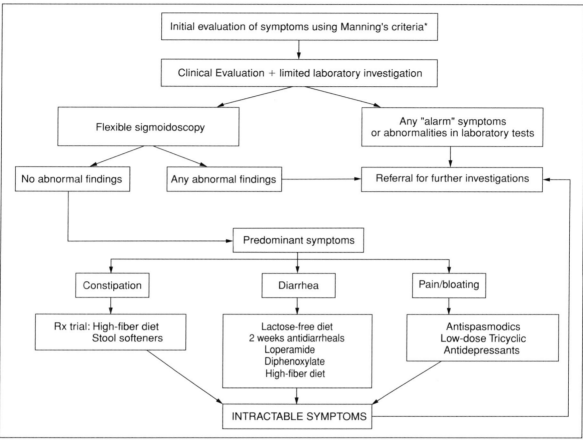

Algorithm: Evaluation of Patients with Irritable Bowel Syndrome. *See text.

Functional gastrointestinal disorders have a strong association with psychological factors. This link is based on various epidemiologic studies, the temporal relation between stressful events and gastrointestinal symptoms, and the response of some symptoms to drugs that modify psychological states or to psychotherapeutic measures. Before considering psychotherapeutic medication or measures, general treatment directed toward various symptoms may be tried.

Functional Dyspepsia

The treatment of functional dyspepsia traditionally starts with the avoidance of offending foods, high-fat diets, coffee, tobacco, and alcohol. Large meals are avoided in favor of four to six small meals, especially if bloating is a major symptom. It must be noted that none of these measures have been established to be of value, but anecdotally they have been effective in many patients.

ANTACIDS

Antacids have been the mainstay of treatment of dyspeptic symptoms for many years. Studies looking at antacid efficacy have not found antacids to be effective in treatment of dyspepsia; but since these studies have not been conducted in the general population, they may not present a true picture of antacid efficacy. Antacids are usually used by patients to treat quite diverse symptoms; and since they are available as over-the-counter medication, their true efficacy may be difficult to estimate.

ACID SUPPRESSION

Inhibitors of acid secretion, H_2 antagonists, are frequently prescribed for dyspeptic symptoms even though their effect according to various studies is equivalent or only slightly superior to a placebo. Treatment with potent proton-pump inhibitors has also not shown significant benefit in the treatment of functional dyspepsia. Those who do respond probably have acid reflux as the main source of their symptoms, and they probably suffer from GERD rather than dyspepsia.

PROKINETICS

Techniques to assess motility of the gastrointestinal tract in patients with functional gastrointestinal disorders have often shown abnormal motor patterns, but no causal relation between dysmotility and symptoms has been established. Prokinetics such as metoclopramide may have some beneficial symptomatic effect in some patients, but this response has not been consistent or sustained.

PSYCHOTHERAPY

The link between psychological factors, stress, and functional gastrointestinal disorders has been established in several studies. Patients with dyspepsia have high scores for depression, anxiety, and somatic complaints. Hence, several researchers have tried various forms of therapy including psychotherapy, relaxation therapy, and cognitive

therapy with significant benefits in some patients. Tricyclic antidepressants have been effective in treating chronic abdominal pain, either by their effect on underlying depression or due to a direct but as yet unknown effect on the gut or pain receptors. Even when nausea and vomiting are the dominant symptoms, response rates of up to 80 percent have been reported with the use of tricyclic antidepressants.

Irritable Bowel Syndrome

The pathophysiology of functional dyspepsia and IBS are very similar. The treatment of IBS also entails the elimination of stress, modifying lifestyle and diet, and judicious use of drugs. The patient must understand the chronic and recurring nature of the disorder and also understand that while symptoms may be controlled they rarely disappear completely.

DIET

While no specific diet causes IBS, patients should avoid food substances that produce excessive bloating. Too much caffeine should be avoided because it stimulates intestinal motility and may increase anxiety. Diets that have a high content of fiber have been advocated for a long time for IBS, and it has been found that psyllium products (e.g., Metamucil) and polycarbophil products (e.g., FiberCon), with their capacity to bind fluid and stool, help both with diarrhea and constipation. If these dietary measures do not work, then medical therapy needs to be considered.

ANTISPASMODICS AND ANTICHOLINERGICS

Antispasmodics and anticholinergics are prescribed for cramping abdominal pain, bloating, and diarrhea. They act by blocking acetylcholine-mediated depolarization of intestinal smooth muscle and act best when taken at the onset of pain. Several agents are available (dicyclomine, propanthaline, and hyoscyamine) and treatment may need to be tailored based on best response and side-effect profile. Dryness of mouth, blurring of vision, tachycardia, and urinary retention are the common side effects. These drugs have little effect on patients with constipation and should be avoided.

PROKINETICS

There are few studies on the use of prokinetics in IBS. Cisapride has been used in patients with constipation-predominant IBS with some reported benefits, but this drug was withdrawn from the market in 1999. Erythromycin and related 14-member macrolide compounds accelerate gastric emptying and shorten oral-cecal transit time. In the large bowel, a significant decrease in transit time with these agents is observed only in the right colon; and, therefore, their use in constipation-predominant IBS appears to be doubtful. Newer compounds derived from the macrolides are being developed, and these drugs may be of use in the treatment of IBS in the future.

ANTIDEPRESSANTS

Psychological factors and visceral hypersensitivity seem to play an important role both in dyspepsia and in IBS. Antidepressants have a beneficial effect though their exact mode of action is not known. They may work by controlling some of the psychological symptoms that accompany functional gastrointestinal disorders, but they also work where no psychiatric diagnosis exists. They may have effects on bowel neuroreceptors, receptors within the central nervous system, or directly on bowel motility. There is often significant reduction in abdominal pain, but constipation-dominant symptoms are less responsive to antidepressant therapy.

PSYCHOTHERAPY

Psychological treatment has been tried quite effectively in functional gastrointestinal disorders with reduction in abdominal pain, bloating, and diarrhea. Cognitive behavioral therapy and hyp-

notherapy have also been shown in noncontrolled trials to be effective in treatment of diarrhea-predominant IBS. However, the efficacy of these treatments has not been established in randomized controlled trials and further treatment evaluation of psychological interventions needs to be conducted. It is quite likely that in the future behavioral therapies and pharmacologic treatments may have to be combined with management that is individualized to patients' specific needs.

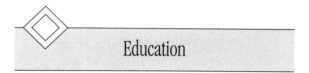
Education

Once the diagnosis is secure based on symptom criteria, physical examination, and targeted tests, patients must be educated about functional gastrointestinal disorders. They must be told that their diagnosis is benign, and although symptoms are likely to be chronic and recurrent, there is very little effect on life expectancy. Patients must be given dietary advice, which should include information concerning regular eating habits; avoidance of aggravating factors such as smoking, alcohol, and excessive coffee; and consumption of a well-balanced diet with adequate dietary fiber. Lifestyle changes, including the awareness of and avoidance of stress, should be emphasized. Patients should be told of the role of psychosocial factors in functional gastrointestinal disorders. Depression, anxiety, panic, and unexpressed fears, including the fear of cancer, should be identified. Patients should be encouraged to address these issues, and appropriate therapy should be instituted.

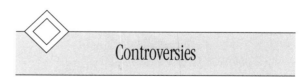
Controversies

A high frequency of sexual and physical abuse in women with functional gastrointestinal disorders was first reported in 1990. Subsequent studies at other centers have also reported similar findings. However, most of these studies have been conducted in referral centers where patients with more refractory symptoms are selectively seen. It is not clear that similar findings would be reported from primary care centers, although one population-based study did show that a high percentage of women with functional gastrointestinal disorders had a history of abuse. Physicians should be aware of this, especially if symptoms are severe and refractory and if an abuse history is suspected. Patients must be encouraged to address these issues with their primary care clinician.

Emerging Concepts

Over the years several researchers have shown that patients who suffer from functional gastrointestinal disorders have altered visceral sensitivity to various stimuli, especially distension. Balloon distension within the colon of patients with IBS produce pain at much lower volumes than it does in healthy subjects. It is now felt that this altered sensation is a part of visceral hyperalgesia. Based on these findings newer forms of pharmacologic treatment are emerging. For example, a peripheral kappa opiate agonist has been developed that seems to decrease gastric sensitivity to distension. In preliminary work, this agent has been found to be effective both in dyspepsia and IBS.

Bibliography

Agreus L, Svardsudd K, Nyren O, Tibblin G: Irritable bowel syndrome and dyspepsia in the general population: Overlap and lack of stability over time. *Gastroenterology* 109:671–680, 1995.

American Gastroenterological Association Medical Position Statement: Evaluation of dyspepsia. *Gastroenterology* 114:579–581, 1998.

Clouse RE: Antidepressants for functional gastrointestinal syndromes. *Dig Dis Sci* 39:2352–2363, 1994.

Dapoigny M, Abitbol JL, Fraitag B: Efficacy of peripheral kappa agonist fedotozine versus placebo in treatment of irritable bowel syndrome. A multicenter dose-response study. *Dig Dis Sci* 40:2244–2249, 1995.

Drossman DA: Diagnosing and treating patients with refractory functional gastrointestinal disorders. *Ann Intern Med* 123:688–697, 1995.

Drossman DA, Leserman J, Nachman G, et al: Sexual and physical abuse in women with functional or organic gastrointestinal disorders. *Ann Intern Med* 113:828–833, 1990.

European *Helicobacter pylori* Study Group: Current European concepts in the management of *Helicobacter pylori* infection. The Mastricht Consensus Report. *Gut* 41:8–13, 1997.

Fraitag B, Homerin M, Hecketsweiler P: Double-blind dose-response multicenter comparison of fedotozine and placebo in treatment of non-ulcer dyspepsia. *Dig Dis Sci* 39:1072–1077, 1994.

Guthrie E, Creed F, Dawson D, Tomenson B: A controlled trial of psychological treatment for the irritable bowel syndrome. *Gastroenterology* 100:450–457, 1991.

Jian R, Ducrot F, Ruskone A, et al: Symptomatic radionuclide and therapeutic assessment of chronic idiopathic dyspepsia. A double-blind placebo-controlled evaluation of cisapride. *Dig Dis Sci* 34:644–657, 1989.

Jones R, Lydeard S: Irritable bowel syndrome in the general population. *Br Med J* 304:87–90, 1992.

Lambert JR: The role of *Helicobacter pylori* in nonulcer dyspepsia. *Gastroenterol Clin North Am* 22:141–151, 1993.

Longstreth GF: Economic considerations in the evaluation of dyspepsia and the irritable bowel syndrome. International Symposium on Functional Gastrointestinal Disorders 103–106, 1999.

Mangel AW, Northcutt AR: The safety and efficacy of alosetron, a 5HT3 receptor antagonist, in female irritable bowel syndrome patients. *Alim Pharmacol Ther* 13 (suppl 2):77–82, 1999.

Manning AP, Thompson WG, Heaton KW, Morris AF: Towards a positive diagnosis of the irritable bowel. *Br Med J* 2:653–654, 1978.

Nyren O, Adami H-O, Bates S: Absence of therapeutic benefit from antacids or cimetidine in non-ulcer dyspepsia. *N Engl J Med* 314:339–343, 1986.

Poynard T, Naveau S, Mory B: Meta-analysis of smooth muscle relaxants in the treatment of irritable bowel syndrome. *Alim Pharmacol Ther* 8:499–510, 1994.

Prakash C, Lustman PJ, Freedland KE, et al: Tricyclic antidepressants for functional nausea and vomiting. Clinical outcomes in 37 patients. *Dig Dis Sci* 43: 1951–1956, 1998.

Prior A, Read NW: Reduction of rectal sensitivity and post prandial motility by granisetron or 5HT$_3$-receptor antagonist in patients with irritable bowel syndrome. *Alim Pharmacol Ther* 2:175–180, 1993.

Ritchie J: Pain from distension of the pelvic colon by inflating a balloon in the irritable colon syndrome. *Gut* 14:125–132, 1973.

Stam R, Akkermans LMA, Wiegant VM: Trauma and the gut: Interactions between stressful experiences and intestinal function. *Gut* 40:704–709, 1997.

Talley NJ, Fett SL, Zinsmeister AR, Melton LJ: Gastrointestinal tract symptoms and self-reported abuse: A population-based study. *Gastroenterology* 107: 1040–1049, 1994.

Talley NJ, Gabriel SE, Harmsen WS: Medical costs in community subjects with irritable bowel syndrome. *Gastroenterology* 109:1736–1741, 1995.

Talley NJ, Meineche-Schmidt V, Pane P, et al: Efficacy of omeprazole in functional dyspepsia. Double-blind, randomized, placebo controlled trial. *Alim Pharmacol Ther* 12:1055–1065, 1998.

Talley NJ, Owen BK, Boyce P, Paterson K: Psychological treatment for irritable bowel syndrome: A critique of controlled treatment trials. *Am J Gastroenterol* 91:277– 286, 1996.

Talley NJ, Piper DW: The association between non-ulcer dyspepsia and other gastrointestinal disorders. *Scand J Gastroenterol* 20:896–900, 1985.

Talley NJ, Stanghellini V, Heading RC, et al: GNJ Rome II: A multinational consensus document on functional gastrointestinal disorders. *Gut* 45 (suppl 2), 1999.

Talley NJ, Zinsmeister AR, Schleck CD, Melton LJ, III: Dyspepsia and dyspepsia subgroups: A population-based study. *Gastoenterology* 102:1259–1268, 1992.

Thompson WG, Creed F, Drossman DA: Functional bowel disorders and functional abdominal pain. *Gastroenterol Int* 5:99–103, 1992.

Tibblin G: Introduction to the epidemiology of dyspepsia. *Scand J Gastrenterol* 20 (suppl 109):29–33, 1985.

Weir RD, Backett EM: Studies of the epidemiology of peptic ulcer in a rural community: Prevalence and natural history of dyspepsia and peptic ulcer. *Gut* 9: 75–83, 1968.

Whorwell PJ, Prior A, Farregher FB: Controlled trial of hypnotherapy in the treatment of severe refractory irritable bowel syndrome. *Lancet* 2:1232–1234, 1984.

Mohan Charan
Steven A. Edmundowicz

Chapter 7

Acute Abdominal Pain

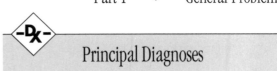

How Common Is Acute Abdominal Pain?

Acute abdominal pain is a common complaint of patients coming to a primary care physician. A primary objective of the initial evaluation is to determine if the presentation requires emergent evaluation and therapy. Localizing a complaint of pain to a region or organ system is useful in the rapid evaluation of patients. An understanding of the neural innervation of the abdominal cavity assists in the diagnostic evaluation of patients with acute abdominal pain.

Abdominal pain can originate from the abdominal viscera or other structures in the abdominal cavity. Acute inflammation, infection, bowel distension, and ischemia can all cause similar abdominal pain. The peritoneum consists of two double-layered sheets of cells that form the visceral and the parietal peritoneal layers. The visceral and parietal peritoneal layers are in continuity, but have separate neural innervation. Autonomic nerves innervate the visceral layer that covers the organs. The visceral pain fibers are bilateral and unmyelinated, and they enter the spinal cord at multiple levels. The pain from these nerves is dull, achy, crampy, and poorly localized. In general, visceral pain from the esophagus, stomach, and proximal duodenum is referred to the epigastric area; the distal duodenum, small bowel, and right colon to the periumbilical area; and the left colon and rectum to the hypogastric or suprapubic area in the abdomen. Somatic nerves originating from the T7 to L2 spinal nerves innervate the parietal peritoneum. The umbilicus is at the level of T10. Pain produced by ischemia, inflammation, or stretch of parietal peritoneum is transmitted through myelinated afferent fibers to specific dorsal root ganglia on the same side and the same dermatomal level as the origin of pain. This type of pain is more sharp, discrete, and localized. It is responsible for the physical findings of tenderness to palpation, guarding, and rebound.

Principal Diagnoses

Acute *upper* abdominal pain may be due to several disorders, including gastric ulcer, duodenal ulcer, acute cholecystitis, acute pancreatitis, or small-bowel obstruction. Acute *lower* abdominal pain may be due to large-bowel obstruction, acute diverticulitis, and acute appendicitis. Acute mesenteric ischemia can involve both the upper and lower abdomen depending on the vessels involved. Rarely, conditions that are considered more chronic may present suddenly with acute abdominal pain, including inflammatory bowel disease, malignancies, infections, and hemorrhage into lesions (hepatic adenomas) or organs. The abdomen contains various organs and any of them can cause abdominal pain. This chapter will focus on the most common causes of abdominal pain originating from the gastrointestinal tract.

Acute Upper Abdominal Pain

GASTRIC ULCER

The peak incidence for gastric ulcer is at age 55 to 65. Most patients with a gastric ulcer have acid secretory rates within normal range. They usually occur on the lesser curve near the angulus, at the junction of oxyntic and antral mucosa. The exact role of *Helicobacter pylori* in this pathogenesis is unclear. There is no definitive evidence that stress, alcohol, corticosteroids, or caffeine causes chronic gastric ulceration. Nonsteroidal anti-inflammatory drugs, aspirin, bile reflux, and smoking predispose to gastric ulceration.

The natural course of a gastric ulcer is healing in 65 to 70 percent of subjects on placebo. On follow-up for 1 year, 55 to 89 percent will have recurrence of gastric ulcer on placebo. Hemorrhage is a common complication, occurring in up to 25 percent. If the ulcer is located in the pyloric channel or most distal antrum, it may cause gastric outlet obstruction. Gastric perforation occurs less frequently than does hemorrhage. Mortality with gastric ulcer perforation is 3 times that with duodenal ulcer. Increased mortality is due in part to increased age of gastric ulcer patients but may also result from uncertainty and delay in diagnosis and from greater soilage of the peritoneum.

DUODENAL ULCER

In the United States, the lifetime prevalence of duodenal ulcer in males is 10 percent and in females is 4 percent. Duodenal ulcers are more common between the ages of 30 to 55; however, their incidence has been declining for the last 30 years. Ninety percent of duodenal ulcer patients have associated *H. pylori* gastritis.

Successful eradication of *H. pylori* decreases duodenal ulcer recurrence to less than 5 percent per year. The risk of duodenal ulcer is increased by aspirin, nonsteroidal anti-inflammatory drugs, and smoking. Hemorrhage is more common with gastric ulcer than it is with duodenal ulcer. Gastric outlet obstruction occurs in 2 percent of all ulcer patients; and in 90 percent of cases, it is due to a duodenal ulcer.

ACUTE CHOLECYSTITIS

Cholecystitis is associated with gallstones in over 90 percent of cases. When a calculus becomes impacted in the cystic duct, inflammation develops, leading to acute cholecystitis. The organisms most frequently isolated by culture of gallbladder bile in these patients include *Escherichia coli, Klebsiella* sp., group D *Streptococcus, Staphylococcus* sp., and *Clostridium* sp. Gallstones are more common in women than they are in men and increase in incidence with aging. In the United States, over 20 percent of men and 35 percent of women have gallstones by age 75. The stones are divided into three major types: cholesterol and mixed stones account for 80 percent of the total and pigment stones comprise the remaining 20 percent. Acute cholecystitis caused by infectious agents (e.g., cytomegalovirus, cryptosporidiosis, or microsporidiosis) may occur in patients with AIDS. Acalculous cholecystitis should be considered when unexplained fever or right upper quadrant pain occurs within 2 to 4 weeks of major surgery or in critically ill patients with multiple injuries, severe burns, or sepsis who have had no oral intake for a prolonged period.

ACUTE PANCREATITIS

Alcohol abuse and gallstone passage are the most common causes of acute pancreatitis seen in the United States. The third most common cause is idiopathic (10 percent). Almost 5 percent of cases are drug related. The drugs most commonly implicated are thiazide diuretics, furosemide, sulfonamides, tetracycline, oral contraceptives, pentamidine, dideoxyinosine (ddi), and azathioprine or 6-mercaptopurine. Other causes of acute pancreatitis include hypercalcemia, hypertriglyceridemia, mumps, and Coxsackie viral infection.

Most patients with acute pancreatitis recover without any sequelae. The overall mortality rate of acute pancreatitis is 5 to 10 percent. *Ranson's criteria* reliably predict mortality in acute pancreatitis and help assess the severity of pancreatitis on admission (Table 7-1). When three or more criteria are present on admission, a severe course, which is often complicated by pancreatic necrosis, can be predicted.

ACUTE SMALL-BOWEL OBSTRUCTION

Mechanical obstruction of the small intestine is a common surgical disorder. The most common causes of obstruction are adhesions (history of prior abdominal surgery), strangulation in a hernia, volvulus, internal hernias, radiation enteritis, Crohn's disease, intestinal wall hematomas (trauma or anticoagulants), and neoplasms. Acute small-bowel obstruction needs to be differentiated from an adynamic ileus and chronic intestinal pseudo-obstruction, which may have a similar appearance.

Acute Upper or Lower Abdominal Pain

ACUTE MESENTERIC ISCHEMIA

The intraabdominal portions of gastrointestinal tract are supplied by three major unpaired arteries

Table 7-1

Ranson's Criteria for the Evaluation of Patients
with Acute Pancreatitis

Age over 55 years
WBC count over 16,000/μl
AST over 250 U/liter.
Serum LDH over 350 U/dl
Blood glucose over 200 mg/dl
IN THE FIRST 48 H, DEVELOPMENT OF THE FOLLOWING INDICATES A WORSENING PROGNOSIS:
Serum calcium <8 mg/dl
Rise in BUN >5 mg/dl
Base deficit over 4 meq/liter
Arterial PO_2 <60 mmHg
Hematocrit drop >10% points
Estimated fluid sequestration >6 liters.
Mortality rates correlate with number of criteria present: if <3, 1%; 3–4 criteria, 15%; 5–6 criteria, 40%; and 7 or more criteria predict >90% mortality.

WBC, white blood cell; AST, aspartate aminotransferase; LDH, lactic acid dehydrogenase; BUN, blood urea nitrogen; PO_2, partial pressure of oxygen.

arising from the abdominal aorta: the celiac artery, superior mesenteric artery, and inferior mesenteric artery. Approximately 30 percent of resting cardiac output flows through these three splanchnic arteries. Mesenteric ischemia results from a critical decrease in blood and oxygen supply to the small or large intestine. Mesenteric infarction represents ischemic necrosis of the small or large intestine. The small bowel, right colon, and proximal transverse colon are often involved when the superior mesenteric artery is involved.

Acute mesenteric ischemia is commonly caused by sudden occlusion or marked decrease in blood flow through the superior mesenteric artery. It could result from embolic occlusion, spontaneous primary thrombosis, isolated dissection of the superior mesenteric artery, or mesenteric vein thrombosis (if venous collaterals are also blocked). Cirrhosis, abdominal infection, and hypercoag-

ulable and low-flow states are the most common predisposing factors. Nonocclusive mesenteric ischemia is usually seen in critically ill elderly patients with markedly diminished cardiac output or hypovolemia or in those elderly who are receiving vasoconstrictive therapy.

Acute Lower Abdominal Pain

ACUTE APPENDICITIS

Acute appendicitis is mainly a condition of young adults but affects all ages (uncommon under 3 years of age). It is the most common surgical emergency, affecting approximately 10 percent of the population. It occurs most commonly in the 20- to 30-year-old age group. Obstruction of the appendix by a fecalith, inflammation, neoplasm, or a foreign body leads to inflammation. If left untreated, gangrene and perforation develop within 36 h. The mortality rate from uncomplicated appendicitis is extremely low. In perforated appendicitis, the mortality rate is 0.2 percent in most groups, but approaches 15 percent in the elderly.

LARGE-BOWEL OBSTRUCTION

The usual cause of large-bowel obstruction is carcinoma of the colon (left side); other causes include sigmoid volvulus (10 percent of cases), diverticulitis, extrinsic obstruction from metastatic carcinoma, stricture, hernia, pseudo-obstruction, adhesions, and fecal impaction.

ACUTE DIVERTICULITIS

Diverticular disease of the colon is common in developed countries. The true incidence of diverticulosis is difficult to measure, as most patients are asymptomatic. The incidence increases with age, varying from less than 10 percent in those under 40 years, to an estimated 50 to 60 percent in patients over 80 years. *Diverticulitis* is defined as inflammation and/or infection associated with diverticula and is seen in 10 to 25 percent of patients with diverticulosis. The diverticulum becomes obstructed by inspissated stool in its neck, ultimately leading to perforation of a single diverticulum. The extent and localization of the perforation determines its clinical behavior.

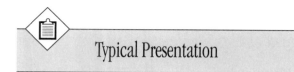

Typical Presentation

Gastric Ulcer

Epigastric pain is the presenting symptom in 80 to 90 percent of cases, which may be precipitated or accentuated by food. The pain is described as gnawing, dull, aching, or hunger-like. The pain is not specific or sensitive enough to serve as reliable diagnostic criteria. Symptom relief with antacids is less consistent than it is with duodenal ulcers. Weight loss may occur due to anorexia or aversion to food due to discomfort produced by eating.

Duodenal Ulcer

Patients have epigastric pain that is described as sharp, gnawing, or burning. It characteristically occurs from 90 min to 3 h after eating and frequently awakens patients at night. The pain is usually relieved in a few minutes by food or antacids. Symptoms tend to be recurrent and episodic. The severity of pain varies from patient to patient. Changes in character of ulcer pain may signal development of complications. For example, ulcer pain that becomes constant, no longer relieved by food or antacids, or radiates to the back or either upper quadrant may indicate penetration of the ulcer, which is often posteriorly into the pancreas.

Acute Cholecystitis

The acute attack is often precipitated by a large or fatty meal. Approximately 60 to 70 percent of patients report having experienced prior attacks that resolved spontaneously. The attack is characterized by sudden appearance of severe, steady epigastric or right upper quadrant pain, which in uncomplicated cases may gradually subside over a period of 12 to 18 h. The pain may radiate to the interscapular area, right scapula, or shoulder. Patients are anorectic and nauseated. Vomiting occurs in about 75 percent of cases and may produce signs and symptoms of vascular and extracellular volume depletion. Jaundice is unusual early in the course but may occur later when edematous inflammatory changes involve the bile ducts. A low-grade fever is characteristically present, but shaking chills or rigors are not uncommon.

Acute Pancreatitis

Patients have abdominal pain, which may vary from mild and tolerable discomfort to severe, constant pain. The pain is steady and boring in character, located in epigastrium and periumbilical region and often radiates to the back, as well as to the chest, flanks, and lower abdomen. Patients often sit up with trunk flexed and knees drawn up to obtain relief from pain. Ingestion of food, alcohol, and supine posture increase the pain.

Nausea, vomiting, and abdominal distension are also noted. Most patients are hypovolemic, because fluid accumulates in the abdomen. In over one-half of patients, some degree of hypoxemia is present and patients may complain of dyspnea. Fever, if present, is low grade rarely exceeding 101° (38.33°C) F in the absence of complications.

Acute Small-Bowel Obstruction

The pain is usually severe and colicky in nature and located in the epigastric and mainly periumbilical region. Spasms occur every 3 to 10 min (according to the level of obstruction) and last about 1 min. Later, pain becomes constant and diffuse as abdominal distension develops. Vomiting follows the onset of pain within minutes in proximal obstruction to hours in distal obstruction. Patients usually develop constipation after the bowel is empty.

Acute Mesenteric Ischemia

Patients are usually older than 50 years of age and appear to be seriously ill. Patients experience sudden onset of severe, colicky, periumbilical abdominal pain at the onset. It later becomes diffuse and constant. Vomiting is seen in 75 percent of patients, and occult or gross blood is found in the gastric contents of 73 percent. Diarrhea is also common and often is heme-positive.

Acute Appendicitis

Appendicitis often begins as a vague, often colicky, periumbilical or epigastric pain. There is often an accompanying urge to defecate or pass flatus. The pain increases in severity, becomes continuous, and shifts to the right iliac fossa usually within 6 h. The pain is aggravated by motion or cough. Almost all patients have nausea with one or two episodes of vomiting. The development of nausea or vomiting before the onset of pain is extremely rare. Low-grade fever is typical; high fever or rigors suggests another diagnosis or appendiceal perforation.

Large-Bowel Obstruction

Patients have a sudden onset of colicky abdominal pain in the midline hypogastric region. Each spasm lasts for less than 1 minute. Vomiting may be absent or late, but constipation with no flatus is usual. The clinical findings in large-bowel obstruction depend on a number of factors: rapidity of onset, degree of obstruction, cause of obstruction, presence of comorbid conditions, and presence of ileocecal valve competency or a closed loop. If a closed loop is present or ileocecal valve is competent, colonic distension is greater, increasing the risk of ischemia and perforation. In patients with a competent ileocecal valve, the areas at risk

for perforation are the cecum and the primary tumor. An incompetent ileocecal valve permits colonic decompression into the small intestine, which may make differentiation from small-bowel obstruction difficult.

Acute Diverticulitis

Patients with localized inflammation or infection have mild to moderate aching abdominal pain usually in the left lower quadrant. The pain may be intermittent or constant and is frequently associated with a change in bowel habit. Anorexia, nausea, and vomiting may occur. Hematochezia is rare. Patients with free perforation present with a dramatic picture of generalized abdominal pain and peritoneal signs.

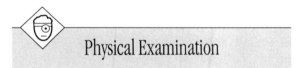

Physical Examination

Physical examination of patients with abdominal pain is of prime importance. A careful examination coupled with a proper history of present condition will frequently secure the diagnosis. The overall appearance of patients is quite helpful. Patients with intestinal perforation and diffuse peritonitis will usually be very still, whereas those with biliary colic will often writhe in agony. The facial expression of patients may indicate whether pain is constant or crampy. Tachycardia and hypotension signify hypovolemia and possible shock, as seen with acute pancreatitis and small-bowel obstruction. The blood pressure should be measured in each arm, as a pressure gradient between arms may signify aortic dissection leading to acute mesenteric ischemia. Patients' respiratory patterns should be observed, as patients with peritonitis would have rapid, shallow breathing. The head and neck should be examined for intraoral lesions, scleral icterus, and fundoscopic signs of emboli. The skin of the abdomen and thorax should be examined for evidence of herpes zoster or other rash. Chest examination may reveal evidence of pneumonia or pleurisy, which may be a cause for referred pain in the upper abdomen.

The abdomen should be examined with patients lying flat, and the abdomen uncovered from the xiphoid to the groin. Patients should be asked to point directly and precisely to the area that hurts the most. If patients cannot localize a point, it indicates that the abdominal process has not markedly inflamed the parietal peritoneum. A visual inspection of the abdomen should be completed looking for distension, hernias, pulsation, and pattern of movement with respiration. Bruising over the flanks (Grey Turner's sign) and periumbilical discoloration (Cullen's sign) suggest severe hemorrhagic pancreatitis. Abdominal auscultation should then be completed, appreciating bowel sounds and bruits. In bowel obstruction, increased bowel sounds are a feature, whereas with perforated peptic ulcer and acute pancreatitis bowel sounds are reduced or absent. The presence of an abdominal bruit is indicative of vascular narrowing; and in the setting of acute abdominal pain it may suggest bowel ischemia.

Following auscultation, abdominal palpation should be performed gently with warm hands to alleviate apprehension and excessive stimulation. Initially, superficial palpation is done to locate a site of maximum tenderness, followed by deep palpation. It is sometimes preferable to ask patients to cough in order to elicit a point of maximum tenderness. All quadrants of the abdomen should be palpated, carefully noting masses, muscle tone, organomegaly, warmth, pulsation, and the presence of hernias. Guarding refers to the contraction of the abdominal wall muscle when it is palpated. If patients can consciously eliminate the muscular response, it is referred to as voluntary guarding. If patients cannot eliminate the response, it is described as an involuntary guarding. If the abdominal wall is tense and boardlike (usually a sign of diffuse peritonitis), it is called rigidity. Sometimes muscle spasm is a result of a process limited to the abdominal wall such as a rectus sheath hematoma. To differentiate this, the ab-

domen is palpated first with the abdominal wall as relaxed as possible. Subsequently, the abdomen is palpated with the abdominal wall forcefully contracted by raising the head toward the chest. If the tenderness elicited on deep palpation is more with the abdominal wall contracted, then the process is likely localized to the abdominal wall (Fothergill's sign). Various signs have been described in patients with inflammation in the pelvis and lower retroperitoneum. The psoas sign is pain on resisted flexion of the leg or on hip extension causing irritation of the psoas muscle region. This is frequently seen with iliopsoas abscess and retrocecal appendicitis. The obturator sign is pain felt in the hypogastrium, elicited by flexing the right thigh at the hip with the knee bent and then internally rotating the hip, which causes irritation of internal obturator muscle. The usual causes are a ruptured appendix, direct injury to the muscle of pelvic floor, or a tuboovarian abscess.

The digital rectal examination is an integral part of the abdominal evaluation. It can allow detection of a pelvic collection or mass. The rectal examination reveals tenderness on the right in cases of pelvic peritonitis or appendicitis. Stool should be examined for occult and gross blood. Visual inspection of the perineum may show hemorrhoids, fistulas, or vesicles. In males, testes are examined for evidence of inflammation or swelling. In adult females, a pelvic examination, including both speculum and bimanual examination is required. The cervix should be checked for motion tenderness, discharge, or bleeding and cultures are obtained for *Chlamydia trachomatis* and *Neisseria gonorrhoeae*. The adnexa are palpated for tenderness or masses.

In patients with uncomplicated peptic ulcer disease, the physical examination is often unremarkable. Mild, localized epigastric tenderness on deep palpation may be present. Patients with perforated peptic ulcers, however, will often be pale, sweating, or ashen with boardlike abdominal rigidity and maximal guarding at the point of perforation. The bowel sounds are reduced and shifting dullness may be present. Vital signs are usually normal at first with tachycardia and shock occurring later. There may be pelvic tenderness on rectal examination.

Patients with acute cholecystitis will demonstrate tenderness in the right upper quadrant or epigastrium associated with muscle-guarding and rebound. Deep inspiration or cough during subcostal palpation of the right upper quadrant usually produces increased pain and inspiratory arrest (Murphy's sign).

Fever is usually present, and jaundice is seen in 25 percent of cases. The bowel sounds may be hypoactive from a paralytic ileus; and there may be abdominal distension. A definable mass in the right upper quadrant, especially if accompanied by minimal tenderness, should raise suspicion of a tumor in the gallbladder or of an enlarged gallbladder secondary to obstruction of the common bile duct.

In acute pancreatitis, patients will have tenderness in the upper abdomen often without guarding, rigidity, or rebound. The abdomen may be distended and bowel sounds may be reduced or absent due to an ileus. Fever and tachycardia are usually present. Tenderness, guarding, and rigidity in the left iliac fossa are often seen in acute diverticulitis. Patients will have a fever and an inflammatory mass can often be palpated.

In acute appendicitis, tenderness can be elicited in the right iliac fossa usually at McBurney's point. The psoas and obturator signs may be positive. Local rigidity, rebound, tenderness, guarding, and superficial hyperesthesia may or may not be present. In small-bowel obstruction, the abdomen is usually soft, but tender when palpated or if focally distended. Increased sharp tinkling bowel sounds are noted.

In large-bowel obstruction, abdominal distension occurs early and is marked. The bowel sounds are increased, especially during pain. The abdomen is rigid with local tenderness; and the rectum is usually empty on rectal examination. Patients with acute mesenteric ischemia will be symptomatic with a paucity of physical examination findings. There is localized tenderness, rigidity, and rebound over the site of infarcted bowel. Stool examination obtained during the digital rectal exam may be positive for frank hemorrhage or occult blood.

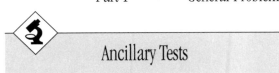

Ancillary Tests

After a detailed history and physical examination, a preliminary differential diagnosis can be formulated. Depending on the condition of patients, further testing can be instituted. In extreme situations, patients may be sent immediately to the emergency room for further evaluation or possibly the operating room for surgical exploration. The laboratory testing that follows can be accomplished in stable or actively resuscitated patients while a definitive treatment plan is developed (see Figures 7-1 and 7-2).

Complete Blood Cell Count

Patients with peptic ulcer disease may be anemic due to chronic blood loss. Hemoconcentration may be seen in patients with acute pancreatitis, mesenteric ischemia, and small-bowel obstruction. A leukocytosis is seen in peptic ulcer penetration, perforation, acute diverticulitis, acute pancreatitis, acute cholecystitis, and small-bowel obstruction.

Blood Chemistry

The serum amylase may be elevated in a number of disorders including acute pancreatitis, acute cholecystitis, bowel ischemia, perforated peptic ulcer, ruptured ectopic pregnancy, ruptured aortic aneurysm, and renal failure. In cases of perforated peptic ulcer, amylase elevation is usually less than twice the normal limit and lipase is normal. In pancreatitis, serum amylase and/or lipase are elevated in excess of three times the upper limits of normal. It is usually not necessary to measure both serum amylase and lipase. Serum lipase measurement is preferable if it can be done as rapidly as serum amylase, because it remains normal in some conditions associated with an elevation of serum amylase, including macroamylasemia, parotitis, and some carcinomas (lung, ovary, esophagus). The height of the serum amylase and lipase does not correlate with the severity of pancreatitis.

Figure 7-1

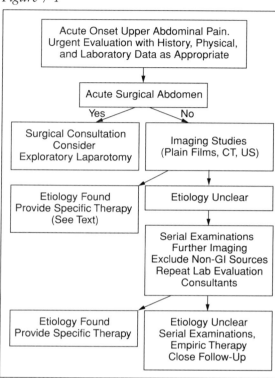

Algorithm for the evaluation and treatment of acute upper abdominal pain. CT, computed tomography; US, ultrasound; GI, gastrointestinal.

Figure 7-2

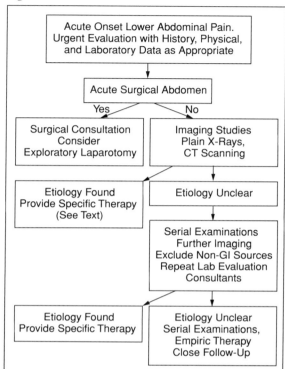

Algorithm for the evaluation of acute lower abdominal pain. CT, computed tomography; GI gastrointestinal.

Elevation of the serum bilirubin may be seen in acute cholecystitis even in the absence of common duct obstruction and in pancreatitis when edema causes obstruction of the common bile duct. There could also be mild elevation of aminotransferases in acute cholecystitis. The blood urea nitrogen and creatinine can be elevated in conditions associated with dehydration such as small-bowel obstruction, acute appendicitis, or with conditions leading to third spacing of fluid as seen in acute pancreatitis.

Abdominal X-Ray (Erect and Supine)

The upright chest film, performed in midexpiration and after positioning patients left side down, has been shown to be highly sensitive in identify-

ing the presence of a pneumoperitoneum. In perforated peptic ulcer, free air under the diaphragm is seen. A dilated loop of bowel over the pancreatic area (sentinel loop) or abrupt cut off of gas in the transverse colon (colon cut off sign) may be seen in acute pancreatitis. Pancreatic calcification indicates chronic pancreatitis. Radiopaque gallstones can be seen in 15 percent of cases. A ladder-like pattern of dilated small bowel with air-fluid levels is often seen in acute small-bowel obstruction. These findings are often minimal if the obstruction is proximal. In complete small-bowel obstruction, the colon and rectum have little or no air. In large-bowel obstruction dilated colon, especially cecal distension with separation of the haustral markings, is seen. The upper limit of normal for cecal size is 9 cm. A cecal diameter greater than 10 to 12 cm is worrisome for the possibility of eventual cecal wall ischemia due to distension. In mesenteric ischemia, a plain abdominal x-ray may show "thumb printing" due to mucosal edema in the gas-filled bowel. In diverticulitis, the plain film may be normal or reveal a localized ileus or large-bowel obstruction.

Barium Radiography

It is useful in evaluation of small-bowel obstruction to confirm the presence and localize site of obstruction. A barium meal can be used for evaluation of peptic ulcer disease in patients who refuse endoscopy. A barium enema is contraindicated during initial stages of an acute attack of acute diverticulitis because there is risk of free perforation. It can be performed after 7 to 10 days in patients who respond to medical therapy to corroborate the diagnosis and to exclude other disorders. The single-contrast barium enema has been used in equivocal cases of acute appendicitis. Filling of the bulbous tip of the appendix with barium essentially excludes appendicitis. Nonfilling of the appendix with an extrinsic mass effect on the cecum is strongly suggestive of appendicitis because of periappendiceal inflammation, phlegmon, or abscess. These features are not diagnostic of appendicitis as they can be seen in other conditions such as Crohn's disease, pelvic inflammatory disease, endometriosis, and appendiceal mucocele.

Ultrasonography

Ultrasonography is very useful in the evaluation of gallbladder disease. Right upper quadrant ultrasound may show the presence of gallstones, but this is not specific for cholecystitis. Associated findings of pericholecystic fluid or wall thickening are suggestive of acute cholecystitis. A sonographic Murphy's sign (pain on manipulation of the gallbladder with the ultrasound transducer) may also suggest the diagnosis. Ultrasonography is less reliable in a diagnosis of acute pancreatitis, because echoes are deflected by gas-filled loops of the duodenum and small intestine. Ultrasound is the initial study obtained when pancreatitis is thought

to be caused by gallstones. It also is useful in evaluation of a pancreatic pseudocyst.

Acute appendicitis can be evaluated by sonography. The normal appendix can rarely be seen. The abnormal inflamed appendix is characterized by an outer diameter greater than or equal to 7 mm in adults and on cross-section by an inner echogenic ring of submucosa and an outer hypoechoic ring of muscularis and serosa. The identification of both these anatomic structures indicates edema and inflammation. Sonography can also identify appendicoliths, periappendiceal fluid, and inflammatory changes in the periappendiceal fat. It can also identify other causes of acute right lower abdominal pain such as ovarian cysts, hemorrhage or torsion, adnexal masses, complications of pregnancy, and pelvic inflammatory disease.

Hepatobiliary Scanning

A hepatobiliary scan or HIDA scan is useful in demonstrating an obstructed cystic duct, which is the cause of acute cholecystitis in most patients. It is reported as positive if the gallbladder is not visualized following excretion of the radioisotope into the bile duct and duodenum. False-positive examinations may occur if the gallbladder is full of bile (as in a prolonged fast) or if the sphincter of Oddi is widely patent (as in following endoscopic sphincterotomy). This test may be unreliable if the serum bilirubin is markedly elevated.

Computed Tomography Scan

Computed tomography (CT) scanning is widely used in patients with acute abdominal pain. In many situations it has allowed physicians to correctly identify pathology that previously was found only at exploratory laparotomy. Dynamic contrast-enhanced CT scan should be performed in those patients who are stable enough to undergo the evaluation and are not at risk for complications due to intravenous contrast (renal insufficiency, allergy, etc.). In patients with suspected pancreatitis it can confirm the diagnosis and distinguish interstitial from necrotizing pancreatitis. Interstitial pancreatitis is characterized by an intact microcirculation and uniform enhancement of the gland. In necrotizing pancreatitis, there is disruption of microcirculation so that large areas of the pancreas are not enhanced. Small areas of nonenhancement could represent the presence of intraparenchymal fluid. The CT scan is considered by many as the procedure of choice in the evaluation of acute diverticulitis. Abdominal and pelvic scanning are generally performed with water-soluble contrast, both orally to opacify the small bowel and rectally to evaluate rectosigmoid. Intravenous contrast is generally used if there are no contraindications. The CT criteria suggestive of diverticulitis include the presence of diverticula with pericolic infiltration of fatty tissue, thickening of colonic wall, and abscess formation. It has high sensitivity (69 to 98 percent) and specificity (75 to 100 percent). CT scanning can confirm the diagnosis of acute appendicitis by visualizing a distended fluid-filled appendix with an outer diameter of 4 to 20 mm, an enhancing wall, and periappendiceal inflammatory changes. Periappendiceal inflammation, phlegmon, or abscess in association with a calcified appendicolith is diagnostic of appendicitis.

Angiography

Angiography is the diagnostic procedure of choice in patients suspected of having acute thrombotic mesenteric ischemia. It may demonstrate the presence of thrombosis, emboli, and mesenteric vasoconstriction, as well as the adequacy of collateral circulation. Patients should be fluid resuscitated before arteriography to avoid false-positive findings. In patients with renal failure, magnetic resonance arteriography (magnetic resonance imaging with magnetic resonance angiography) may be an option.

Endoscopy

Upper or lower endoscopy can be utilized to evaluate selected patients with abdominal pain. It is useful in the diagnosis of peptic ulcer disease and ischemic bowel disease with associated heme-positive stool. It provides better diagnostic accuracy than does barium radiography. Endoscopy also provides the ability to biopsy *for H. pylori* and malignancy.

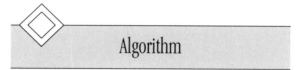

An algorithm for the evaluation and treatment of acute upper abdominal pain is depicted in Figure 7-1. A similar algorithm for lower abdominal pain is depicted in Figure 7-2.

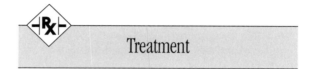

Peptic Ulcer

Patients should be encouraged to eat a balanced diet. Smoking should be discouraged as it retards the rate of ulcer healing and increases the frequency of recurrences. If patients have *H. pylori* infection, it should be eradicated.

Proton-pump-inhibitor-based regimen (any of the proton-pump inhibitors at equivalent dosages should be effective with this regimen):

Omeprazole 20 mg bid or lansoprazole 30 mg bid for 14 days with one of following:
Amoxicillin 1 g bid and clarithromycin 500 mg bid or
Metronidazole 500 mg bid and clarithromycin 500 mg bid or
Bismuth subsalicylate 2 tablets qid, tetracycline 500 mg qid, and metronidazole 250 mg qid.

After completion of the regimen, the omeprazole 20 mg qd or lansoprazole 30 mg qd is continued for an additional 2 weeks in patients with duodenal ulcer. For gastric ulcer, omeprazole 40 mg qd or lansoprazole 60 mg qd is continued for an additional 6 weeks. After completion of a 2-week course of *H. pylori* eradication, H$_2$-receptor antagonist or sucralfate can be given for 6 to 8 weeks. Confirmation of *H. pylori* eradication is not necessary in patients with uncomplicated ulcer. Successful eradication of *H. pylori* infection reduces the rate of ulcer recurrence to less than 10 percent. Reinfection rate is 0.5 percent per year following successful eradication of *H. pylori*.

Acute Pancreatitis

In patients with mild pancreatitis, treatment is largely supportive. It includes effective pain control, fluid resuscitation, and nutritional support. Patients should not be given any food or fluids orally until they are free of pain and recover normal bowel sounds. A diet composed of carbohydrates stimulates the pancreas less than does fat or protein; small feedings of carbohydrate-containing foods should be used. Total parenteral nutrition or tube feedings into the jejunum beyond the ligament of Trietz should be considered in patients who have severe pancreatitis and who will not be able to resume oral nutrition for 7 to 10 days. Lipids should be included in total parenteral nutrition unless serum triglycerides are elevated to a level of more than 500 mg/dl. Pain control usually requires narcotic analgesics. Adequate intravenous fluid replacement is required to prevent hypovolemia caused by third-space losses and vomiting. A nasogastric tube is usually not helpful in mild acute pancreatitis, but it is useful for treating either gastric or intestinal ileus and preventing aspiration of gastric contents in severe acute pancreatitis. Hypocalcemia may occur and should be recognized and corrected with calcium replacement. Patients with severe pancreatitis are best managed in intensive care units with monitoring of central venous pressure and blood gases. Broadspectrum intravenous antibiotic coverage is usually utilized in this setting. Urgent endoscopic retrograde cholangiopancreatography may benefit those patients with severe gallstone pancreatitis exhibiting three or more Ranson's criteria or with suspected cholangitis. If urgent endoscopic retrograde cholangiopancreatography is to be completed, it is recommended within the first 3 days. If gall-

stones are found in the common bile duct, they are removed and a sphincterotomy is performed. In patients with necrotizing pancreatitis who demonstrate improvement in organ failure and general systemic toxicity, medical treatment is continued. If there is no clinical improvement in the first 7 to 14 days, a CT-guided percutaneous aspiration of pancreatic necrosis should be performed to distinguish sterile from infected necrosis. If infection is documented, surgical debridement should be performed. If there is no evidence of infection (sterile necrosis), patients should be managed medically as long as possible with the hope that systemic toxicity will eventually resolve.

Acute Diverticulitis

Most patients can be managed with conservative measures. Patients with mild symptoms, no peritoneal signs, supportive home network, and the ability to take fluids orally can be managed as outpatients. Appropriate patients for outpatient treatment should be treated with a clear liquid diet and a broad-spectrum antibiotic with activity against anaerobes and gram-negative rods, particularly *Escherichia coli* and *Bacteroides fragilis*. Amoxicillin plus clavulanic acid, sulfamethoxazole-trimethoprim with metronidazole, or a quinolone with metronidazole have all been recommended. Patients should be instructed to call the physician for fever, inability to tolerate oral fluids, or increasing pain, which may necessitate hospitalization. The antibiotics are continued for 7 to 10 days. Patients should notice symptomatic improvement in 2 to 3 days, at which time the diet may be advanced slowly.

Patients hospitalized for diverticulitis should be placed on intravenous fluids to restore or maintain intravascular volume and ensure adequate urine output. Intravenous antibiotics should be given; choices include metronidazole or clindamycin for anaerobic coverage and aminoglycoside (gentamycin, tobramycin) and third-generation cephalosporin (ceftazidime, ceftriaxone, cefotaxime) for gram-negative coverage. The beta-lactamase inhibitor combination such as ampicillin-sulbactam, ticarcillin-clavulanate, or second-generation cephalo-sporins, such as cefotetan-cefoxitin, can be used as single agents to treat acute diverticulitis. In 2 to 4 days, symptomatic improvement is usually noticed with decreasing fever and leukocytosis; at that point, diet can be advanced. Antibiotics are continued for a period of 7 to 10 days. Most patients admitted for acute diverticulitis will respond to conservative medical therapy, but it has been estimated that 15 to 30 percent will require surgery during the admission. Most commonly, resection of the involved segment of the colon with a proximal end colostomy and closure of rectal stump (Hartmann's procedure) is performed. The colostomy is closed in 2 to 3 months, restoring continuity of colon. The recurrence rate after an attack of acute diverticulitis ranges from 7 to 62 percent, with half of these second attacks within a year and 90 percent in 5 years. Recurrent attacks respond less favorably to medical therapy and have a high mortality rate. Most authorities agree that elective resection is indicated after two attacks of uncomplicated diverticulitis.

Acute Cholecystitis

Acute cholecystitis will usually subside with conservative management including withholding oral feeding, intravenous alimentation, analgesics, and antibiotics. Meperidine is preferable to morphine for pain because of less spasm of sphincter of Oddi. In high-risk patients, ultrasound-guided aspiration and drain placement into the gallbladder (percutaneous cholecystostomy) may postpone or even avoid need for surgery. If there is evidence of gangrene or perforation, cholecystectomy is mandatory. The risk of recurrent attacks is 10 percent in the first month and up to 30 percent in 1 year following the first attack. Cholecystectomy should be performed within 3 days after hospitalization in the otherwise stable patient.

Acute Mesenteric Ischemia

Patients with mesenteric ischemia should have nothing by mouth and be resuscitated with intra-venous fluids. A nasogastric tube placement is indicated in patients with vomiting, ileus, signs of peritonitis, and in preparation for surgery. A surgical consultation should be obtained early in the course as urgent laparotomy is often necessary. Broad-spectrum antibiotics are given to the patients with peritonitis, sepsis, and radiographic evidence of bowel necrosis or perforation, and in preparation for surgery. Some clinicians advocate thrombolytic therapy in highly selected patients with an early diagnosis of superior mesenteric artery embolus unassociated with bowel necrosis. Exploratory laparotomy is indicated without delay in patients with evidence of perforation or bowel necrosis. In the patients with nonocclusive mesenteric ischemia, selective arterial vasodilator therapy may be initiated through arteriography catheter. Intraarterial papaverine, 30 to 60 mg bolus, followed by 30 to 60 mg/h continuous infusion is given until resolution of symptoms or surgical intervention.

Large-Bowel Obstruction

The management of large-bowel obstruction will depend on the underlying cause. Patients suspected of having perforation or ischemia require urgent laparotomy. For patients who do not have such indications, laparotomy may still be required if they do not improve or if cecal distension continues during 12 to 24 h with nonoperative treatment. All patients are kept without food or drink, with intravenous fluid replacement to maintain intravascular volume. In patients with sigmoid volvulus, early nonoperative decompression followed by surgery is performed. The decompression can be performed with a colonoscope or flexible sigmoidoscope. A rectal tube may be left in the sigmoid colon through the area of volvulus to prevent recurrence. In cecal volvulus, decompression can be attempted with colonoscope. Patients with acute colonic pseudoobstruction should be managed conservatively if there are no peritoneal signs and cecal diameter is less than 12 cm. The underlying illness should be treated aggressively. A nasogastric and rectal tube should be placed. Patients should be asked to change position periodically. All drugs that reduce intestinal motility should be discontinued. If a large amount of stool is noted on radiographs, enemas can be given. If patients show progressive dilatation of the colon, decompression with a colonoscope can be attempted. In patients with unsuccessful colonoscopy, a tube cecostomy can be performed.

Small-Bowel Obstruction

Patients with small-bowel obstruction require nasogastric suction to relieve vomiting and abdominal distension. Intravascular volume depletion is corrected with isotonic fluids. If patients are suspected of having strangulation, broad-spectrum antibiotics with gram-negative and anaerobic coverage are given. Patients with partial obstruction may respond to conservative measures. All patients with complete obstruction require surgery.

Acute Appendicitis

The treatment of uncomplicated appendicitis is surgical appendectomy. Patients are given antibiotics prior to surgery to reduce incidence of postoperative wound infection. In patients with perforated appendicitis with generalized peritonitis, an emergency appendectomy is performed. The appendectomy can be performed through laparotomy or by laparoscopy. In patients with perforated appendicitis and contained abscess, treatment is controversial. Some recommend percutaneous CT-guided drainage of the abscess, with intravenous fluids and antibiotics to allow inflammation to subside. An interval appendectomy can be performed after 6 weeks to prevent recurrent appendicitis.

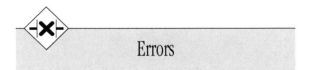

Errors

Most causes of an acute abdomen are serious and early diagnosis is mandatory to reduce mortality and morbidity. The abdomen contains various organ systems, in addition to the gastrointestinal tract, that could produce abdominal pain. A careful history and physical examination with appropriate diagnostic tests and frequent reevaluations are clearly important to arrive at a correct diagnosis. Conditions such as a ruptured abdominal aortic aneurysm are life-threatening and if not diagnosed early would lead to fatality. The risk factors for aortic aneurysm are male gender, age greater than 65 years, hypertension, history of tobacco smoking, atherosclerotic peripheral vascular disease, Marfan's syndrome, Ehlers-Danlos syndrome, chronic obstructive pulmonary disease, and a first-degree relative with history of abdominal aortic aneurysm. Patients have abdominal, flank, or back pain or syncope. It can be diagnosed rapidly by abdominal CT scan, ultrasound, or arteriography. Patients who are clinically unstable should go directly to the operating room.

If patients have history of urinary symptoms, various conditions giving rise to abdominal pain would include renal calculi, pyelonephritis, cystitis, or clot colic. A urine microscopy for red blood cells, white blood cells, and calcium oxalate crystals would help define the etiology.

In female patients, history of missed menstrual periods, with lower abdominal or suprapubic pain, could be due to ruptured ectopic pregnancy. The pain associated with the menstrual cycle could be due to dysmenorrhea or endometriosis. Pain associated with rupture of an ovarian cyst is often acute and without any prodrome. A serum beta human chorionic gonadotropin level should be obtained to exclude pregnancy. Finally, medical conditions including diabetic ketoacidosis, acute intermittent porphyria, and familial Mediterranean fever may initially present with abdominal pain.

Bibliography

Abi-hanna P, Gleckman R: Acute abdominal pain: A medical emergency in older patients. *Geriatrics* 52 (7):72, 1997.

Banks PA: Practice guidelines in acute pancreatitis. *Am J Gastroenterol* 92:3, 377–386, 1996.

Brazaitis MP, Dachman AH: The radiologic evaluation of acute abdominal pain of intestinal origin. *Med Clin North Am* 77(5):939, 1993.

Friedman LS: Liver, biliary tract, and pancreas. *Current Medical Diagnosis and Treatment 1999,* 38th ed. Norwalk; Appleton & Lange, 1999, 538–677.

Khoo SK: Lower abdominal and pelvic pain in women. *Aust Fam Physician* 17:3, 147, 1988.

Koo KP, Thirlby RC: Laparoscopic cholecystectomy in acute cholecystitis. *Arch Surg* 131:540, 1996.

Lanza FL: A guideline for treatment and prevention of NSAID-induced ulcers. *Am J Gastroenterol* 93(11): 2037, 1998.

Lopez-Kostner F, Hool GR, Lavery IC: Management and causes of acute large bowel obstruction. *Surg Clin North Am* 77(6):1265, 1997.

Martin RF, Rossi RL: The acute abdomen. *Surg Clin North Am* 77(6):1227, 1997.

McKinsey JF, Gewertz BL: Acute mesenteric ischemia. *Surg Clin North Am* 77(2):307, 1997.

McQuaid K: Alimentary tract. *Current Medical Diagnosis and Treatment 1999,* 38th ed. Norwalk; Appleton & Lange, 1999.

Murtagh J: Acute abdominal pain: A diagnostic approach. *Aust Fam Physician* 23(3):358, 1994.

Soll AH: Medical treatment of peptic ulcer disease. *JAMA* 275(8):622, 1996.

Stollman NH, Raskin JB: Diverticular disease of colon. *J Clin Gastroenterol* 29(3):241, 1999.

Viggiano TR, Poterucha JJ: Gastroenterology. *Mayo Internal Medicine Board Review 1996–1997.* Rochester, MN, Mayo Foundation for Medical Education and Research, 1996, pp. 271–333.

Walker JS, Dire DJ: Vascular abdominal emergencies. *Emerg Med Clin North Am* 14(3):571, 1996.

Mary F. Chan

Chapter 8

Acute Upper Gastrointestinal Bleeding

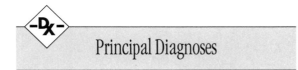

Incidence and Background

Gastrointestinal (GI) bleeding is the most common problem addressed by gastroenterologists in hospitals. However, patients with GI bleeding rarely go to a specialist. Rather they go to primary care physicians or local emergency rooms, and the gastroenterologist becomes involved as a consultant. Therefore, it is imperative that primary care clinicians know how to assess patients with gastrointestinal bleeding. The clinician must rapidly and accurately assess disease severity over the telephone, in the office, or at the hospital, so that appropriate management decisions can be made. Before the gastroenterologist becomes involved, an initial evaluation must have been performed, and the primary care clinician must have already made a decision about the triage and disposition. This chapter reviews common causes of upper GI bleeding, initial assessment, diagnostic evaluation, management decisions, treatment strategies, emerging concepts, technologies, and therapies.

Principal Diagnoses

Acid-Peptic Disease

Peptic ulcer disease is the most common cause of upper GI bleeding, and has remained so, despite the availability of good therapy with histamine$_2$-receptor antagonists, proton-pump inhibitors, and antibiotic regimens for *Helicobacter pylori* infection. As many as 95 percent of duodenal ulcers and 80 percent of gastric ulcers are associated with *H. pylori* infection (see Chapter 5), but the use of aspirin and other nonsteroidal anti-inflammatory drugs (NSAIDs) is the major risk factor for perforation and bleeding from peptic ulcers. Prostaglandins play a cytoprotective role in the gut. Aspirin and NSAIDs cause GI ulcers by inhibiting prosta-

glandin synthesis. Esophagitis, gastritis, and duodenitis may also cause bleeding, but the blood loss is usually trivial and hemodynamically insignificant.

Varices and Portal Hypertensive Gastropathy

Portal hypertension is the most important risk factor for massive upper GI hemorrhage in patients with chronic liver disease. Patients are at risk for bleeding from varices and portal hypertensive gastropathy when the pressure gradient between the portal vein and inferior vena cava exceeds 12 mmHg. Cirrhotic patients with coagulopathy from liver dysfunction and thrombocytopenia from hypersplenism are also at increased risk for bleeding from any other GI lesions, including peptic ulcers and Mallory-Weiss tears.

Mallory-Weiss Tears and Other Uncommon Lesions

Mallory-Weiss tears (mucosal rents at the gastroesophageal junction) cause acute, upper GI bleeding less frequently than do ulcers or varices. Nonetheless, Mallory-Weiss tears are recognized more often than in the past as a cause of bleeding. Other lesions, including aortoenteric fistulae, Barrett's ulcers, malignancy, hemobilia, and hemosuccus pancreaticus, occur much less frequently than do ulcers, varices, and Mallory-Weiss tears and are classified as rare causes of acute upper GI hemorrhage (Table 8-1).

Table 8-1

Frequency of Endoscopic Findings in Patients Who Have Upper Gastrointestinal Bleeding

ENDOSCOPIC FINDINGS	FREQUENCY (%)
Peptic ulcer (gastric or duodenal)	50
Varices (esophageal or gastric)	25
Esophagitis, gastritis, or duodenitis	15
Mallory-Weiss tear	5
All other findings	5

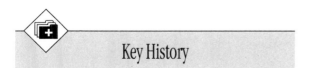

Typical Presentation

Patients with acute, upper GI bleeding typically have complaints of emesis, diarrhea, melena, or a combination of these. Patients with red and maroon hematemesis or hemochezia almost always recognize that they are bleeding and will report the bleeding to paramedics and physicians. Patients with melena or coffee-ground emesis may not realize that they are bleeding and, therefore, may not report the blood loss. Thus, health care providers and their office personnel must be astute enough to ask the right questions to detect GI bleeding. This is especially true when patients telephone their clinicians with complaints of nausea, vomiting, and diarrhea.

Patients with significant, acute bleeding will also complain of postural hypotension, near-syncope, or syncope. Abdominal pain is variably present and is associated with the lesion that is bleeding, not with the bleeding per se. Peptic ulcers may cause pain; Mallory-Weiss tears and varices do not.

Patients with red or maroon hemochezia from an upper GI lesion will have signs of hemodynamic compromise or collapse. The red color correlates with a rapid rate of bleeding and a significant intravascular volume loss. Less hemodynamically significant upper GI bleeding causes melena. Patients with hemochezia and no hemodynamic compromise will most likely have a lower GI source of bleeding.

Key History

The clinician obtaining the medical history for patients with GI bleeding must obtain a great deal of information in a short period of time, so that appropriate management can be initiated expeditiously. Questions need to be directed at quanti-fying the blood loss, assessing risk factors for ongoing or recurrent bleeding, and identifying poor prognostic indicators and comorbid conditions that can adversely affect outcome (Table 8-2). This information needs to be rapidly incorporated into a prognostic assessment, a triage decision, and a management plan.

Acuity and Severity

The acuity of the bleed and the amount of blood lost can be estimated from questions in the history regarding frequency, volume, and color of emesis and stool. The number of episodes of hematemesis, melena, and hemochezia; the volume of each bloody emesis and bowel movement; and the color of the emesis and stool are all used to quantify the blood loss. The presence or absence of near-syncope and syncope corroborates the estimated blood loss and its acuity. When a significant percentage (>15 percent) of intravascular volume is lost acutely, patients will have hemodynamic compromise. The resultant decrease in central nervous system perfusion causes postural dizziness or loss of consciousness.

Risk Factors and Comorbid Conditions

The etiology for acute upper GI bleeding needs to be sought during patient interviews. Past medical history may provide clues. Questions are asked

Table 8-2

Factors Associated with High Mortality from Acute Upper Gastrointestinal Bleeding

Age over 60 years
Comorbid medical conditions
Persistent hypotension
Need for emergency surgery
Endoscopic features
   Hemorrhage from malignancy
   Variceal hemorrhage
   Actively bleeding visible vessel
   Nonbleeding visible vessel

regarding prior GI bleeding, peptic ulcer disease, gastroesophageal reflux, chronic liver disease, and varices. Risk factors for ongoing and recurrent bleeding include use of aspirin and other NSAIDs, heparin, or coumadin; a history of coagulopathy or thrombocytopenia; portal hypertension; and alcohol and tobacco use. Comorbid conditions, such as cardiac, pulmonary, renal, rheumatologic, hematologic, and liver diseases may all negatively influence outcome. Older (age over 60 years) hospitalized patients, who bleed while in the hospital for another reason, are at particularly high risk for rebleeding and for poor outcomes. Patients with coagulopathy, hemodynamic compromise, portal hypertension, advanced age, and significant comorbid diseases should be admitted to intensive care units. Young patients who are hemodynamically stable without portal hypertension may be admitted to a hospital ward and, on occasion, may be evaluated in the emergency room and discharged home.

Physical Examination

General Condition and Postural Vital Sign Changes

Physical examinations of patients with acute upper GI bleeding begin as soon as the clinician enters the room. The history taking and physical examination may occur simultaneously in very ill patients. The clinician first notes general condition of patients, noting whether or not patients are distressed, pale, or jaundiced.

Vital signs should first be taken with patients in the supine position. Patients with hypotension and tachycardia in the supine position have lost at least 20 to 25 percent of their intravascular volume. Taking postural vital signs is unnecessary and should not be done.

If the vital signs are normal in the supine position, they should be taken in the sitting position and, if indicated, in the standing position. Changes

in postural vital signs occur in a predictable sequence as the blood loss increases. The first change is an increase in resting heart rate, followed by a drop in diastolic, and then systolic, blood pressure in the upright position. Next the resting, supine heart rate increases, again followed by a decrease in diastolic, then systolic, blood pressure. Thus, it is unnecessary and dangerous to have patients sit or stand if they are tachycardic and relatively hypotensive while lying supine.

A postural drop in systolic blood pressure of >10 mmHg, or an increase in heart rate of >10 beats per minute is indicative of 15 to 20 percent loss of blood volume. The absence of postural vital sign changes is indicative of less than 15 percent intravascular volume loss (Table 8-3).

Multiorgan System Examination

After the vital signs are taken, a complete multiorgan system physical examination is then performed to elicit clues about the etiology of the bleed and to assess prognosis. Pale conjuctivae and nailbeds suggest severe anemia. Scleral icterus suggests liver disease, alerting the examiner to the possibility of underlying portal hypertension. Conjuctival hemorrhage may be seen with forceful emesis, suggesting the possibility of a Mallory-Weiss tear at the gastroesophageal junction. Blood in the

Table 8-3

Hemodynamic Severity of Acute Bleeding

SEVERITY	ACUTE VOLUME LOSS
Shock on presentation	Minimum 20 to 25% blood loss
Postural vital sign changes*	15 to 20% blood loss
No postural vital sign loss	Less than 15% blood changes

*Sequence of postural vital sign changes with acute blood loss: First the heart rate increases, then the diastolic blood pressure falls, and last the systolic blood pressure falls. These changes occur first in the upright position, and later (with ongoing hemorrhage) in the supine position.

nose, mouth, and hypopharynx may suggest a naso-pharyngeal source of blood loss, especially if patients have melena and deny hematemesis. The neck examination may reveal flat jugular veins confirming a significant blood loss. Jugular venous distension suggests underlying chronic congestive heart failure, acute high-output heart failure, or possible myocardial infarction due to acute, severe anemia. Rales, cardiac gallops, abnormal precordial examination, and peripheral edema may confirm the diagnosis of congestive heart failure.

Abdominal and Rectal Examinations

The abdominal examination should note the presence and location of abdominal tenderness, signs of peritoneal irritation, masses, hepatosplenomegaly, ascites, and evidence of trauma. Digital rectal examination is a mandatory part of the patient evaluation for GI bleeding. The color and consistency of the stool must be noted, as well as the presence or absence of blood. Red blood on rectal examination will be associated with postural hypotension or shock if the source of the red blood is in the upper GI tract. Black (melanotic) stools suggest an upper GI blood loss of at least 500 ml. The color of the stool at presentation needs to be compared with the information given in the history to determine if the bleeding is slowing or accelerating. For example, red blood on a rectal examination in patients with the presenting complaint of melena suggests that the rate of blood loss has increased. Melena on a rectal examination in patients who complained of hemochezia would suggest that the bleeding has slowed or stopped.

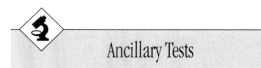

Ancillary Tests

Laboratory tests provide essential data in the evaluation of bleeding patients. Complete blood counts (CBCs), prothrombin time, partial thromboplastin time, and blood type and screen must be ordered.

The hemoglobin and hematocrit are the least sensitive indicators of the severity of bleeding. Patients with chronic blood loss may have a low hematocrit without any hemodynamic compromise, and patients with a normal hematocrit who have an exsanguinating hemorrhage may die. Serial hematocrits are necessary to assess ongoing blood loss. To interpret the changes in hematocrit, the physician must take into account volume resuscitation with crystalloid and blood products.

Elevation of the blood urea nitrogen (BUN) to creatinine ratio may provide evidence of upper GI bleeding when it is not clear if the source of blood loss is in the upper or lower GI tract. Blood in the upper GI tract will be partially digested and the urea nitrogen from the protein catabolism will be absorbed. The BUN level may rise before equilibrium with renal excretion is achieved. However, many factors may affect BUN and creatinine, thus any interpretation of the laboratory results must take into account the entire medical condition of each patient.

Liver enzymes, serum bilirubin, serum protein levels, and clotting parameters should be measured, if patients are suspected of having underlying liver disease and portal hypertension. Abdominal radiographs are rarely helpful in the evaluation of acute GI bleeding. However, abdominal films should be ordered when signs or symptoms suggest concomitant illnesses or complications that would otherwise be evaluated radiographically. For example, patients with GI bleeding and peritonitis should be assumed to have a perforated viscus and free air should be excluded with radiography.

Chest radiographs and electrocardiograms should be performed to exclude complications of acute GI bleeding such as aspiration pneumonia and cardiac ischemia. Computed tomography, magnetic resonance imaging, or angiography may be indicated if aortoenteric fistula, pseudoaneurysm, or other vascular abnormality is suspected.

Once patients are stabilized, endoscopy is the diagnostic and therapeutic test of choice in acute upper GI bleeding. Endoscopy is contraindicated in patients with known or suspected bowel perforation, and when the risks to their health or life are judged to outweigh the most favorable benefits of the procedure. Upper endoscopy is performed prior to full resuscitation if, and only if, patients are exsanguinating, in which case, surgical and angiographic support must be immediately available.

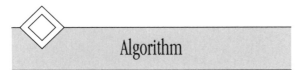

Algorithm

An algorithm for the diagnosis and management of acute upper GI bleeding is presented in Figure 8-1.

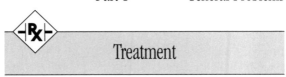

Treatment

Resuscitation

Management of patients with acute upper GI bleeding begins even before a diagnosis is made (Table 8-4). Initial management begins with stabilization. Two large-bore (≥18 gauge) intravenous catheters should be inserted. Peripheral lines are preferable to central lines, because the shorter catheters have less resistance and allow for more rapid infusion of blood products and crystalloid.

Figure 8-1

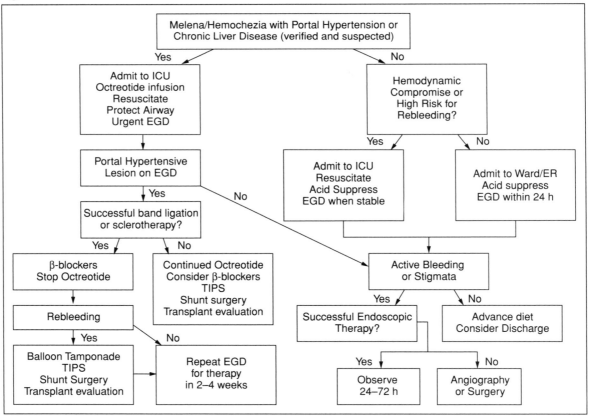

Algorithm for diagnosis and management of acute upper gastrointestinal bleeding. ICU, intensive care unit; EGD, esophagogastroduodenoscopy; ER, emergency room; TIPS, transjugular intrahepatic portosystemic shunt.

Protect the airway, if necessary.
Place at least 2 large-bore (18 gauge or larger)
   intravenous catheters.
Resuscitate with crystalloid and blood products,
   as indicated by vital signs and laboratory
   values.
Correct coagulopathy.
Admit patients with hemodynamic compromise or
   comorbid conditions to an intensive care unit.
Treat empirically with acid suppression.
Add octreotide, if chronic liver disease is
   suspected.
Remember it is never too early to call the
   reinforcements: the gastroenterologist,
   surgeon, and interventional radiologist.

Volume resuscitation with isotonic fluids, such as normal saline or lactated Ringer's solution, begins immediately in the emergency room. Patients with an estimated blood loss of 15 percent or more should be blood-typed and cross-matched for transfusion. Transfusion of packed red blood cells to keep the hemoglobin level at least 8 g/dl is usually recommended. Patients with cardiovascular disease may need a hemoglobin level of 10 g/dl or greater. Resuscitation efforts usually occur simultaneously with the initial and ongoing evaluation.

Patients with acute GI bleeding must not be given anything by way of the mouth, except medications. Aspirin, NSAIDs, heparin, and coumadin should be withheld and, if feasible, any coagulopathy should be corrected with supplemental vitamin K, fresh frozen plasma, or platelet transfusions. Therapeutic endoscopy will be unsuccessful and may actually exacerbate bleeding in patients with coagulopathy.

Empiric Therapy

All patients should be treated empirically with acid suppression. Histamine$_2$-receptor antagonists and proton-pump inhibitors are acceptable choices. Cytoprotective agents, such as sucralfate and antacids, should be avoided initially as they may interfere with subsequent endoscopy. Patients with suspected liver disease and portal hypertension should be treated with octreotide 50 μg IV bolus, followed by 25 to 50 μg/h infusion until therapeutic endoscopy is performed.

Endoscopy

Managing patients with GI bleeding is a process that requires constant readjustment as clinical parameters change. As laboratory values become available, additional management strategies are implemented. The treatment chosen will depend upon the nature of the lesion and the local expertise.

Coagulopathy is corrected. Cross-matched blood products are transfused, if indicated. Stabilized patients undergo endoscopy as soon as is feasible.

Endoscopy may be diagnostic, therapeutic, and prognostic. Active bleeding sites and visible vessels within peptic ulcers may be treated with injection or coagulation. Injection into and around bleeding sites with epinephrine, hypertonic saline, and sclerosants are all equally efficacious. Coagulation may also be achieved with heater probe therapy, bipolar electrocoagulation, argon plasma coagulation, and laser therapy. Mechanical hemostasis may be achieved with hemostatic clips and suturing devices, but this technology is not widely available. Variceal hemorrhage is controlled with variceal band ligation or sclerotherapy.

The endoscopic findings have prognostic implications as well. Clean-based ulcers have a low (1 to 5 percent) likelihood of rebleeding. Stigmata of recent bleeding, including an adherent clot that cannot be washed off and hemosiderin staining of the ulcer base, are associated with a 10 to 15 percent risk of rebleeding. Visible vessels seen in the ulcer base and actively bleeding ulcers have a risk of recurrent and ongoing bleeding that has been reported to be as high as 50 percent (Table 8-5).

Most rebleeding occurs within 72 h. Thus, patients with visible vessels or active bleeding at

Table 8-5

Natural History of Peptic Ulcers
with Stigmata of Recent Hemorrhage

ENDOSCOPIC FINDING	RISK OF REBLEEDING (%)
Active arterial bleed	90
Visible vessel	50
Adherent clot	15
Oozing; no other stigmata	10
Flat spot	7
Clean ulcer base	3

the time of the initial endoscopy should be monitored in the hospital for at least 72 h. Patients who must resume heparin, coumadin, aspirin, and other NSAIDs, in contrast to those who do not, are at an even greater risk of rebleeding and should be monitored for a longer period of time.

When peptic ulcers are found as the cause of GI bleeding, the endoscopist should obtain antral biopsies from the lesser curve of the stomach to diagnose *H. pylori* infection, if present. One- or two-tissue samples can be used for a rapid urease test (CLO test® or hpfast). Two-tissue samples can be placed in formalin and the specimens reserved pending the results of the urease test. Because acute GI bleeding can cause a false-negative urease test, the formalin-preserved specimen should be processed for *H. pylori* if the urease test is negative. To increase the diagnostic yield of histopathology, special stains for *H. pylori* can be utilized. If the urease test is positive, there is no need to process the formalin-preserved specimen for the purpose of diagnosing *H. pylori* infection. A positive urease test is specific for the presence of the organism. Alternatively, serology can be used to complement the rapid urease test to diagnose *H. pylori*. Like the histopathology, the serology is used when the urease test is negative, despite the presence of peptic ulcer disease. *H. pylori* antibodies are sensitive for past exposure, but do not indicate active infection. How-

ever, when positive serology is found in patients with ulcers who have never received antibiotic therapy for *H. pylori*, a presumptive diagnosis of active infection can be made and treatment should be initiated.

Postendoscopy Treatments

PEPTIC ULCER DISEASE

Patients with bleeding ulcers should be treated with a proton-pump inhibitor for at least 4 weeks or with H_2-receptor antagonists for 6 to 8 weeks. If *H. pylori* infection is found in association with peptic ulcer disease it should be treated with a multidrug regimen (Table 8-6), and eradication of the organism should be documented 2 to 6 months after the antibiotic course is completed. Aspirin and NSAID use must be avoided, whenever possible, by patients who have bled from peptic ulcers. If these medications have to be used, patients must be treated simultaneously with acid suppression therapy or misoprostol.

PORTAL HYPERTENSION

Hemodynamically stable patients with a history of variceal hemorrhage or portal hypertensive gastropathy should be treated with beta-blockers or nitrates to decrease the risk of rebleeding. These medications work by decreasing portal vein pressure. A 20 percent decrease in resting heart rate has been shown to correlate fairly well with a decrease in portal vein pressure; thus propranolol or nadolol must be titrated to a dose that achieves a 20 percent decrease in resting heart rate.

Patients with hemorrhage from esophageal varices should undergo subsequent endoscopy with band ligation or sclerotherapy until variceal obliteration is achieved. Patients with gastric varices due to splenic vein thrombosis are best treated with splenectomy. Patients with recurrent bleeding from esophageal and gastric varices are best treated with portosystemic shunts or liver trans-

Table 8-6

FDA-Approved Antibiotic Regimens for *H. Pylori* Infection

DRUG REGIMEN	DOSES	DURATION OF TREATMENT	EFFICACY (%)
1. Bismuth	2 Tablets qid	14 days	>90
Tetracycline	500 mg qid		
Metronidazole	500 mg qid		
H_2RA or PPI	Usual doses		
2. Bismuth	2 Tablets qid	14 days	>90
Tetracycline	500 mg qid		
Clarithromycin	500 mg tid		
H_2RA or PPI	Usual doses		
3. PPI	Usual bid	14 days	75-90
Clarithromycin	500 mg bid		
Amoxicillin	1000 mg bid		
4. PPI	Usual bid	14 days	75-90
Clarithromycin	500 mg bid		
Metronidazole	500 mg bid		
5. RBC	400 mg bid	14 days	>90
Clarithromycin	500 mg bid		
Amoxicillin	1000 mg bid		
6. RBC	400 mg bid	14 days	>90
Clarithromycin	500 mg bid		
Metronidazole	500 mg bid		
7. RBC	400 mg bid	14 days	>90
Clarithromycin	500 mg bid		
Tetracycline	500 mg bid		
8. RBC	400 mg bid	14 days	>90
Metronidazole	500 mg bid		
Amoxicillin	1000 mg bid		
9. RBC	400 mg bid	14 day	>90
Clarithromycin	500 mg bid		
Tetracycline	500 mg bid		
10. PPI	Usual qam	14 days	70–80
Clarithromycin	500 mg tid		
11. PPI	Usual tid	14 days	20–70
Amoxicillin	1000 mg tid		
12. RBC	400 mg bid	14 days	70–80
Clarithromycin	500 mg tid		
then			
RBC	1000 mg bid	14 days	
13. PPI	Usual bid	14 days	>90
Bismuth	2 tablets qid		
Tetracycline	500 mg qid		
Metronidazole	500 mg tid		

Bismuth, bismuth subsalicylate or subcitrate; H_2RA, histamine$_2$-receptor antagonist; PPI, proton-pump inhibitor; RBC, ranitidine bismuth subcitrate.

plantation. If subsequent liver transplantation is a consideration, transjugular intrahepatic portosystemic shunts (TIPS) or distal splenorenal shunts are preferred over portocaval or mesocaval shunts.

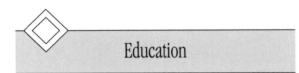

Education

Anti-Inflammatory Medications

Education is important for patients at risk for GI bleeding. Preventing the first episode of bleeding may be difficult to achieve, because aspirin and NSAIDs are so widely available. However, patients need to be told that increasing age, dose of NSAID, and duration of NSAID use all contribute to the risk of complicated peptic ulcer disease. It is important that patients understand that symptoms of dyspepsia and pain do not correlate with endoscopic findings. Many patients have silent ulcerations until they present with bleeding or perforation. Patients must be aware that aspirin and NSAIDs are in many over-the-counter preparations, and they must be encouraged to read all labels before using a product. Prolonged use of anti-inflammatory medications should be minimized whenever possible.

Helicobacter pylori

Patients with *H. pylori* infection need to understand the pathophysiologic role this organism plays in peptic ulcer disease. Patients must be told how difficult it is to eradicate the organism; the importance of completing the prescribed antibiotic regimen, despite side effects and complicated dosing schedules, must be stressed. For patients who have bled from ulcers caused by *H. pylori*, the need to document eradication must be explained. Patients who understand these concepts will be more compliant with therapeutic regimens and subsequent testing.

Portal Hypertension

Patients should be given an explanation of how portal hypertension and chronic liver disease predispose them to acute GI bleeding. Understanding the association between portal hypertension and bleeding will help them understand how preventive measures work to their benefit. Patients who understand the rationale for therapy are more likely to allow titration of beta-blockers to achieve target heart rate, despite experiencing constitutional side effects, such as fatigue and malaise.

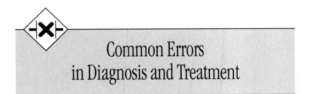

Common Errors in Diagnosis and Treatment

Diagnostic Errors

COMPLETE BLOOD COUNT AND INAPPROPRIATE TRIAGE

One of the most common errors made by clinicians assessing patients with acute GI bleeding is to rely on the first CBC to determine the severity of the bleed. This is particularly dangerous if postural vital signs are not measured. If there has not been sufficient time for equilibration or volume resuscitation when the initial hemoglobin and hematocrit are measured, these levels may be normal and the significance of the bleeding may be underestimated. Such patients may be inappropriately discharged home. Patients, even those who have lost up to 15 percent of their intravascular volume, may have normal supine vital signs. Thus, postural vital sign changes can be used to estimate the volume of blood loss in patients with normal hemoglobin and hematocrit values and normal supine vital signs. Incomplete assessment and failure to recognize risk factors for recurrent or ongoing bleeding may result in inappropriate triage to a nursing floor rather than to an intensive care unit.

UPPER GASTROINTESTINAL BLEEDING MISTAKEN AS LOWER GASTROINTESTINAL BLEEDING

Another common error in diagnosing GI bleeding is to confuse an upper GI bleed for a lower GI bleed. This occurs more often with duodenal ulcers than it does with gastric lesions. Patients with duodenal ulcers may have edema of the pylorus that prevents blood from refluxing into the stomach. Patients may have red, maroon, or black stools, and the gastric aspirate from a nasogastric tube may fail to show any blood. Patients might then be incorrectly diagnosed with a lower GI bleed, and the algorithm for lower GI bleeding might be inappropriately followed. Such patients may undergo nuclear medicine tagged red blood cell scans and angiography, before an upper GI source is excluded by endoscopy. Thus, esophagogastroduodenoscopy is recommended for any patients in whom it is not absolutely clear that the bleeding is from a lower GI source. If the esophagogastroduodenoscopy is negative, then the lower GI bleeding algorithm can be followed.

DELAY OF ENDOSCOPY

Another common error in diagnosing GI bleeding is failure to keep patients nil per os (NPO). Patients who are stable enough to delay endoscopy should be NPO for solids for at least 8 h, for full liquids for 4 h, and for clear liquids for 2 h to minimize the risk of aspiration during the procedure. Similarly, barium radiographs should not be performed, because barium interferes with endoscopy by obscuring the view and by clogging the suction channel of the endoscope. Sucralfate and liquid antacids cause the same difficulties and should not be given until after the endoscopy has been performed.

Treatment Errors

FAILURE TO ERADICATE *HELICOBACTER PYLORI*

Patients with peptic ulcer disease and *H. pylori* infection should be treated with antibiotics. Eradication of *H. pylori* appears to prevent recurrent peptic ulcer disease and presumably its complications, although there are few studies to support this hypothesis.

Many antibiotic regimens are less than 90 percent effective in eradicating *H. pylori*. Therefore, it is recommended that eradication be documented for all patients who have had complicated (bleeding or perforation) peptic ulcer disease.

For patients diagnosed with peptic ulcer disease, a positive serology for *H. pylori* can be used to make a presumptive diagnosis of *H. pylori* infection, provided that patients have not been previously treated for *H. pylori* infection. Even though many patients lose the antibody for *H. pylori* after it has been eradicated, it is not uncommon for the antibody test to remain positive for years. Therefore, serology alone cannot be used to prove eradication. Paired antibody titers drawn before treatment and 6 months later can be useful, because the antibody titer will decrease over time once *H. pylori* has been eradicated, even if the antibody persists. However, there is so much variation in test results from laboratory to laboratory and from test kit to test kit that this is not a reliable strategy. For the best results, the first serum sample should be frozen and banked until the second sample is obtained months later and the paired-samples should be submitted together for testing. Because this is not feasible, it is not common practice.

Functional tests that take advantage of the urease produced by this organism provide much better tests for documenting eradication. The rapid urease test and the urea breath test are much better for this purpose than is serology; however, these tests have inherent disadvantages as well. The rapid urease test requires endoscopy and the breath test is quite expensive. Neither test should be performed sooner than 2 months after the antibiotic regimen is complete, as false-negative tests are common during that immediate, posttreatment period.

FAILURE TO TITRATE BETA-BLOCKER THERAPY

Patients with portal hypertension who are treated with beta-blockade must have the dose titrated upward until a 20 percent decrease in resting heart rate is achieved. Many patients are placed on an initial dose of propranolol, and the dose is never increased. Failure to achieve a decrease in resting heart rate correlates with failure to achieve a decrease in portal pressure. Patients with portal hypertension are at increased risk of bleeding when the portosystemic pressure gradient is greater than 12 mmHg. For patients who have already bled from portal gastropathy or varices, it is imperative that a decrease in portal pressure be achieved. Adding propranolol without achieving a decreased heart rate and portal pressure simply adds to the number of medications patients are taking without adding efficacy.

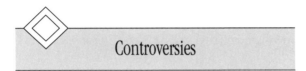

Controversies

Everyone agrees that patients with acute upper GI bleeding should be treated with acid suppression, because in vitro data show that clots are more stable at neutral pH. However, there is controversy over how to achieve the acid suppression. H_2-receptor antagonists are available in intravenous and tablet formulations. Intravenous therapy can be administered as boluses or as continuous infusion. Proponents of continuous infusion argue that gastric pH can be maintained at ≥ 4, whereas the gastric pH may fall below 4 between boluses. There are no good data to argue for either approach. Furthermore, neither approach has been shown to be superior to oral dosing. Proton-pump inhibitors are longer acting than H_2-receptor antagonists and maintain a more sustained elevation in gastric pH. There are some data to suggest that high-dose proton-pump inhibitor therapy is more efficacious than usual dose therapy in preventing recurrent bleeding.

Another area of controversy involves aspirin use by patients with severe arteriosclerotic disease who are at high risk for GI bleeding. These patients are at risk for thrombotic events such as cerebro-vascular accidents and myocardial infarction, but these same people are at risk for ischemic cerebrovascular accidents and myocardial infarctions when they hemorrhage. Thus, the clinician must weigh the relative risks and benefits of antiplatelet therapy and make recommendations to the patients. Patients who have had GI bleeding or peptic ulcer disease in the past and who must be treated with aspirin or NSAIDs should be treated simultaneously with H_2-receptor blockers, proton-pump inhibitors, or prostaglandins (misoprostol) in an attempt to minimize the risk of ulceration and GI bleeding from the aspirin or NSAIDs. Selective inhibitors of cyclooxygenase$_2$ (COX_2) may offer a safer alternative for patients requiring anti-inflammatory medications, but COX_2 inhibitors do not have the antiplatelet activity of aspirin and nonselective NSAIDs . Therefore, COX_2 inhibitors are not alternatives to aspirin for patients with atherosclerotic disease.

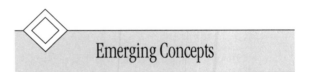

Emerging Concepts

NSAIDs predictably cause gastropathy and are associated with a significantly increased risk for GI bleeding. NSAIDs inhibit COX, a rate-limiting enzyme in the pathway of prostaglandin and thromboxane synthesis. This enzyme, COX, exists as two isoforms: COX_1 and COX_2. Platelets produce COX_1 only. COX_2 is expressed in inflamed tissues as part of a response to cytokines and local injury. Nonselective NSAIDs inhibit both isoforms. The inhibition of COX_1 is responsible for most of the organ-specific toxicity of NSAIDs and for the antiplatelet effect. Selective COX_2 inhibitors, therefore, are intended to retain the anti-inflammatory effect of NSAIDs without the gastrointestinal toxicity. Studies have shown that COX_2-selective NSAIDs are less injurious to the gastric mucosa than are nonselective NSAIDs, but long-term studies are not yet available, and it cannot be assumed that they are totally without adverse effects.

Bibliography

Berardi RR, Welage LS: Proton-pump inhibitors in acid-related diseases. *Am J Health Syst Pharm* 55:2289, 1998.

Cook DJ, Guyatt GH, Salena BJ, Laine LA: Endoscopic therapy for acute nonvariceal upper gastrointestinal hemorrhage: A meta-analysis. *Gastroenterology* 102:139, 1992.

Lanas A, Hirschowitz BJ: Toxicity of NSAIDs in the stomach and duodenum. *Eur J Gastroenterol & Hepatol* 11:375, 1999.

Mandell BF: COX 2-selective NSAIDs: Biology, promises, and concerns. *Cleve Clin J Med* 66:285, 1999.

Peterson WL, Cook DJ: Antisecretory therapy for bleeding peptic ulcer. *JAMA* 280:877, 1998.

Rollhauser C, Fleischer DE: Nonvariceal upper gastrointestinal bleeding: An update. *Endoscopy* 29:91, 1997.

Rollhauser C, Fleischer DE: Upper gastrointestinal nonvariceal bleeding: A review covering the years 1996–1997. *Endoscopy* 30:114, 1998.

Roth S: NSAID gastropathy: A new understanding. *Arch Intern Med* 156:1623, 1996.

Storey DW, Bown SG, Swain P, et al: Endoscopic prediction of recurrent bleeding in peptic ulcers. *N Engl J Med* 305:915, 1981.

Swaim MW, Wilson JA: GI emergencies: Rapid therapeutic responses for older patients. *Geriatrics* 54:20, 1999.

Wara P: Endoscopic prediction of major rebleeding—A prospective study of stigmata of hemorrhage in bleeding ulcer. *Gastroenterology* 88:1209, 1985.

Chandra Prakash

Chapter

9

Acute Lower Gastrointestinal Bleeding

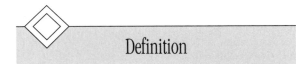

How Common Is Acute Lower Gastrointestinal Bleeding?

Approximately 80 percent of patients with gastrointestinal (GI) bleeding will pass blood in some form through the rectum. The lower GI tract accounts for up to one-third of all cases of GI bleeding; the upper tract accounts for the remainder. The annual incidence of acute lower GI bleeding (LGIB) has been estimated at 20 to 27 cases per 100,000 population. In comparison, the annual incidence of upper GI bleeding is significantly higher: 100 to 200 cases per 100,000 of the population are at risk. The incidence rate increases 200-fold from the third to the ninth decade of life. For unclear reasons, LGIB occurs significantly more often in men than it does in women. The mortality rate from acute LGIB is <5 percent, while that from acute upper GI bleeding can be as high as 10 percent. Mortality rates are higher (~23 percent) among patients who develop bleeding after hospital admission.

Definition

Lower GI bleeding has traditionally been defined as bleeding originating distal to the ligament of Treitz. Therefore, the definition includes both small-bowel and colonic sources of bleeding. The percentage of small-bowel bleeding contributing to rectal bleeding with hemochezia ranges from <1 to 9 percent, while that of upper GI bleeding can be up to 10 percent.

Typical Presentation

The typical presentation consists of the passage of blood in the stool, resulting in discoloration of

the stool to varying shades of red. There is lack of uniformity in the nomenclature of the color of bloody stool, both on the part of the patients and their treating physicians. Objective stool-color testing using standardized colors has been shown to assist in differentiating between lower and upper GI bleeding; stool colors matching the brightest shades of red have high positive predictive value for LGIB, while black stool or melena predicts an upper GI source. Rapid blood loss from the upper GI tract can result in stool colors approaching bright red, but this is almost invariably associated with hemodynamic compromise.

About 50 percent of patients with LGIB have both a decrease in hemoglobin concentration and hemodynamic disturbance in some form at presentation. About one-third of patients have orthostatic changes, defined as a drop in systolic blood pressure of >10 mmHg or an increase in heart rate of >15 beats/min with the assumption of the upright position from the supine position. About 10 percent of patients have cardiovascular collapse and another 10 percent have syncope. The degree of hemodynamic disturbance is a reflection of the amount of circulating volume lost with the bleeding episode. Patients with acute LGIB generally require less blood transfusion and are less likely to have hemodynamic compromise than are those with upper GI bleeding. The pattern of bleeding is characteristically intermittent, with spontaneous cessation of bleeding in 80 to 85 percent of cases.

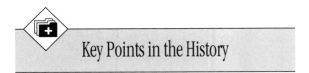

Key Points in the History

The initial evaluation of patients is performed concurrently with resuscitative measures, as described later. History taking is directed toward determining the anatomic level of bleeding, the quantity of blood lost, the etiology of the bleeding, and the precipitating factors.

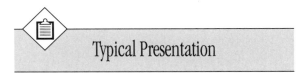

Anatomic Level of Bleeding

Bleeding from the anorectal area typically results in bright blood coating the exterior of formed stool and can be associated with distal colonic symptoms including rectal urgency and pain during defecation. A history of constipation and straining at stool may be obtained from patients with stercoral ulcers (induced by the passage of hard stool), hemorrhoids, or anal fissures. Clots can be passed when bleeding rates are slower and when bleeding originates from the distal colon.

Bleeding from more proximal parts of the colon results in varying degrees of mixing of blood within stool; the stool color becomes progressively darker red the more proximal the bleeding site. Melena has been reported with right colonic and small-bowel bleeding.

Quantity of Blood Lost

Loss of 10 to 20 percent of the circulating blood volume can result in orthostatic symptoms such as dizziness and lightheadedness on standing up. Up to 10 percent of patients with acute LGIB can present with syncope. Patients' estimates of amounts of blood lost can be inaccurate as even a small quantity of blood can discolor the water in a toilet bowl enough to suggest a larger volume of blood loss.

Etiology of Bleeding

Ingestion of nonsteroidal anti-inflammatory drugs (NSAIDs) may result in mucosal damage throughout the GI tract—not just in the stomach. Evidence suggests that these medications may have a significant role particularly in diverticular bleeding, by causing erosions at the mouths of diverticula.

A recent history of hypotension and hypovolemic shock may suggest ischemic colitis as the etiologic bleeding lesion. Radiation therapy to the prostate or pelvis can result in radiation proctitis and intermittent LGIB months to years later. A history of aortic graft surgery should bring to mind the possibility of an aortoenteric or aortocolonic fistula. Chronic constipation may suggest stercoral or stool-induced ulceration of the rectum as a cause for bleeding, while recent colonoscopy and polypectomy may suggest postpolypectomy bleeding. Patients with chronic renal disease and/or on hemodialysis are more prone to develop GI arteriovenous malformations, as are patients with aortic valvular disease.

Precipitating Factors

When there is a potential bleeding source in the small bowel or colon, abnormalities of the coagulation mechanism from any cause can result in clinically evident bleeding. Therefore, the history should include inquiries about medications that are known to affect coagulation, including warfarin, heparin, aspirin, NSAIDs, and thrombolytic agents. Disorders of coagulation can also influence the course of bleeding; liver disease, von Willebrand's disease, and vitamin K deficiency are examples.

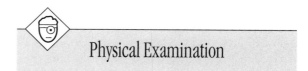

Physical Examination

The initial physical examination should be directed toward assessment of the degree of blood loss. Hypotension with a systolic blood pressure <100 mmHg or baseline tachycardia suggests significant hemodynamic compromise and signals the need for urgent volume resuscitation. If baseline pulse and blood pressure are within normal limits, sitting patients up or having patients stand may result in a drop of systolic blood pressure or a rise in the heart rate. These orthostatic changes are useful in identifying patients with mild-to-moderate volume loss needing volume resuscitation.

Direct examination of the bloody stool may provide important clues to the etiology and anatomic level of bleeding. As noted earlier, distal colonic or rectal sources can result in bright blood coating the outside of formed stool. More proximal bleeding sources result in stool mixed with altered blood. Blood may be mixed with loose stool with mucus, suggesting an inflammatory colitis. Large amounts of bright blood suggest rapid and ongoing bleeding, while clots suggest slow bleeding rates.

The rectal examination is an essential adjunct to physical examination in acute LGIB. In addition to accurate assessment of the color of bloody stool, it may also reveal evidence to suggest an anorectal source of blood loss. Hemorrhoids are typically not palpable, though external hemorrhoids can be visualized on examination of the anal area. Anal fissures can result in extreme pain during a rectal examination and may be identified on careful examination of the anal area. In addition, rectal cancer may be palpated by the examining finger in rare instances. The remainder of the physical examination is typically unrevealing, although systemic manifestations of GI diseases may be evident.

Nasogastric aspiration may help rule out an upper GI source of bloody stool. Although nasogastric tube placement is easy and safe, it is not popular with patients. However, it is an essential part of initial evaluation, especially in patients with evidence of hemodynamic compromise and apparent LGIB as up to 10 percent of these patients can have bleeding sources in the upper GI tract. It is important to remember that a small fraction of patients with bleeding duodenal ulcers may have a nonbloody nasogastric aspirate. There is no utility of hemoccult testing of nasogastric aspirate.

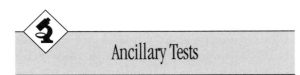

Ancillary Tests

Laboratory Studies

At presentation, blood should be sent to the laboratory for complete blood count (CBC), coagulation parameters (prothrombin time, activated partial thromboplastin time, and platelet count), blood group, and cross-matching of 2 to 4 units of blood as appropriate. A chemistry profile including liver and renal function will help stratify risk in case invasive intervention is required and may assist with differential diagnosis.

Sigmoidoscopy and Anoscopy

In a nonemergent setting, anoscopy can be useful in the detection of internal hemorrhoids. Both anoscopy and sigmoidoscopy are simple, expedient procedures that can be performed in unsedated patients without formal bowel purge. The utility of these procedures is mainly in an outpatient or emergency room setting where a rapid diagnosis may assist patient triage. However, even if a potential source of bleeding is evident, subsequent full colonoscopy is still required in patients whose age puts them at risk for colorectal cancer.

Colonoscopy

The concept of early colonoscopy after rapid bowel preparation is relatively new. Rapid bowel purge using a balanced electrolyte solution (e.g., GoLYTELY, Braintree Labs, MA) has been proved to be safe in hemodynamically stable patients with acute LGIB. Patients unable to drink the large volumes required can have the electrolyte solution infused into the stomach using a nasogastric tube.

The yield of finding a potential bleeding source is estimated to be highest if colonoscopy is performed early in the clinical course, preferably within the first 24 h after hospital admission. While continued active bleeding increases the diagnostic yield of the procedure, it can make visualization of the colonic wall difficult and interfere with conscious sedation by causing hemodynamic instability.

Resuscitation always takes precedence over bowel preparation and conscious sedation for colonoscopy. The test is best performed in patients who appear to have clinically stabilized and have tolerated an adequate bowel purge. All patients with LGIB from an unknown source should eventually undergo endoscopic evaluation during their initial hospitalization or soon thereafter.

Reports of finding a potential source of bleeding at colonoscopy range from 50 to 90 percent. However, nonbleeding lesions visualized during colonoscopy do not necessarily represent the source of blood loss. This is particularly true with diverticulosis, a common finding in elderly individuals. Adoption of specific criteria for definitive endoscopic identification of a bleeding source decreases

the diagnostic yield but can increase the level of confidence in the diagnosis (Table 9-1). The criteria include finding an actively bleeding lesion, a nonbleeding visible vessel, and adherent clot. These criteria were initially developed for identification of bleeding peptic ulcers and have been used in studies of acute LGIB. Other endoscopic criteria specific to the colon include ulceration at the mouth of a diverticulum and fresh blood localized to a short segment of colon. It is important to remember that LGIB can originate from the small bowel as well as the colon; finding fresh blood within the terminal ileum has sometimes been considered to indicate small-bowel bleeding.

Table 9-1

Levels of Diagnostic Certainty in the Investigation of Acute Lower Gastrointestinal Bleeding

Level I: Definitive diagnosis

A: Actively bleeding lesion found at endoscopy or angiography

B: Stigmata of recent bleeding noted in association with a lesion at endoscopy

Nonbleeding visible vessel

Adherent clot

C: Positive tagged red blood cell (TRBC) scan if associated with one of the above

Level II: Presumptive diagnosis and circumstantial evidence

A: Fresh blood localized to a colon segment inhabited by a potential bleeding source

B: Positive TRBC scan, with endoscopy showing a potential bleeding site in the same area as TRBC scan localization

C: Bright red blood per rectum confirmed by objective color testing, colonoscopy showing a single potential bleeding site, and negative upper endoscopy

Level III: Equivocal diagnosis

A: Hemochezia or blood in the rectum not objectively confirmed, with endoscopy demonstrating one or more potential bleeding sites

Adapted with permission from Zuckerman GR, Prakash C: Acute lower intestinal bleeding: Part II: Etiology, therapy and outcomes. Gastrointest Endosc 49:228–238, 1999.

Tagged Red Blood Cell Scan

Red blood cells (RBC) labeled with 99m-technetium remain in circulation for as long as 48 h and extravasate into the bowel lumen with active bleeding. Bleeding can therefore be identified by pooling of the radioactive tracer within the gut on scanning using a gamma camera (Figure 9-1). Bleeding rates as low as 0.1 ml/min can be detected in research settings. The advantages of tagged red blood cell (TRBC) scanning include simplicity and portability of the test, lack of complications, and ease of performance without requirement for bowel preparation or sedation. However, the test is only positive about 45 percent of the time, probably because of the intermittent nature of acute LGIB. When TRBC scan localization is verified by an alternative test such as angiography, endoscopy, or surgery, it is accurate in 78 to 80 percent. The false localization rate of about 20 percent makes this an unreliable test to direct surgical resection. Therefore, current use of the TRBC scan is mainly to screen patients prior to angiography, a more invasive test that requires a higher bleeding rate than does the TRBC scan. A positive TRBC scan identifies a population likely to have high in-hospital morbidity and mortality, with a high requirement for invasive intervention including surgery. Conversely, a negative TRBC scan implies better short-term prognosis, with less blood transfusion requirement or surgery.

Figure 9-1

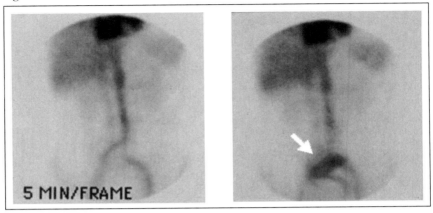

Sequential images from a tagged red blood cell scan showing active bleeding in the sigmoid colon (arrow). The pattern of peristaltic flow of the extravasated blood assists in identification of the location of bleeding.

There is evidence to suggest that the diagnostic yield of TRBC scanning is highest when performed while patients are actively bleeding, though hemodynamic compromise and number of units of blood transfused have not been found to predict test positivity. One study found the yield highest when patients were actively passing fresh blood per rectum during the test. Delayed scans performed several hours after injection of labeled RBC can be misleading due to peristaltic movement of the extravasated blood in the gut. The TRBC scans that demonstrate extravasation of blood immediately on initiation of scanning have been found to be associated with the highest yield of a positive diagnosis at subsequent angiography. Scans that become positive after >2 h of scanning have a low yield at angiography.

Angiography

Angiography may demonstrate extravasation of contrast into the intestinal lumen at bleeding rates exceeding 0.5 ml/min and, therefore, localize the site of bleeding. Angiography may also delineate the anatomy of the bleeding lesion and provide information regarding the etiology, especially bleeding diverticula and angiodysplasia. Sometimes other findings such as the late draining vein of an angiodysplasia or a tumor blush may be identified even in nonbleeding patients. Angiography is the most common confirmatory test after a positive TRBC scan. Patients who have an immediate blush on TRBC scan have the highest yield of localizing the bleeding source upon angiography.

When performed for acute LGIB, about 47 percent of angiograms are positive, with a range 27 to 77 percent. Preselection criteria including patients requiring >4 units of blood within 2 h and patients with positive TRBC scans help increase the diagnostic yield. In stable patients with bleeding that is difficult to localize, infusion of anticoagulants (e.g., heparin) or thrombolytic agents (e.g., streptokinase and urokinase) during a bleeding episode may increase the diagnostic yield of angiography. Intravenous vasodilators may also prolong the bleeding episode and increase the chance of finding the bleeding lesion. These provocative measures can be associated with excessive bleeding and should only be used in specialized centers in stable patients without comorbid illnesses.

Angiography is associated with complications in about 10 percent of patients. Major complications are hematoma formation, femoral artery thrombosis, contrast reactions, renal failure, and transient ischemic attacks.

Esophagogastroduodenoscopy

Since about 10 percent of patients with bright blood in the rectum can have an upper GI source of bleeding, an esophagogastroduodenoscopy (EGD) may be indicated in certain situations in patients with apparent acute LGIB. There is evidence to suggest that when a bleeding upper GI tract lesion results in bright blood in the rectum, it is almost invariably associated with hemodynamic compromise. An EGD is invaluable for diagnosis and endoscopic therapy in this situation. An EGD has also been recommended in cases where massive bleeding necessitates blind total colectomy, to be absolutely sure an upper GI source of bleeding is not overlooked.

Small-Bowel Enteroscopy

When radiological evaluation suggests a jejunal or distal ileal source of bleeding, endoscopic examination of the small bowel may be possible using dedicated enteroscopes (jejunum) or at colonoscopy (retrograde ileoscopy). The entire small bowel can be examined endoscopically with the surgeon advancing the endoscope during laparotomy. This procedure is reserved only for patients with recurrent bleeding of presumed small-bowel origin, in whom the risk of recurrent bleeding is thought to be higher than is the risk of a surgical procedure.

Barium Studies

Barium studies have no role in the initial evaluation of acute LGIB. In fact, barium enemas have been reported to be misleading in the work-up of acute LGIB. Moreover, barium can interfere with visualization of the colonic mucosa at subsequent endoscopy. After bleeding as ceased, barium enemas may be ordered to complement an incomplete colonoscopy or flexible sigmoidoscopy. Small-

bowel follow-through x-rays can sometimes help delineate small-bowel lesions, especially tumors.

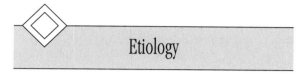

Etiology

Diverticulosis

Diverticulosis accounts for up to 55 percent of acute LGIB. The prevalence of diverticula on routine colonoscopy ranges from 35 to 57 percent. Bleeding is thought to occur from rupture of the branches of the marginal artery at the dome of the diverticulum, due to unclear reasons, although trauma from the fecal stream is thought to play a role. Two-thirds of bleeding diverticula found upon colonoscopy are in the left colon or sigmoid in location, while two-thirds of bleeding diverticula identified upon angiography are in the right colon.

A large proportion of the cases of LGIB-designated diverticular bleeding after colonoscopy have a presumptive rather than a definitive diagnosis. In fact, when definitive criteria are used in designating potential bleeding lesions in the colon, diverticulosis accounts for only 15 to 20 percent of cases of acute LGIB. Bleeding spontaneously ceases in as many as 80 percent of cases of diverticular bleeding. Recurrent bleeding may be seen in approximately 40 percent.

Angiodysplasia

The term *angiodysplasia* is used to describe mucosal vascular ectasias in the GI tract. They can be identified upon endoscopy as discrete, flat or raised, bright red lesions with a stellate or fern-like appearance, usually <10 mm in size.

Angiodysplasia has a prevalence of <1 percent on routine colonoscopy and accounts for up to 3 to 12 percent of acute LGIB, although some series report numbers as high as 37 percent. A higher incidence of GI angiodysplasia than that found on routine colonoscopy has been reported in patients with aortic stenosis, chronic renal disease, atherosclerotic disease, collagen vascular disease, von Willebrand's disease, cirrhosis of the liver, and chronic obstructive pulmonary disease. Use of meperidine during colonoscopy may mask angiodysplasia by reducing mucosal blood flow, and narcotic antagonists such as naloxone have been used by some investigators to enhance the size of the angiodysplastic lesion during the withdrawal phase of colonoscopy when angiodysplasia are strongly suspected.

Neoplasia

Colonic polyps and neoplasia account for 2 to 26 percent of acute LGIB. Polyps that cause bleeding are usually >1 cm in size. Cancers are thought to bleed from erosions or ulceration in the luminal surface of the tumors. Clinically significant bleeding occurs in 0.2 to 0.6 percent of cases after endoscopic polypectomy. Delayed bleeding can occur as late as 2 weeks after initial polypectomy.

Medications

Aspirin, NSAIDs, and anticoagulants can potentiate bleeding by altering mechanisms for hemostasis. Patients with acute LGIB are twice as likely to have taken NSAIDs when compared to patients without acute LGIB. NSAIDs can cause mucosal damage anywhere in the GI tract, resulting in mucosal erosion, ulceration, and even bowel perforation. Patients with diverticular bleeding on NSAIDs have been noted to demonstrate erosion or ulceration at the mouths of the diverticula. The expected incidence of acute LGIB related to NSAID use has been estimated at 7 per 100,000. It remains to be seen whether widespread use of cyclooxygenase$_2$ (COX$_2$) inhibitors will reduce this incidence.

Other Causes

Idiopathic, infectious, and ischemic colitides can account for 3 to 30 percent of cases of acute LGIB. Life-threatening bleeding is rare in idiopathic inflammatory bowel disease. Bloody diarrhea can be seen with infections with *Salmonella, Shigella,*

Campylobacter, Yersinia, and *Escherechia coli* O157:H7. Other infectious causes include amebiasis, cytomegalovirus colitis, and pseudomembranous colitis. Graft-versus-host disease can also result in inflammatory colitis and bloody diarrhea. Ischemia to the colonic mucosa from decreased mucosal blood flow can result in mucosal erosion and ulceration that can also result in acute LGIB.

Hemorrhoids can account for up to 10 percent of cases of acute LGIB, although it is often difficult to establish hemorrhoids as a definite etiologic diagnosis. This is partly due to the extremely high prevalence rate of hemorrhoids on routine colonoscopy. Anal fissures, stercoral or stool-induced ulcers, and solitary rectal ulcers can also result in acute LGIB.

Less frequent causes of acute LGIB that need to be considered include radiation-induced changes, vasculitis, aortoenteric fistula, and endometriosis. Other rare causes are listed in Table 9-2.

Table 9-2
Etiology of Acute Lower Gastrointestinal Bleeding

Common conditions
Colonic diverticulosis
Angiodysplasia
Neoplasia (polyps and cancer)
Colitis (idiopathic, infectious, and ischemic)
Anorectal lesions (hemorrhoids, anal fissures, and idiopathic rectal ulcers)
Less common conditions
Postpolypectomy bleeding
Radiation-related injury
Endometriosis
Vasculitis
Upper gastrointestinal bleeding manifesting as hemochezia
Rare conditions
Aortoenteric fistula
Gastrointestinal bleeding in athletes
Meckel's diverticulum
Small-bowel diverticular bleeding
Colonic varices and portal colopathy
Dieulafoy's lesion of the colon
Intussusception

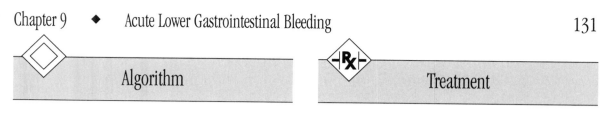

Algorithm

Treatment

A diagnostic and treatment algorithm for lower gastrointestinal bleeding is depicted in Figure 9-2.

Initial Resuscitation

Frequently, initial evaluation and resuscitation will proceed simultaneously in patients with

Figure 9-2

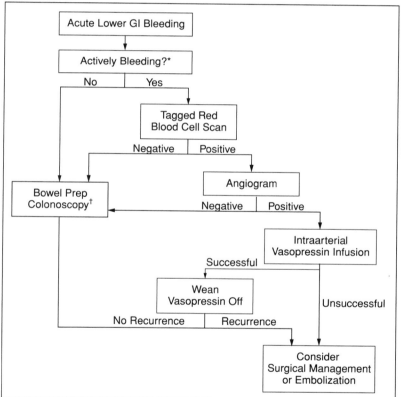

Algorithm for work-up of acute lower gastrointestinal bleeding. Volume resuscitation and correction of coagulopathy always takes precedence over investigative procedures.

*Some investigators would proceed to bowel preparation and colonoscopy even with active bleeding; the decision to order radiologic tests may depend on the level of radiologic expertise and institutional bias.

†Specific management depends on the colonoscopic findings; upper endoscopy, small-bowel enteroscopy, and/or small-bowel radiographs may be indicated depending on individual situations.

acute LGIB. All patients with clinically significant bleeding should have adequate peripheral or central intravenous access. Initial blood tests should include a complete blood count; coagulation parameters including prothrombin time, partial thromboplastin time, and platelet count; blood group and cross-match; and a chemistry profile including liver and renal function.

Initial volume resuscitation can be performed with normal saline or lactated Ringer's solution; blood transfusion may subsequently be necessary. Coagulopathy should be corrected whenever possible in addition to discontinuation of anticoagulant medication. Fresh frozen plasma and/or parenteral vitamin K may be required for elevated prothrombin time, while platelet transfusion is generally reserved for active bleeding with a platelet count <50,000/mm^3. Desmopressin (DDAVP) may be considered at a dose of 15 μg/kg of body weight to improve platelet function in patients with chronic renal insufficiency.

Specific Treatment

Patients with massive bleeding and exsanguination may require urgent surgery without further evaluation to save their life. Frequently, however, acute LGIB is intermittent and ceases spontaneously, allowing for intervention in a less emergent setting. Specific management may involve endoscopic, angiographic, and surgical therapy, alone or in combination.

Endoscopic Therapy

While endoscopic therapy is used over 50 percent of the time in upper GI bleeding, only 12 to 27 percent of patients with acute LGIB undergo endoscopic therapy. Lesions most amenable to endoscopic therapy are angiodysplasia and postpolypectomy bleeding. Angiodysplasia can be successfully ablated using thermal contact probes or laser in the majority of instances. As noted, the use of narcotic analgesics for conscious sedation may mask angiodysplasia by causing decrease in mucosal blood flow, and some investigators recommend avoiding narcotics or using narcotic antagonists when these lesions are a consideration. Early postpolypectomy bleeding can sometimes be controlled by re-snaring the polypectomy stalk and holding pressure for a few minutes. Epinephrine injection and thermal contact probes are routinely used when the bleeding polypectomy site can be identified.

Other lower GI bleeding lesions are less amenable to endoscopic therapy. Bleeding diverticula are difficult to localize during colonoscopy, even if patients are actively bleeding. Epinephrine injection and thermal contact probes have been successfully used when the bleeding diverticulum can be identified. Hemorrhoidal bleeding can be controlled with band ligation, and metallic clip placement has been used for visible vessels noted in association with colonic ulceration.

Angiotherapy

When selective mesenteric angiography demonstrates extravasation of contrast, vasoconstrictor therapy in the form of intraarterial vasopressin infusion can be applied to the bleeding vessel. Intraarterial vasopressin therapy controls bleeding in >60 percent of cases, but rebleeding can occur when the infusion is weaned off. Efficacy is higher in colonic bleeding when compared to small-bowel bleeding. Major complications of intraarterial vasopressin include serious arrhythmias, myocardial ischemia, hypertension, and pulmonary edema. Minor complications are more common and include fluid retention, hyponatremia, transient hypertension, and transient arrhythmias.

Transcatheter embolization can also be performed during angiography for control of massive bleeding. This technique is usually reserved for patients who are poor surgical risks or in situations where vasopressin infusion is contraindicated or has failed. Embolic agents used include gelatin-sponge pledgets, polyvinyl alcohol particles, microcoils, and detachable balloons. Methylene blue staining of the bleeding bowel segment at angiography may direct the surgeon at subsequent laparotomy.

Surgery

Emergency surgery for acute LGIB may be required when bleeding is severe or continuous, usually from a source that is not identified. Elective surgery is considered when bleeding is recurrent from an identified source.

Since blind segmental bowel resection or subtotal colectomy are associated with significant morbidity and mortality, preoperative localization of the bleeding site should be attempted whenever possible. Morbidity, mortality, and rebleeding rates have been demonstrated to be significantly lower when accurate preoperative localization of the bleeding source enables limited intestinal resection. However, when massive ongoing blood loss becomes life-threatening, emergent blind subtotal colectomy may be life saving.

Certain lesions (e.g., colonic neoplasia and Meckel's diverticulum) are surgically resected for a cure. In situations where bleeding is recurrent, several criteria have been utilized for recommending surgical resection of the bleeding bowel segment. Transfusion requirements exceeding 4 U over 24 h or 10 U overall, as well as two (sometimes three) recurrent bleeding episodes from the same source, have been considered indications for surgical therapy. The extent of comorbid medical conditions and the degree of bleeding are other clinical variables that need to be included in the therapeutic equation.

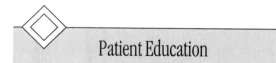

Patient Education

Patients prone to episodes of acute LGIB need to be forewarned about medications that can alter hemostasis, including aspirin, NSAIDs, and anticoagulants. In particular, several over-the-counter cold and flu medications can contain aspirin or NSAIDs. In fact, a significant number of patients with recurrent diverticular bleeding take NSAIDs. Patients with stercoral ulcers, hemorrhoids prone to bleeding, and radiation proctitis can have bleeding precipitated by passing hard stool and need to be advised to avoid constipation. Certain endoscopic procedures, especially endoscopic polypectomy, may be associated with a risk for late rebleeding, up to 10 to 14 days after the procedure. Patients with aortic vascular grafts need to be aware of the potential for developing aortoenteric fistula, which can cause torrential bleeding. These patients should be told to present themselves for evaluation at the earliest sign of blood in the stool. Chronic alcohol use can result in derangement of coagulation mechanisms due to chronic liver disease.

Common Errors in Diagnosis and Treatment

An accurate history and physical examination, stressing the color of bloody stool, are essential to determine the level of bleeding. The multiplicity of terms used by physicians to describe bloody stool sometimes confuses the initial work-up. The term *melena* should be reserved for black, tarry, foul-smelling stool typically seen with an upper GI bleeding source. This finding is significant in that an upper endoscopy is safe, easy, and can be therapeutic in acute upper GI bleeding. Rather than use general terms such as *bloody stool* or *hemochezia*, a precise description of the color (e.g., bright red, dark red, maroon, or black) may be easier to interpret in communicating with other clinicians through medical notes. In one study, the use of a simple pocket-sized card with 5 stool colors (bright red, dark red, maroon, black, and brown) was found to be useful in differentiating upper GI bleeding from colonic bleeding.

Bright blood can be passed in the stool with brisk upper GI bleeding, but this clinical scenario is almost invariably associated with hemodynamic compromise. Nasogastric aspiration is often performed in patients with bloody stool, and this practice can help pinpoint the few situations wherein upper GI bleeding masquerades as acute

LGIB. However, when the pylorus is closed, a duodenal bleeding source may not result in a positive nasogastric aspirate. Endoscopic assessment is essential when an upper GI source is even remotely considered, regardless of the color or content of the nasogastric aspirate.

When a patient with acute LGIB undergoes bowel preparation for colonoscopy, old blood and clots are evacuated from the colon. This is often mistaken for recurrent bleeding. In fact, it is often impossible to distinguish recurrent bleeding from passage of old blood with a bowel preparation. In this situation, monitoring of hemodynamics and serial blood counts are the only reliable indicators of recurrent bleeding. Also, TRBC scanning may not be accurate when bowel preparation is in progress, as the pattern of flow of extravasated blood is an essential aspect of TRBC localization of the bleeding source.

In the outpatient setting, patients may have scant red blood in the stool without other symptoms or hemodynamic compromise. This is often dismissed as hemorrhoidal bleeding, especially if patients give a past history of hemorrhoids. However, ascribing LGIB to hemorrhoids without performing a complete examination of the colon can be potentially hazardous, especially in elderly patients who may be at risk for colonic neoplasia. In young patients not at high risk for colon cancer, if the pattern of bleeding suggests a distal source, a flexible sigmoidoscopy may help rule out other anorectal conditions that cause bleeding.

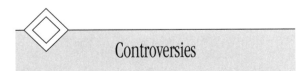

Controversies

Use of Imaging versus Endoscopic Studies

The decision regarding whether to use a radiological or endoscopic test for further intervention initially can be a difficult one. There are no randomized studies addressing this issue. However, almost all patients initially investigated using radiological studies such as TRBC scanning and angiography eventually undergo endoscopy for definitive identification of the bleeding site. There is evidence to suggest that the diagnostic yield of TRBC scanning and angiography are highest when patients are actively bleeding at the time of the study. However, since acute LGIB can be intermittent, determination of whether patients are actively bleeding at the time of the test may be difficult. The presence of bright blood in the stool with a clinical picture compatible with volume loss suggests ongoing bleeding and may be associated with the highest diagnostic yield with radiologic localization. Patients who appear to be stable without evidence of demonstrable volume loss or drop in blood count are best served by bowel preparation and endoscopy within 24 h of presentation.

Identification of the Bleeding Site

The finding of a potential bleeding site at colonoscopy does not necessarily indicate that the lesion found is the bleeding source. One study noted that 42 percent of patients undergoing colonoscopy for acute LGIB had more than one potential bleeding site. Nonbleeding angiodysplasia and diverticula may be wrongly designated as the bleeding source. In order to improve diagnostic certainty and to reduce false localization of the bleeding source, several criteria have been utilized to determine if a given lesion is indeed the bleeding source. The most definitive finding designating a lesion as the bleeding source is active bleeding during colonoscopy. Other definitive criteria suggested include the presence of a nonbleeding visible vessel or an adherent clot. When a TRBC scan localizes to a particular bowel segment, finding a potential bleeding site in the same segment at colonoscopy may provide strong circumstantial evidence in identifying the source of bleeding. The various levels of diagnostic certainty with combinations of radiologic and endoscopic findings are listed in Table 9-1.

Identifying Small-Bowel Bleeding

Investigative procedures in acute LGIB, especially colonoscopy, are directed toward finding a colonic bleeding source. As many as 9 percent of patients presenting with bright blood in the stool could have a small-bowel source of bleeding. Therefore, blind segmental or total colectomy without definitive localization of the bleeding source may be associated with rebleeding episodes if the actual bleeding site is in the small bowel. A combination of TRBC scanning and angiography may be the most efficient method of isolating a small-bowel bleeding source. Conventional endoscopy is useful in this situation only when the bleeding source is in the most proximal small bowel or terminal ileum. Small-bowel enteroscopy may help in visualizing lesions as far down as the mid-jejunum. In intractable cases, Sonde enteroscopy or intraoperative enteroscopy may be required for definitive diagnosis of the bleeding source, but these procedures can be associated with significant complications. Anticoagulants such as heparin and streptokinase have been used to propagate bleeding in difficult cases, followed by TRBC scan or angiography to localize the bleeding source. Patient selection is critical for these provocative measures, as uncontrolled bleeding could result in significant complications in patients with comorbidities. These measures should only be undertaken in specialized centers with facilities for urgent angiotherapy or surgery should bleeding become uncontrolled.

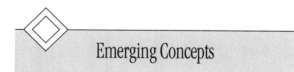

Emerging Concepts

The concept of urgent colonoscopy in patients presenting with acute LGIB is relatively new, first introduced into clinical practice 10 to 12 years ago. Early colonoscopy after rapid bowel preparation has been demonstrated to have a high yield for identification of a bleeding source, especially if performed early in patients' hospital courses. Rapid bowel preparation has been demonstrated to be safe in hemodynamically stable patients. Moreover, an actively bleeding lesion found at colonoscopy may be amenable to endoscopic

therapy. However, the potential for overlooking a bleeding site due to incomplete colon preparation or rapid bleeding has to be considered. Resuscitation and volume repletion take precedence over bowel preparation and conscious sedation for colonoscopy.

Studies have also focused on trying to improve the diagnostic yield of radiologic studies. The diagnostic yield of TRBC scanning has been demonstrated to be highest when patients are actively passing bright blood at the time of the procedure. The yield of angiography is highest when a preceding TRBC scan demonstrated immediate radionuclide extravasation upon initiation of scanning. Requirement for multiple units of blood within a short time and hemodynamic compromise may also help predict patients who may show contrast extravasation upon angiography.

Bibliography

Baker R, Senagore A: Abdominal colectomy offers safe management for massive lower GI bleed. *Am Surg* 60:578–582, 1994.

Breen E, Murray JJ: Pathophysiology and natural history of lower gastrointestinal bleeding. *Semin Colon Rect Surg* 8:128–138, 1997.

Browder W, Cerise EJ, Litwin MS: Impact of emergency angiography in massive lower gastrointestinal bleeding. *Ann Surg* 204:530–536, 1986.

Chalasani N, Wilcox CM: Etiology and outcome of lower gastrointestinal bleeding in patients with AIDS. *Am J Gastroenterol* 93:175–178, 1998.

Davies NM: Toxicity of nonsteroidal anti-inflammatory drugs in the large intestine. *Dis Colon Rectum* 38: 1311–1321, 1995.

Fouch PG: Colonic angiodysplasia. *Gastroenterologist* 5:148–156, 1997.

Fouch PG: Diverticular bleeding: Are nonsteroidal anti-inflammatory drugs risk factors for hemorrhage and can colonoscopy predict outcome for patients? *Am J Gastroenterol* 90:1779–1784,1995.

Gibbs DH, Opelka FG, Beck DE, et al: Postpolypectomy colonic hemorrhage. *Dis Colon Rectum* 39:806–810, 1996.

Jensen DM: Current management of severe lower gastrointestinal bleeding. *Gastrointest Endosc* 41:171–173, 1995.

Jensen DM, Machicado GA: Colonoscopy for diagnosis and treatment of severe lower gastrointestinal bleeding: Routine outcomes and cost analysis. *Gastroenterol Endosc Clin North Am* 7:447–498, 1997.

Kollef MH, Canfield DA, Zuckerman GR: Triage considerations for patients with acute gastrointestinal hemorrhage admitted to a medical intensive care unit. *Crit Care Med* 23:1048–1054, 1995.

Kollef MH, O'Brien JD, Zuckerman GR, Shannon W: BLEED: A classification tool to predict outcomes in patients with upper and lower gastrointestinal hemorrhage. *Crit Care Med* 25:1125–1132, 1997.

Krevsky B: Detection and treatment of angiodysplasia. *Gastrointest Endosc Clin North Am* 7:509–524, 1997.

Longstreth CF: Epidemiology and outcome of patients hospitalized with acute lower gastrointestinal hemorrhage: A population-based study. *Am J Gastroenterol* 92:419–424, 1997.

Machicado GA, Jensen DM: Acute and chronic management of lower gastrointestinal bleeding: Cost-effective approaches. *Gastroenterologist* 5:189–201, 1997.

McGuire HH: Bleeding colonic diverticula. A reappraisal of natural history and management. *Ann Surg* 220:653–656, 1994.

Miller LS, Barbarevech C, Friedman LS: Less frequent causes of lower gastrointestinal bleeding. *Gastroenterol Clin North Am* 23:21–52, 1994.

Muldoon JP, Rusin LC: The initial care and evaluation of the patient with lower gastrointestinal bleeding. *Semin Colon Rect Surg* 8:139–145, 1997.

Peura DA, Lanza FL, Gostout CJ, et al: The American College of Gastroenterology bleeding registry: Preliminary findings. *Am J Gastroenterol* 92:924–928, 1997.

Rantis PC, Harford FJ, Wagmer RH, Henkin RE: Technetium-labeled red blood cell scintigraphy: Is it useful in acute lower gastrointestinal bleeding? *Int J Colorect Dis* 10:210–215, 1995.

Richter JM, Christensen MR, Kaplan LM, Nishioka NS: Effectiveness of current technology in the diagnosis and management of lower gastrointestinal hemorrhage. *Gastrointest Endosc* 41:93–98, 1995.

Rosen RJ, Sanchez G: Angiographic diagnosis and management of gastrointestinal hemorrhage: Current concepts. *Radiol Clin North Am* 32:951–967, 1994.

Teshima T, Hanks GE, Hanlon AL, et al: Rectal bleeding after conformal 3D treatment of prostate cancer: Time to occurrence, response to treatment and duration of morbidity. *Int J Radiat Oncol Biol Phys* 39: 77–83, 1997.

Zuccaro G: Management of the adult patient with acute lower gastrointestinal bleeding. *Am J Gastroenterol* 93:1202–1208,1998.

Zuckerman GR, Prakash C: Acute lower intestinal bleeding. Part I: Clinical presentation and diagnosis. *Gastrointest Endosc* 48:606–616, 1998.

Zuckerman GR, Prakash C: Acute lower intestinal bleeding. Part II: Etiology, therapy and outcomes. *Gastrointest Endosc* 49:228–238, 1999.

Zuckerman GR, Trellis DR, Sherman TM, Clouse RE: An objective measure of stool color for differentiating upper from lower gastrointestinal hemorrhage. *Dig Dis Sci* 40:1614–1621, 1995.

Chapter

10

Occult Bleeding and Iron Deficiency Anemia

Occult bleeding refers to the chemical detection of blood in stools without any grossly visible blood. Such a chronic loss of small volumes of blood via the gastrointestinal (GI) tract will eventually result in iron deficiency anemia. Iron deficiency anemia can also occur with problems not related to the gut (e.g., due to excessive menstrual losses or poor long-term iron intake). Barring such circumstances, patients who have iron deficiency anemia and/or occult bleeding should be evaluated for a GI source of blood loss.

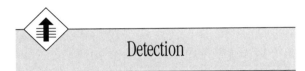

Detection

The normal loss of blood from the GI tract is 2 ml per day. This corresponds to a daily loss of 1 mg of iron. The GI tract normally maintains the iron balance by absorbing 1 to 2 mg of iron per day. A study performed in volunteers revealed that more than 200 ml of ingested blood is required to consistently cause melena. Consequently, it is possible for significant amounts of silent or occult upper GI tract bleeding to occur, without grossly visible blood or melena. Hemorrhoidal bleeding, in contrast, in amounts as small as 1 to 2 ml is visible as hemochezia. When significant occult bleeding occurs, erythropoiesis is stimulated. Intestinal absorption of iron is increased and iron stores are mobilized. Prolonged low-grade bleeding, resulting in a negative iron balance, will eventually deplete the iron stores and result in iron deficiency anemia, which is a continuum of the process of occult GI bleeding.

Blood from the stomach and small bowel undergoes significant degradation by the time it exits the colon. In contrast, heme and globin are much more readily detected in the stool when the source of blood loss is in the distal small bowel or colon. Table 10-1 illustrates the blood degradation product found in stool depending on the site of bleed.

Three types of occult blood test kits are currently commercially available. Due to differences in degree of degradation of hemoglobin, depending on the site of bleeding, each of the tests, theoretically, may help localize the site of bleeding to either the upper or lower GI tracts.

1. Guaiac test: This is the most widely used test. The oxidation by peroxidase (from hemoglobin) and any other oxidants in the stool turns guaiac blue. Since the test is more likely to be positive in the presence of fecal heme, it is best at detecting larger and more distal lesions.
2. Immunochemical tests use antibodies to detect human globin epitopes. Theoretically, these tests are more likely to detect bleeding from the colon.
3. Heme-porphyrin test: measures porphyrin spectrofluorometrically. This test has a limited role clinically.

Table 10-1

Blood Degradation Product Found in Stool Based on Site of Bleeding

| | | Hb Components in Stool | | |
Bleeding Site	Hb Insults During Luminal Transit	Globin	Heme	HDPS
Upper GI tract	Globin completely digested, minimal heme absorption, colonic flora convert heme to HDP	0	+	+++
Distal ileum, proximal colon	Globin altered by peptidases of colonic flora, colonic flora converts heme to HDP	+	+	++
Rectosigmoid colon	Minimal alteration of hemoglobin molecule	++++	+++	0/+

GI, gastrointestinal; Hb, hemoglobin; HDP, heme-derived porphyrius.

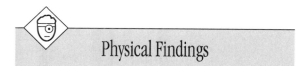

Chapter 10

Clinical Presentation

Occult bleeding is often detected by fecal occult blood testing in asymptomatic individuals during routine annual physical examination. Current colon cancer screening guidelines advise annual fecal occult blood testing after 50 years of age. Mild anemia is often asymptomatic. However, due to the chronic nature of the blood loss, albeit in small volumes, patients may have severe symptomatic anemia, including congestive heart failure or angina. Use of nonsteroidal anti-inflammatory drugs and anticoagulants for other medical conditions may further increase the amount of daily blood loss. First-degree relatives with either colon polyps or colon cancer identify those at a higher risk for colonic neoplasms as compared to the general population. Individuals with a family history of hereditary hemorrhagic telangiectasia may experience chronic blood loss from the widespread telangiectatic lesions in the gut.

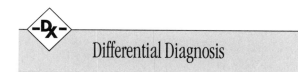

Physical Findings

Besides pallor, physical examination may reveal physiologic changes that occur in anemia. Depending on the severity of anemia, these findings include tachycardia, wide pulse pressure, and hyperdynamic precordium. An ejection systolic murmur is often heard over the precordium, particularly at the pulmonic area. These cardiac findings disappear when anemia is corrected. Koilonychia (spoon-shaped nails) may be evident. Also, physical examination may reveal findings suggestive of rare causes of GI bleeding. Such findings include dermatitis herpetiformis (celiac sprue), Kaposi sarcoma (AIDS), koilonychias, atrophic tongue (Plummer-Vinson syndrome) and tylosis (esophageal cancer). Occasionally, glossitis, cheilitis, or atrophic rhinitis may result from iron deficiency.

Laboratory Data

There is normally 14 to 18 g/dl of hemoglobin in males and 12 to 16 g/dl of hemoglobin in females. Normal serum iron is 80 to 180 μg/dl and iron-binding capacity is 250 to 460 μg/dl. Normal saturation is 20 to 45 percent. The anemia may be detected incidentally on laboratory studies or during evaluation of symptomatic anemia. Iron deficiency anemia is classically microcytic, with the mean corpuscular volume (MCV) less than the 83 fl. Other coexisting deficiencies (B_{12} and folate) or the presence of an underlying chronic disease may render the MCV inaccurate. Reticulocytosis may be seen as a result of the release of an increased number of immature red blood cells from the bone marrow. Iron deficiency anemia is characterized by low iron and elevated total iron-binding capacity (TIBC). Serum iron and transferrin levels are depressed by conditions such as inflammation, cancer, and liver disease, leading at times to skewed ratios. If a bone marrow biopsy is performed as part of the work-up, marrow iron stores will be undetectable.

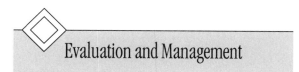

Differential Diagnosis

The differential diagnosis of occult GI bleeding with or without iron deficiency is broad (Table 10-2).

Evaluation and Management

Given that nutritional lack of iron is uncommon in developed countries, as are parasitic infections (e.g., hookworm infestation), an anatomic etiology in the GI tract as a cause of iron deficiency should be considered once patients are identified with iron deficiency anemia. Documenting of

Table 10-2

Differential Diagnosis

Inflammatory causes	Acid-peptic diseases, Cameron's erosions (ulcerations associated with large hiatal hernias), inflammatory bowel disease, Whipple's disease, sprue, eosinophilic gastroenteritis, and solitary colon ulcers
Infectious causes	Hookworm, strongyloidosis, ascariasis, amebiasis, and tuberculous enterocolitis.
Vascular causes	Vascular ectasias and angiodysplasia, hereditary hemorrhagic telangiectasia, gastroesophageal varices, congestive gastropathy, hemangiomas, watermelon stomach, and blue rubber bleb nevus syndrome
Neoplasms	Any primary or metastatic malignant tumor involving the GI tract; ulcerated benign lesions, e.g., leiomyoma and lipoma
Drugs	NSAIDs
Artifactual causes	Hemoptysis, epistaxis, hematuria, and menstrual bleeding
Miscellaneous	Long-distance running, coagulopathies, gastrostomy tubes, and other devices

GI, gastrointestinal; NSAIDs, nonsteroidal anti-inflammatory drugs.

occult blood in the stools doubly justifies pursuing an endoscopic evaluation of the gut in this situation, even if the stools are heme-negative; however, in the appropriate clinical setting with postmenopausal females or any males, evaluation for GI sources should be performed. Patients are usually given three or more guaiac cards to smear stool on separate occasions. The test should be performed without rehydration to avoid a high rate of false positivity. Any instance of occult blood

positivity in the stool or symptoms suggestive of a problem in the gut (weight loss, abdominal pain, nausea, vomiting, early satiety, dysphagia, recent change in bowel habits, or GI bleeding) should trigger an endoscopic evaluation. Iron studies will confirm the need for replacement iron therapy.

In evaluating patients with occult blood in the stools or with iron deficiency anemia, the initial endoscopic examination is usually directed at the colon if no site-specific (upper GI tract or lower GI tract) symptoms are present (see Figure 10-1). If this exam is unrevealing, then the upper endoscopy is subsequently performed. Some studies, however, have found a bleeding lesion at least as often in the upper GI tract as in the lower GI tract. Upper endoscopy resulted in a change in the management in up to 49 percent of the patients. However, those individuals with upper tract symptoms such as dyspepsia, heartburn, or early satiety should have upper endoscopy in this setting regardless of the findings on colonoscopy. A small-bowel biopsy in individuals with iron deficiency anemia and overtly normal endoscopies may reveal villous atrophy consistent with celiac sprue.

About 30 to 50 percent of cases of occult bleeding will not have a source identified on upper and lower endoscopy. In such situations, it is reasonable to give oral iron supplements and monitor patients clinically. In the vast majority of patients, this will result in the permanent resolution of the problem. If the anemia or occult blood in the stools persists, consideration should be give to further evaluation of the problem.

In individuals with chronic GI blood loss that results in significant anemia, with unrevealing esophagogastroduodenoscopy and colonoscopy, the next step in the evaluation involves performing a push enteroscopy. At the same time, a careful examination of the esophagus, stomach, and duodenum can also be carried out. Depending on operator expertise and patient anatomy, a variable length of the small bowel can be examined—usually the proximal and middle thirds of the small bowel. Often, lesions will be found in the stomach that were not appreciated at the time of the index endoscopy. These include Cameron's lesions, peptic ulcers, or angiodysplasia (see Figure 10-2).

Figure 10-1

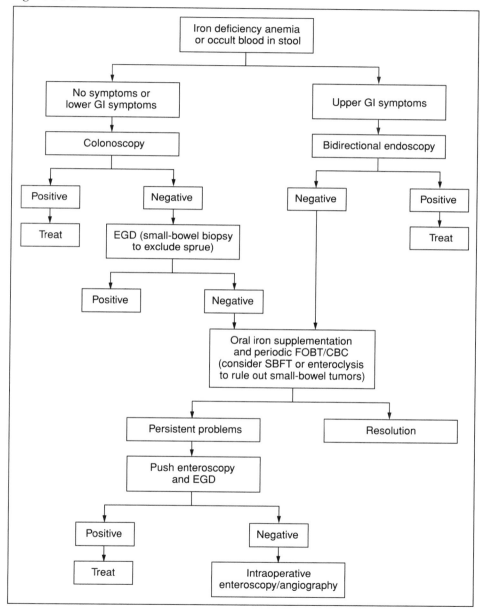

EGD, esophagogastroduodenoscopy; CBC, complete blood count; FOBT, fecal occult blood test; SBFT, small-bowel follow through.

Figure 10-2

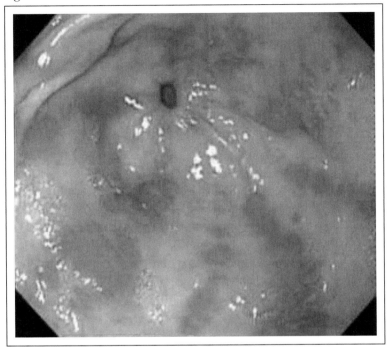

Gastric angio vascular ectasia in a patient with iron deficiency anemia.

Careful examination of the small bowel may demonstrate vascular malformations or, in rare instances, tumors. Heater probes, bipolar electrocautery units, Nd:YAG lasers, and argon plasma coagulators can be used to deliver thermal energy to cauterize these lesions. In one trial of the Nd:YAG laser, 100 percent of patients with angiodysplasia, 75 percent of patients with gastric antral vascular ectasia, and 66 percent of patients with hereditary hemorrhagic telangiectasia had a sustained decrease in transfusion requirements. If a small-bowel neoplasm is identified, biopsies can be taken and further surgical management can be appropriately planned.

While an endoscopic approach is customary, in individuals who are unable to undergo conscious sedation, unable to discontinue anticoagulation, or are reluctant to undergo endoscopy, the radiographic alternatives are upper GI series, small-bowel follow-through, or enteroclysis and barium enema. In one study, the combination of air-contrast barium enema (ACBE) and flexible sigmoidoscopy had a sensitivity of 98 percent for carcinomas and 99 percent for adenomas. However, smaller mucosal lesions are not well detected by ACBE. Also, ACBE lacks therapeutic capability, and flat lesions such as angiodysplasia, which are often seen in this group of patients, will not be appreciated radiographically.

In a small minority of patients with documented persistent significant GI bleeding of an unknown source, an intraoperative enteroscopy may have to be performed. This is performed under general anesthesia, and the small bowel is accessed via a laparotomy. The surgeon advances the small bowel over the endoscope, which is introduced into the small bowel orally or via an enterotomy; this allows for the entire length of the small bowel to be examined. Any necessary resections can be performed at the same time.

Abdominal angiography is more commonly performed for overt unexplained upper or lower GI bleeding (see Figure 10-3). However, in patients with persistent, severe iron deficiency with documented blood in the stools and dependent on red blood cell transfusions, abdominal angiography may reveal the presence of previously undetected angiodysplasia or neoplasm in the small bowel. Lesions detected during angiography may be embolized. It has also been reported that methylene blue dye was injected into the bleeding vessel in order to stain the small-bowel mucosa and direct the surgeon. It is a more common practice, however, to perform an intraoperative enteroscopy in this setting. Tagged red cell scans are not of significant use in the evaluation of occult blood in the stool or iron deficiency anemia unless the rate of bleeding is over 0.1 ml/min.

In individuals with diffuse vascular lesions, lesions in areas not accessible to endoscopic therapy, or with failed endoscopic or surgical therapy, medical therapy may have a role. Gastrointestinal blood loss associated with angiodysplasia in a setting of chronic renal failure, hereditary hemorrhagic telangiectasia, and Von Willebrand's disease, in various clinical trials, has been effectively controlled by combination estrogen-progesterone therapy. While in some studies, estrogen in a dose of 0.035 mg with norethisterone, 1 mg, has been shown to be effective, others have suggested that combination therapy with a higher dose of estrogen (ethinyl estradiol, 0.05 mg) may be needed if the lower dose therapy fails. The exact duration of therapy prior to considering patients treatment failures is unclear; however, some investigators recommend a 6-month course of therapy with intermittent pauses in an

Figure 10-3

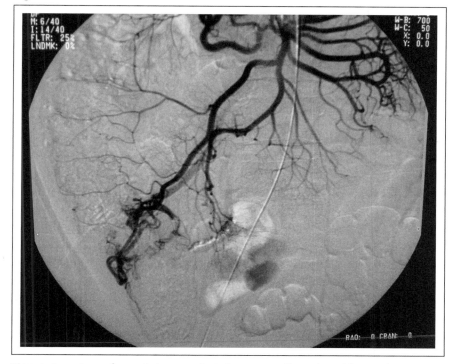

Mesenteric angiogram demonstrates a cecal arteriovenous malformation with an early draining vein.

effort to reduce the incidence of side effects. Octreotide (0.05 to 0.1 mg subcutaneously) has also been reported to decrease blood loss from intestinal angiodysplasia. The exact mechanism of action is, however, unclear.

Surgical therapy for occult bleeding is usually directed against bleeding tumors or in concert with either intraoperative enteroscopy or angiography. In one study, bowel palpation and transillumination allowed for 65 percent of patients with obscure bleeding undergoing surgical exploration to receive targeted surgery.

In another study of 44 patients with recurrent occult gastrointestinal bleeding, a site-specific source was seen in the small bowel in 31 patients; 27 patients had lesions amenable to segmental resection. However, 23 patients had recurrent bleeding despite this surgical intervention. This led to the conclusion that intraoperative enteroscopy in select patients with occult GI bleeding correctly identifies a treatable source and prevents recurrent bleeding in 41% of patients.

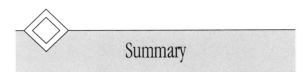

Summary

The presence of occult blood in the stool or of iron deficiency anemia should trigger a thorough evaluation of the GI tract for sources of blood loss. When the causative lesions are identifiable, further loss of blood can usually be averted by endoscopic therapy. In the appropriate clinical setting, individuals with an unidentifiable source of blood loss may need push enteroscopy, intraoperative enteroscopy, or angiography.

Bibliography

Ahlquist DA: Approach to the patient with occult gastrointestinal bleeding, in Yamada T et al (eds). *Textbook of Gastroenterology*, 2nd ed. Philadelphia, Lippincott, 1995, pp 699–717.

Anthanasoulis C, Moncure A, Greenfield A: Intraoperative localization of small bowel bleeding sites with the combined use of angiographic methods and methylene blue injection. *Surgery* 87(1):77–84, 1980.

Baird IM, Dodge O, Palmer F, et al: The tongue and esophagus in iron deficiency anemia and the effect of iron therapy. *J Clin Pathol* 14:603–609, 1961.

Barkin JS, Ross BS: Medical therapy for chronic gastrointestinal bleeding of obscure origin. *Am J Gastroenterol* 93(8):1250–1254, 1998.

Bronner MH, Pate MB, Cunningham JT: Estrogen-progesterone therapy for bleeding gastrointestinal telangiectasias in chronic renal failure. *Ann Intern Med* 105(3):371–374, 1986.

Jacobs A, Cavill I: The oral lesions of iron deficiency anemia: Pyredoxine and riboflavin status. *Br J Hematol* 14(3):291–295, 1968.

Kewenter J, Brevinge H, Engaras B, et al: The yield of flexible sigmoidoscopy and double contrast barium enema in the diagnosis of neoplasms in the large bowel in patients with a positive hemoccult test. *Endoscopy* 27(2):159–163, 1995.

Lau WY, Fan ST, Won SH, et al: Preoperative and intraoperative localization of gastrointestinal bleeding of obscure origin. *Gut* 28(7):869–877, 1987.

Reis AM, Benacii JC, Sam MG: Efficacy of intraoperative enteroscopy in diagnosis and prevention of recurrent occult gastrointestinal bleeding. *Am J Surg* 163(1):94–98, 1992.

Rockey D, Koches J, Cello J, et al: Relative frequency of upper gastrointestinal and colonic lesions in patients with positive fecal occult blood tests. *N Engl J Med* 339(3):153–159, 1998.

Rossini FP, Arrigan A, Pennazio M: Octreotide in the treatment of bleeding due to angiodysplasia of the small intestine. *Am J Gastroenterol* 88(9):1424–1447, 1993.

Sargeant IR, Loizou LA, Rampton D, et al: Laser ablation of upper gastrointestinal vascular ectasia: Long-term results. *Gut* 34(4):470–475, 1993.

Van Cutsem E, Rutgerts P, Coremans G, et al: Dose response study of hormonal therapy in bleeding gastrointestinal malformations. *Gastroenterology* 104: A286, 1993.

Van Cutsem E, Rutgerts P, Van Trappen G: Treatment of bleeding gastrointestinal vascular malformations with estrogen-progesterone. *Lancet* 335:953–955, 1990.

Zuckerman G, Benitez J: A prospective study of bidirectional endoscopy in the evaluation of patients with occult gastrointestinal bleeding. *Am J Gastroenterol* 87(1):62–66, 1992.

Anita C. Lee

Chapter

11

Flatulence

A fabis abstinetes. (Eat no beans)
—Pythagoras

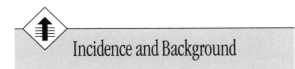

Incidence and Background

Flatulence, a universal physiologic process, is occasionally a source of satisfaction, but more a source of anxiety or worry for people. Its importance in daily life has been documented through the centuries from as early as 1550 B.C. Pythagoras, in his pointed quote above, suggests one of the mainstays of empiric treatment for flatulence: dietary manipulation. Flatulence is generally diet-dependent, but can in rare cases be a symptom of more serious disease. It is a common general medical complaint and is most often treated empirically unless the history and physical dictate otherwise. Other common symptoms that may be described with flatulence include cramping, bloating, chest pain, nausea, belching, dyspepsia, "wind," and gas.

Definition of Normal

What defines *normal* flatulence varies from person to person. Studies from young, healthy male volunteers suggest that there is approximately 100 to 200 ml of gas in the digestive tract at a time. On average, 600 ml of gas per 24 h is expelled per person, but it can range from 500 to 3000 ml, derived from colonic bacterial fermentation of fiber or undigested polysaccharides. The frequency of flatus is also quite varied, with an average of 14 times a day (range of 7 to 25). Flatus is passed more in the first 5 hours after a meal and less during the night. The amount of flatus can drop by two-thirds with a low-fiber diet.

The social acceptance of flatus is also varied. A small survey of patients participating in a healthy volunteer trial in the United States found that 47 percent thought flatus was a natural event and were comfortable with it; 21 percent did not like flatus,

but thought it was accepted in society; and 32 percent were embarrassed by the topic and event.

Composition of Flatus

Flatus is composed of swallowed air (oxygen and nitrogen) and endogenously produced gases (hydrogen, carbon dioxide, methane, and trace gases). The relative composition of flatus varies widely among the population depending on diet and intrinsic bacterial fermentation. For example, patients with aerophagia may have flatus that mimics inhaled air (20% oxygen, 70 to 80% nitrogen). Patients with severe lactose intolerance may have 40 to 60% hydrogen in their flatus.

Oxygen (O_2) is derived purely from swallowed air and is not produced in the intestinal lumen. It is regurgitated by belching, diffused into the bloodstream, used in bacterial metabolic processes, and expelled in generally small quantities in flatus.

Nitrogen (N_2) concentration in flatus is also mostly from air. Trace amounts may be generated from bacterial colonic fermentation or from lumenal absorption from blood.

Hydrogen (H_2) is produced almost exclusively in the colon from bacterial fermentation of undigested carbohydrates. The measurement of hydrogen concentration via mouth forms the basis for hydrogen breath testing, used to detect malabsorptive states in which the volume and production rate of hydrogen are increased.

Carbon dioxide (CO_2) is usually excreted in small concentrations in flatus. It is produced during the neutralization of acid by bicarbonate, in reactions of food and pancreatic secretions during digestion of fat and protein, and in largest quantities from bacterial fermentation.

Methane (CH_4) is produced by fermentation of undigested carbohydrates by specific anaerobic bacteria, *Methanobrevibacter smithii*. Methane production occurs in approximately one-third of the population. It has both genetic and environmental influences. The causes of environmental influences are unclear but are demonstrated in certain populations of patients. For example, a larger percentage of institutionalized patients are methane producers. It also endogenously produced from glycoproteins and proteins.

Other gases in trace amounts include hydrogen sulfide (H_2S), methanethiol, and dimethyl sulfide. These three are thought to be the most odor-producing gases. Ammonia, amines, skatoles, and indols may contribute to odor as well. Hydrogen sulfide in as little as three parts per million may lead to detectable odor.

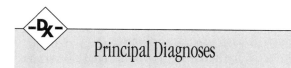

Principal Diagnoses

There are many causes of excessive flatulence (Table 11-1). However, a few diagnoses comprise the majority of cases: aerophagia, carbohydrate malabsorption, irritable bowel syndrome, and dysmotility.

Aerophagia

Aerophagia, or air swallowing, is an often unsuspected and underdiagnosed cause for flatulence. In most people, the amount of flatus depends on bacterial fermentation in the colon. However, in aerophagia, the large majority of flatus is a direct result of swallowing, and the gas contents of flatus would be similar to ambient air. Many risk factors have been proposed for aerophagia (Table 11-2). These range from talking while eating to drinking carbonated beverages to anxiety and hyperventilation with subsequent air swallowing. Aerophagia can sometimes be seen with gastroesophageal reflux disease as well.

Carbohydrate Malabsorption

Carbohydrate malabsorption is an extremely common cause for flatulence. It is present in 25 percent of the U.S. population, and up to 75 percent

of the world population, more commonly in Asians and blacks. It is a result of incomplete digestion of carbohydrates, usually from specific enzyme deficiencies such as lactase. There is increased delivery of the undigested carbohydrate to the colon resulting in more bacterial fermentation and production of endogenous gases. Sprue, inflammatory bowel disease, and lymphoma may also contribute to malabsorption.

Most carbohydrates are derived from plants except for small amounts of glycogen, found in meats, and lactose, found in milk. Carbohydrates

Table 11-1
Causes of Flatulence

Most common
Aerophagia
Lactose malabsorption
Other carbohydrate malabsorption—sucrose, fructose
Irritable bowel syndrome
Dysmotility
Gastroparesis
Drugs
Narcotics
Calcium channel blockers
Anticholinergics
Antibiotics
Protease inhibitors
α-Glucosidase inhibitors (Acarbose)
Fibric acid derivatives
Antidiarrheals
Less common
Bacterial overgrowth
Malignancy: gastric, small bowel, colonic
Peptic ulcer disease
Obstruction or pseudoobstruction
Inflammatory bowel disease
Infection—giardiasis or amebiasis
Cholelithiasis
Hypothyroidism
Diabetes mellitus
Anorexia nervosa

Table 11-2

Causes of Aerophagia

Eating in the recumbent position
Eating or drinking too quickly
Chewing gum or eating hard candy
Smoking cigarettes, cigars, and pipes
Drinking through straws
Drinking carbonated beverages
Oral irritation or dentures
Postnasal drip
Dry mouth
Anxiety or hyperventilation

are divided into monosaccharides, disaccharides, oligosaccharides, and fiber. Monosaccharides include glucose and fructose. Fructose in high doses can be poorly absorbed even in healthy volunteers. Disaccharides, such as sucrose and lactose, are ubiquitous in the American diet and in dairy products. Lactase (β-galactosidase) deficiency is the single most common enzyme deficiency in carbohydrate malabsorption. Tri- to octo- (oligo) saccharides include fructans found in onion and artichoke. Stachyose, raffinose, and verbascose, three other oligosaccharides found in numerous vegetables, are broken down by α-galactosidase. Fiber is an undigested carbohydrate, and the amount of dietary fiber correlates well with flatus production. Pectins and gums are two kinds of fiber that are extensively metabolized in the colon and are found as additives in many foods.

Even in the healthy volunteer, there can be excessive flatus production with a high-percentage carbohydrate diet. With large quantities of ingested carbohydrates, the rate-limiting factor of the amount of enzyme available for breakdown of carbohydrate is exceeded.

Lactose intolerance often presents with flatus, but can also be accompanied by abdominal pain, distension, loose watery stools, and cramping. It is diagnosed principally by dietary history and response to empiric therapy. Hydrogen breath testing is the standard for diagnosis; jejunal biopsy is rarely used. The amount of lactase decreases with age: 10 percent of lactase enzyme activity is lost by

age 20. Lactose intolerance is both over- and under-diagnosed. One study of patients with lactose intolerance showed that small quantities of milk (8 oz) were well tolerated with no change in bloating, diarrhea, and flatus symptoms over placebo.

Irritable Bowel Syndrome

Irritable bowel syndrome (IBS) is a common functional multifaceted syndrome of abdominal pain, bloating, flatulence, and irregular bowel habits that occurs in 20 percent of the population. There may be more gas production in these patients from a variety of mechanisms, including prolonged transit time and, therefore, more bacterial exposure to carbohydrates. Patients with IBS often produce and maintain the same total volumes of flatulence; however, they may be more sensitive to colonic distension with these volumes. Patients with IBS also have a reported 20 to 60 percent incidence of lactose intolerance, which may present with identical symptoms.

Dysmotility

Dysmotility is another less common cause of flatulence. It may be idiopathic, but is more often associated with diabetes and gastroparesis. Neuromuscular disorders such as muscular dystrophy or spinal cord injury may also contribute to dysmotility. Pseudoobstruction, bacterial overgrowth, and anorexia nervosa are also causes.

Other Causes

There are numerous other causes of flatulence. Drugs can be a common cause of flatulence by decreasing motility, changing bacterial flora, creating malabsorption, and causing aerophagia. These include calcium channel blockers, narcotics, anticholinergics, antibiotics, protease inhibitors, acarbose (a α-glucosidase inhibitor), and fibric acid derivatives.

Small-bowel bacterial overgrowth, from dysmotility disorders as earlier or small-bowel surgery, may also present with flatulence. Sprue, any achlorhydric state, inflammatory bowel disease, and antibiotic therapy are all underlying causes. Gas bloat syndrome (in which there is retention of gas in the stomach), hepatic flexure, and splenic flexure, can lead to flatulence. Peptic ulcer disease including that from *Helicobacter pylori*, gastric outlet obstruction, adhesions and hernias, and neoplasms of the stomach and small and large intestines are uncommon causes.

Infections, especially parasitic diseases such as that caused by *Giardia lamblia*, must be considered in patients with the appropriate travel and ingestion history. Patients with fecal incontinence or decreased rectal tone may present with flatulence. There are also variations in normal menstrual cycles in women, who report more flatulence in the luteal phase.

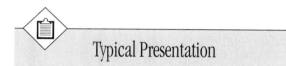

Typical Presentation

Flatulence is a straightforward symptom, but what compels people to seek medical attention may relate to the frequency, amount, and smell of the flatus. As mentioned previously, norms for flatus are quite varied from individual to individual. It is generally agreed that 25 or fewer episodes of flatus are "normal." Case reports of "extremely flatulent" patients have documented up to 140 episodes of flatulence in a 24-h period. It is also difficult to evaluate the amount of flatus that a person expels, as measuring techniques are quite cumbersome and rarely used. The rate of gas production may cause explosive flatus, which may be more uncomfortable to patients than the amount of flatus. Also, what constitutes discomfort before expelling gas varies with different individual sensitivities to amounts of gas in the rectum. The symptoms of rectal distension are relieved with the passage of flatus or a bowel movement. Smell of the flatus also makes people seek medical attention, but a single symptom is not suggestive of any particular pathologic etiology. Benign flatulence rarely wakens people at night, although flatus is still expelled.

Flatulence is closely related to belching and bloating. Belching, or eructation, is the retrograde passage of esophageal or gastric gas across the upper esophageal sphincter and out the oral cavity. This sequence of relaxation of the lower esophageal sphincter then upper esophageal sphincter, then expelling of gas after meals, especially those high in onions, tomatoes, or mints, or after a carbonated beverage, is generally physiologic.

Belching often relieves postprandial epigastric fullness and bloating—a phenomenon known as magenblase syndrome. Belching in other situations is almost always a voluntary event, but in a small minority of patients, it can represent a functional disorder.

Bloating or distension and flatulence are tightly linked, and the differential diagnosis for these symptoms is the same. In bloating, areas of the colon can trap air and may be distended on exam and on plain films. Diffuse abdominal pain may also be present. Patients may typically relate either loose stools or constipation or both.

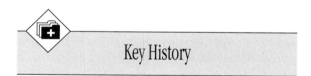

Key History

General

The comprehensive history is the cornerstone for diagnosis of serious versus nonserious disease in flatulence and should focus on how the flatulence bothers the patient: whether there is a change in the flatulence pattern, frequency, or smell. Although there is a general perception that the elderly and males produce more flatus, in fact, the amount and frequency of flatus production is not significantly different in people on the same diets. The perception of the flatus changes with age, as the elderly tend to report more awareness of flatus. One caveat is that the elderly do have more comorbid conditions that could lead to increased flatus. In irritable bowel syndrome, patients are sensitive to small amounts of rectal and colonic distension.

A thorough history for systemic disease is also necessary, asking specifically for any history of diabetes, inflammatory bowel disease, or neuromuscular disease. Abdominal surgery may affect gastric or colonic motor functions and may predispose to adhesions and obstruction, and any surgical blind loops may contribute to bacterial overgrowth.

A comprehensive gastrointestinal history will aid in the elimination of serious pathology from the differential diagnosis. Besides the previously mentioned bloating and belching, other associated symptoms may include borborygmi—a loud rumbling abdominal noise—and constipation. Patients should be asked about the quality of their stools: hard, soft, brown, acholic, or floating. Although floating stools are often associated with steatorrhea, in actuality, patients who produce large amounts of methane may also produce floating stools from the amount of methane gas trapped in stool. Since one-third of Americans are methane producers, floating stools are more likely to be from gas and not fat. Inquiry about abdominal pain and its quality and location may pinpoint an underlying disorder.

Important other associated symptoms include weight loss, change in bowel habits, dysphagia, and anorexia. These and the age of patients will prompt an in-depth evaluation for malignancy. Fever points toward an infectious etiology. Any nocturnal diarrhea, bloody diarrhea, or rectal bleeding will prompt an endoscopic evaluation; and jaundice will lead to liver function testing. Other key parts of the history include diet history, family history, and medications.

Dietary

The average American diet is composed of 40 to 50 percent carbohydrates (200 to 300 g). This percentage may be increasing since fiber is being touted as having possible beneficial effects on coronary artery disease, gastrointestinal malignancy, and regulation of bowel habits.

A detailed history of the consumption of carbohydrates is essential. Specifically, inquire about tolerance to different cereals. Rice is rarely flatulogenic because its lack of protein binding helps its degradation in the small bowel. However, most other grains (oat, bran, and wheat) produce moderate flatulence. The removal of all fiber in the diet can lead to a dramatic decrease in flatus. Patients should be asked about any intolerance to dairy or sugar products with focus on the timed relation between ingestion of the food and any subsequent diarrhea, bloating, belching, or flatulence. Often a sugar substitute, sorbitol is used frequently by diabetics. Chocolate may contain maltitol, another undigested polysaccharide. Olestra, a nonabsorbable sucrose fatty acid ester, may also increase flatulence. In addition, vegetarians may have a large percentage of carbohydrate and fiber intake, with possibly increased flatulence as well.

A social history should focus on travel or ingestion of contaminated water, keeping in mind *Giardia* or *Entamoeba,* which may present with flatulence as well as diarrhea. An occupational history may often give a surprising answer for excess flatulence. Submariners, scuba divers, miners, astronauts, and elevator operators all may have excess flatulence because of reverse diffusion of carbon dioxide from the bloodstream into the intestinal lumen. A family history for gastrointestinal malignancy, inflammatory bowel disease, celiac disease, and lactose or other dietary intolerance is sometimes helpful.

Medications are often culprits in flatulence and have been listed. Also sodium bicarbonate, used in various household and folk remedies for halitosis or heartburn, can produce excessive flatulence. A one-half teaspoon of sodium bicarbonate can generate 475 ml carbon dioxide flatus.

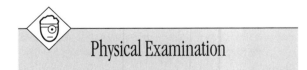

Physical Examination

The physical exam is generally unremarkable in patients who have flatulence as a presenting complaint. Patients should be assessed for anxiety, air swallowing, and belching. Longitudinal observation for weight loss is important. Nutritional status can be evaluated from temporal, interosseous, or thenar wasting.

The abdominal exam helps to exclude serious disease. The abdomen should be evaluated for distension and ascites. A succussion splash, or splashing sound, heard with the stethoscope during palpation of the upper abdomen and gastric area, can indicate gastric outlet obstruction. A digital rectal examination should be routinely included, and any positive hemoccult should be further evaluated.

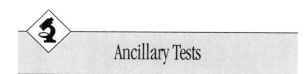

Ancillary Tests

Ancillary tests should be directed at a specific question, and the history and physical exam should help to avoid many unnecessary tests.

Blood Tests, Stool Tests, Plain X-Rays, and Endoscopy

Serum blood testing, including a complete blood cell count and levels of electrolytes and glucose, calcium, liver-associated enzymes, albumin, and total protein should help in excluding diabetes, malignancy, malabsorption, cirrhosis, and possible infection. If clinically indicated, stool should be evaluated for ova and parasites, *Clostridium difficile* or bacterial studies, possibly including *H. pylori*. Steatorrhea may be evaluated with fecal fat collections.

Radiographs of the abdomen are rarely helpful in the evaluation of isolated flatulence, although they may show colonic distension around the hepatic or splenic flexure or reveal obstruction, ascites, and free air. Endoscopy is indicated when there are symptoms such as dysphagia, weight loss, or change in bowel habits, and tissue and/or direct visualization is desired. Duodenal or jejunal biopsy can help with the diagnosis of a malabsorptive state. Colonoscopy may exclude inflammatory bowel disease, masses, anatomic abnormalities such as redundant colon, or other forms of colitis.

Breath Tests

Breath tests are rarely used in the primary care setting, but are diagnostic for many disorders of carbohydrate malabsorption, as well as bacterial overgrowth and detection of *H. pylori*. In the evaluation of flatulence, they are generally reserved after an empiric dietary change has been tried.

HYDROGEN

The hydrogen breath test measures expired hydrogen after administration of an oral dose of the carbohydrate that is suspected to cause the patient's flatulence. This is usually lactose or other sugars (2 g/kg in a 20% solution). The test can also be performed with certain foods such as yogurt.

Hydrogen in the breath is measured at timed intervals, usually 30 min, at baseline and after the administration of the substrate for at least 3 h. It is collected in syringes or mylar bags and is measured by gas chromatography. If patients have carbohydrate malabsorption, undigested carbohydrate will continue on to the colon from the small intestine and be fermented by colonic bacteria to produce, among other gases, hydrogen, which will be expelled via breath and flatus.

The results are expressed as the concentration of hydrogen excreted in parts per million (ppm) over time (see Figure 11-1). For lactose deficiency, a 10- to 20-ppm increase over baseline within 120 min of the test is a positive response and is positive in over 90% of patients with lactose malabsorption. Bacterial overgrowth is implied if the amount of hydrogen expired increases by 10 to 20 ppm within 30 min, and stasis and bacterial overgrowth are likely if the fasting hydrogen expired is greater than 42 ppm.

CARBON DIOXIDE

Carbon dioxide breath testing, using a radiolabelled inhaled substrate, is also used for many different reasons, including bacterial overgrowth and bile absorption, but it is less commonly used for flatulence than is hydrogen breath testing. It may also be used in the diagnosis of fat malabsorption or testing of hepatic drug metabolism.

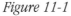

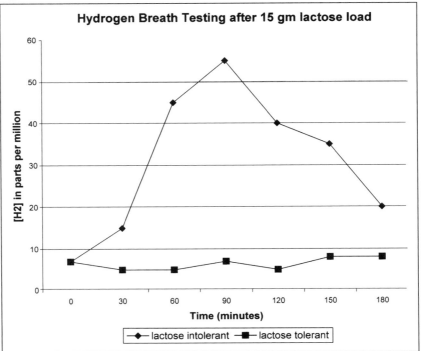

Hydrogen breath test profile in lactose intolerance.

Other Studies

Manometry, both esophageal and rectal, can be helpful in evaluating reflux disease or fecal incontinence. Motility studies, such as gastric emptying studies or intestinal transit studies, may aid in discovering gastrointestinal motor dysfunction. Abdominal ultrasound can evaluate cholelithiasis and ascites.

Flatus gas analysis is extremely rare, not routinely available, and cumbersome, and empiric treatment is generally first used. It is helpful in delineating the etiology of flatus from swallowed air (mostly nitrogen and oxygen) or from intrinsic bacterial formation of gases (mostly hydrogen, carbon dioxide, and methane).

Given the multitude of ancillary tests available to evaluate flatus, the challenge for the primary care physician is to use them to help confirm or exclude specific diagnoses that are suggested from the history.

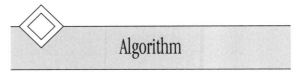

Algorithm

A simplified algorithm for the incorporation of testing is suggested in Figure 11-2. It emphasizes a stepwise approach based on history and physical exam, with initial minimal testing if the flatulence is not associated with other worrisome symptoms (systemic symptoms, weight loss, nocturnal or bloody diarrhea, change in bowel habits, localized abdominal pain).

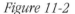

Treatment

If the history and physical exam suggest a benign etiology for flatulence, many empiric treatments can be tried, including dietary modification and medications.

Dietary and behavior modifications are the most successful therapies for patients with flatulence.

This is obviously dependent on the food or behavior that has been identified to produce the flatulence. For example, chronic aerophagia is always a voluntary process. Biofeedback can be helpful. Reviewing eating habits may identify someone who drinks or eats quickly, drinks many carbonated beverages, or chews gum all day; these habits can easily be modified. Chronic belching will also increase aerophagia and should be avoided.

Dietary manipulation is essential, and patients should be advised concerning foods that are gas

Figure 11-2

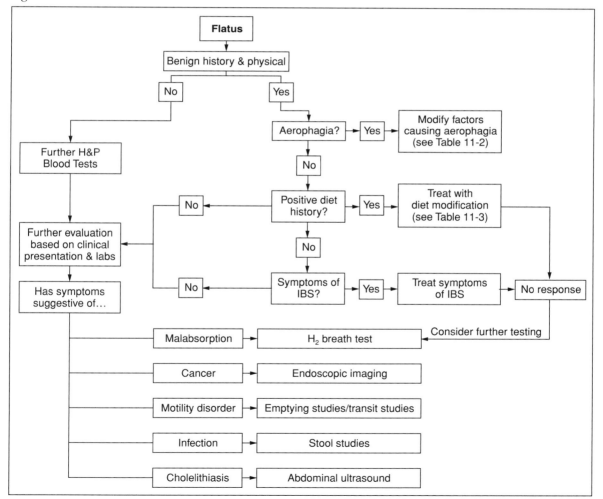

Algorithm for management of flatulence. H&P, history and physical; IBS, irritable bowel syndrome.

and odor-producing (Table 11-3) and foods that are not (Table 11-4). Elimination diets, in which different foods are excluded from the diet in a stepwise manner, can help identify a food source of flatus.

Table 11-3

Foods That Cause Flatulence

Milk Products	Eggplant
Fruits	Garlic*
Apples	Onions*
Apricots	Cereals
Bananas	Bran
Peaches	Wheat with
Pears	gluten
Prunes	Sweeteners
Raisins	Fructose-
Vegetables	containing
Artichokes,	foods
Jerusalem	Maltitol
Beans*	Sorbitol
Broccoli	Other
Brussel sprouts	Olestra
Cabbage*	Nuts*
Carrots	Soybeans
Cauliflower	Additives to beer
Celery	and bread*

*Signifies food causing significant odor.

Table 11-4

Foods That Cause Minimal Flatulence

Red meat	Zucchini
Chicken	Fruits
Fish	Berries
Vegetables	Cantaloupe
Asparagus	Rice
Avocado	Corn meal
Lettuce	Popcorn
Okra	Eggs
Olives	Nonmilk chocolate
Pepper	

Medications: Do They Work?

There are a host of mostly over-the-counter time-honored medications that are said to work for flatulence, sometimes with little data to support their use. However, most of these medications are well tolerated and can be tried without many side effects. Most medications work by either decreasing intestinal gas or regulating bowel function.

DECREASING INTESTINAL GAS

Activated charcoal, a substance used for flatus since 1000 B.C., may reduce hydrogen and hydrogen sulfide excretion by adsorbing and binding the gases. Its efficacy is unclear; however, in some small studies it decreased flatus odor and amount. It can be taken as 2 tablets (520 mg) 30 min before meals.

Bismuth subsalicylate (Pepto-Bismol) and Bismuth subgallate (Devron) may decrease odor by binding to hydrogen sulfide. They do not change significantly the amount of flatulence. Hydrogen sulfide is also considered a possible toxic substance to the lumen of the gut in patients with ulcerative colitis. Therefore, theoretically, bismuth can be good for these patients as well. Bismuth can induce neurotoxicity if used for long periods, so recommended use does not exceed 8 weeks. Typical doses are 2 tablets with each meal.

Simethicone (Gas-X, Mylicon, and Phazyme) is a silicon polymer that changes the elasticity of gas bubbles, making them coalesce. There are no adverse effects to simethicone; however, its effectiveness is unclear. Doses range from 40 mg to 125 mg before meals. Often, medications with simethicone contain other ingredients such as peppermint oils, calcium, or aluminum hydroxide which may or may not help alleviate bloating or flatulence.

α-Galactosidase (Beano) is an enzyme derived from *Aspergillus niger*. It decreases bacterial fermentation by degrading oligosaccharides, found in beans, vegetables, and cereals, to simple sugars, especially galactose. It may have some effectiveness. It should be avoided in patients with galactosemia. Typical doses are 5 to 15 drops on the first bite of food, or 2 to 3 tablets per cup of food.

β-Galactosidase (Lactaid) enzyme, derived from *A. oryzae,* is available for lactose-intolerant patients. It is used in conjunction with dietary manipulation. Its effects can be varied with minimal to full resolution of patients' symptoms, depending on the degree of lactose intolerance and effectiveness of the dose of lactase. It can be incubated in milk overnight: 5 drops in 8 oz of milk provides 70 percent hydrolysis; 15 drops, 100 percent hydrolysis. There are also preincubated milk products. Also, the enzyme can be dosed as 1 to 2 tablets, typically 4500 to 6000 U, taken with dairy products. The amount varies and is titrated according to symptoms. Other enzymes are available (lipase, trizyme, and pancreatic enzymes) and should be used judiciously.

Antibiotics such as metronidazole, fluoroquinolones, and tetracycline are used for the treatment of bacterial overgrowth. By changing or eliminating different types of bowel flora, they can change the proportion of gases produced and decrease flatulence and possibly odor.

REGULATING BOWEL FUNCTION

Isphagula husk (Fybogel, Regulan) is a non-starch polysaccharide fiber that helps regulate bowel movements and may be helpful in patients with IBS. It is a bulk-former and causes additional flatulence in the first week of use. However this decreases over time, and patients may actually have less flatulence as their bowel habits become regular. Other fibers such as psyllium, a derivative of isphagula husk, or methylcellulose (Citrucel) can help in constipation and IBS, but their use must be balanced with the increased flatulence they produce.

Prokinetic agents such as metoclopromide are useful in patients with motility disorders (which should be documented by motility testing) or IBS. Many other miscellaneous drugs have also been tried. Zinc and chlorophyllin copper complex solution (derefil, Rystan) may decrease flatus odor. Peppermint oil may relieve belching and decrease air swallowing. Smooth muscle relaxants, such as hyoscine or dicyclomine, may also relieve bloating. Laxatives and stool softeners should be used in patients with constipation.

Figure 11-3

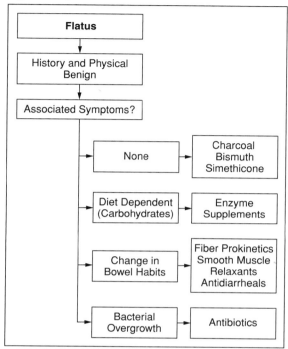

Drug therapy for benign flatulence.

These medications are generally all benign and can be given empirically if no serious etiology has been elicited in history, physical exam, and laboratory investigations. Recommendations on which medications to initially try can be based on the patients' primary symptoms, excluding flatulence, or on the context in which the flatulence occurs (Figure 11-3).

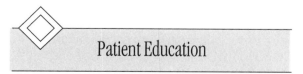

Patient Education

Patients should understand the important role their diet has in the management of flatulence. Patients should be taught to use a symptom and food diary, in which all foods consumed are listed and any symptoms are correlated to the time that food was ingested. A list of foods that are flatulogenic (Table 11-3) can be provided. This often helps to identify a specific food causing excess flatulence. Patients should also be counseled on how, in a stepwise fashion, to eliminate certain foods from their diet. A dietitian may be helpful. If patients are found to be air swallowers, they should be educated on maneuvers to avoid this.

Patients should also be told that "normal" amounts, frequency, and odor of flatulence vary considerably and that isolated flatulence rarely suggests an underlying pathologic process. Patients can be counseled concerning the different types of medications that may be appropriate for them.

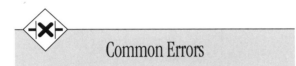

Common Errors

The main error in the evaluation of flatulence is overtesting. History and physical exam with concomitant empiric therapy should direct testing. The main reason to pursue tests other than blood tests are any associated symptoms, especially those of change in bowel habits, anorexia, chronic diarrhea, weight loss, and rectal bleeding.

Another common assumption by both physician and patients is that symptoms are from only one source. For example, in one study of patients that were self-described as lactose intolerant, one-third were not actually lactose intolerant based on hydrogen breath testing, and the incidence of bloating, diarrhea, and flatus was not different between people taking 8 oz of lactose-hydrolyzed milk versus those taking regular milk. These patients may have had an overlap with IBS or another etiology. Dietary logs should be kept in a rigorous fashion to make sure that a food is definitely the reason for flatulence. However, in general, enzyme deficiency is an underdiagnosed phenomenon.

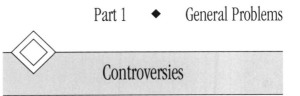

Controversies

Most of the controversies about flatulence have been mentioned, including the definition of norms of flatus and the appropriateness of laboratory testing. There is not much literature on the best way to manage patients with flatus; as a result, the discretion and judgment of each individual physician is still most important. Also, medical therapy relies on mostly unproven drugs.

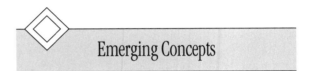

Emerging Concepts

Flatulence is a universal phenomenon, written about throughout thousands of years, and yet, the treatments are not extremely sophisticated. The main advances of the twentieth century have been in the area of breath testing and flatus analysis. Also, many of the dietary etiologic factors have been teased out and the lists of foods to avoid get longer....

In summary, flatulence has a long history with fairly well-defined norms. Most people with flatulence without associated symptoms of weight loss, anorexia, and rectal bleeding will have aerophagia, carbohydrate enzyme deficiency, or IBS. Treatment is largely empiric, with a large proportion of it consisting of dietary and behavior modifications. For the most part, flatulence is "full of sound and fury, signifying nothing" (Shakespeare), but for those who have symptoms of concern, laboratory tests and further diagnostic tests, whether breath tests, endoscopy, or motility studies, are indicated.

Bibliography

Bassotti G, Germani U, Morelli A: Flatus-related colorectal and anal motor events. *Dig Dis Sci* 41(2):335, 1996.

Behall KM, Scholfield DJ, van der Sluijs AM, et al: Breath hydrogen and methane expiration in men and women after oat extract consumption. *J Nutr* 128:79, 1998.

Bolin TD, Stanton RA: Flatus emission patterns and fibre intake. *Eur J Surg* (Suppl) 582:152, 1998.

Curless R, French J, Williams GV, James OFW: Comparison of gastrointestinal symptoms in colorectal carcinoma patients and community controls with respect to age. *Gut* 35:1267, 1994.

Davies GJ, Dettmar PW, Hoare RC: The influence of ispaghula husk on bowel habit. *J R Soc Health* 118(5):267, 1998.

Furne JK, Levitt MD: Factors influencing frequency of flatus emission by healthy subjects. *Dig Dis Sci* 41(8): 1631, 1996.

Ganiats RG, Norcross WA, Halverson AL, et al: Does Beano prevent gas? *J Fam Pract* 39:441, 1994.

Jain NK, Patel VP, Pitchumoni CS: Efficacy of activated charcoal in reducing intestinal gas: A double-blind clinical trial. *Am J Gastroenterol* 81(7):532, 1986.

Kamal N, Chami T, Andersen A, et al: Delayed gastrointestinal transit times in anorexia nervosa and bulimia nervosa. *Gastroenterology* 101:1320, 1991.

Kapadia CR: Motor abnormalities, in Spiro HM (ed): *Clinical Gastroenterology*, 4th ed. New York, McGraw-Hill, 1993, p 577.

King TS, Elia M, Hunter JO: Abnormal colonic fermentation in irritable bowel syndrome. *Lancet* 352:1187, 1998.

Levitt MD, Furne J, Aeolus MR, et al: Evaluation of an extremely flatulent patient. *Am J Gastroenterol* 93(11):2276, 1998.

Levitt MD, Lasser RM, Schwartz JS, Bond JH: Studies of a flatulent patient. *N Engl J Med* 295:260–262, 1976.

Liu J, Chen G, Yeh H, et al: Enteric-coated peppermint oil capsules in the treatment of irritable bowel syndrome: A prospective, randomized trial. *J Gastroenterol* 32:765, 1997.

Malagelada JR: Lactose intolerance (editorial). *N Engl J Med* 333:53, 1995.

Perman JA, Boatwright DN: Approach to the patient with gas and bloating, in Yamada T (ed): *Textbook of Gastroenterology*, 3rd ed. Philadelphia, Lippincott, Williams & Wilkins Company, 1999, p 815.

Pray WS: Excessive gas: What can be done? *U.S. Pharmacist* 23(6):22, 1998.

Rao SC: Belching, bloating, and flatulence. *Postgrad Med* 101(4):263, 1997.

Shaw AD, Davies GJ: Lactose intolerance. *J Clin Gastroenterol* 28(3):208, 1999.

Simethicone for gastrointestinal gas. *The Med Lett* 38 (977):57, 1996.

Spiro HM: Fat, foreboding, and flatulence. *Ann Intern Med* 130:320, 1999.

Storey DM, Koutso GA, Lee A, et al: Tolerance and breath hydrogen excretion following ingestion of maltitol incorporated at two levels into milk chocolate consumed by healthy young adults with and without fasting. *J Nutr* 128:587, 1998.

Suarez FL, Furne J, Springfield J, Levitt MD: Failure of activated charcoal to reduce the release of gases produced by the colonic flora. *Am J Gastroenterol* 94(2):208, 1999.

Suarez FL, Furne JK, Springfield JR, et al: Bismuth subsalicylate markedly decreases hydrogen sulfide release in the human colon. *Gastroenterology* 114:923, 1998.

Suarez FL, Furne JK, Springfield JR, et al: Identification of gases responsible for the odor of human flatus and evaluation of a device purported to reduce this odor. *Gut* 43:100–104, 1998.

Suarez FL, Savaiano DA, Levitt MD: A comparison of symptoms after the consumption of milk or lactose-hydrolyzed milk by people with self-reported severe lactose intolerance. *N Engl J Med* 333:1, 1995.

Suarez FL, Springfield J, Furne JK, et al: Gas production in humans ingesting a soybean flour derived from beans naturally low in oligosaccharides. *Am J Clin Nutr* 69:135, 1999.

Tomlin J, Lowis C, Read NW: Investigation of normal flatus production in healthy volunteers. *Gut* 32(6): 665, 1991.

Traber P: Carbohydrate assimilation, in Yamada T (ed): *Textbook of Gastroenterology*, 3rd ed. Philadelphia, Lippincott, Williams & Wilkins Company, 1999, p 404.

David D. K. Rolston

Acute Diarrhea in Adults

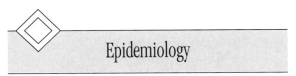

Definition

Acute diarrhea is an increase in stool liquidity or a decrease in consistency, often associated with an increase in stool frequency and volume compared with patients' usual bowel habits. Thus, individuals who normally are constipated and pass one hard stool per day should be regarded as having diarrhea if they start passing 2 semisolid stools per day. Diarrhea persisting beyond 4 weeks is regarded as chronic.

Normal stool weight in adult residents of industrialized countries is defined as less than 200 g/24 h. Individuals who pass stools in excess of 200 g/24 h have diarrhea. This latter definition has been questioned and is clearly not helpful for the practicing physician.

Epidemiology

Diarrheal illness in developing countries is known to cause approximately 3 million deaths in children younger than 5 years of age. Although there are no precise data available on diarrhea-related deaths in adults in these countries, there is no question that diarrhea does result in deaths and considerable morbidity.

In the United States, the estimated incidence of acute diarrhea in adults is 99 million per year, or approximately 1 episode per adult per year. Of these, approximately 8 million are seen by a physician and approximately 250,000 are hospitalized, making acute diarrhea an illness often seen by both primary care physicians and gastroenterologists.

The death rate for children and young adults with diarrhea is 2 to 3 per 100,000. It is dramatically higher in the elderly at 15 per 100,000 adults over the age of 74 years, making this group of individuals truly at risk of death from diarrheal illness.

Table 12-1

Causes of Acute Diarrhea

Bacteria
  Toxin producing
    Staphylococcus
    Vibrios
    Clostridium
    Escherichia coli, enterotoxigenic
  Predominantly invasive
    Salmonella
    Shigella
    E. coli
    Campylobacter
    Aeromonas
    Yersinia
    V. vulnificus
Viruses
  Norwalk virus
  Adenovirus
  Rotavirus, type B
  Astrovirus
  Small round virus
Parasites
  Predominantly small bowel
    Giardia
    Cyclospora
    Isospora belli
  Predominantly large bowel
    Entamoeba histolytica
    Cryptosporidium
    Balantidium coli
Medications (see Table 12-6)
Food toxins
  Ciguatoxin from carnivorous reef fish
  Scombroid
  Tetrodotoxin from puffer fish
  Fungi, *Amanita phalloides*
  Chemicals
Neuropeptides
  Vasoactive intestinal polypeptide
  Gastrin
  Glucagon
Inflammatory bowel disease
  Ulcerative colitis
  Microscopic colitis
Pseudodiarrhea
Factitious diarrhea

Most cases of diarrhea are due to an infectious agent (Table 12-1) and occur following ingestion of foods or water contaminated with the infective organism. Adults who work in day care centers, travelers to subtropical or tropical countries, immunosuppressed individuals, homosexuals, hospitalized individuals, residents of nursing homes and mental institutions, and those living in unsanitary environments are particularly prone to infections that cause diarrhea.

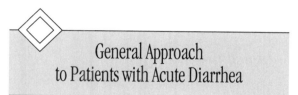

General Approach to Patients with Acute Diarrhea

In patients with diarrhea, it is important to first ascertain whether the diarrhea has its origin in the small or large intestine. Despite some degree of overlap, the etiology, mechanisms involved, and metabolic effects are different in each case. The history should help the clinician assess the severity of the diarrhea and determine the degree of intravascular volume depletion. The history can also give a clue to the etiology of the diarrhea. Knowing the origin of the diarrhea (small versus large intestine), severity, and probable cause are basic to planning treatment.

Small-Bowel versus Large-Bowel Diarrhea

Features that help distinguish acute diarrhea of small-bowel origin from that of the large bowel are given in Table 12-2. It is important to categorize the diarrhea as originating predominantly from the small intestine or predominantly from the large intestine. Most infectious diarrheal illnesses with predominant small-bowel involvement are due to bacterial toxins (e.g., staphylococcal toxin), viruses,

Table 12-2

Differentiation between Small-Bowel and Large-Bowel Diarrhea

	SMALL-BOWEL DIARRHEA	LARGE-BOWEL DIARRHEA
	CLINICAL FEATURES	
Volume	Large	Small
Consistency	Watery	Soft, jelly-like
Blood and mucus	Rare	Often present
Pain	Periumbilical or right lower quadrant, intermittent; often persists after defecation	Hypogastrium and left lower quadrant, relieved by defecation
Fever	Mild, <101°F, (38.33°C)	Usually >101°F (38.33°C)
Tenesmus	Absent	May be present
	INVESTIGATIONS	
Stool		
White blood cell count	−	+
Lactoferrin	−	+
Blood	−	+
Sigmoidoscopy	Normal	Ulcers/erythema/friable mucosa

NOTE: −, absent; +, present.

Table 12-3

Mechanisms of Diarrhea

> Secretory diarrhea
> Caused by mediators of intestinal secretion
>   Bacterial toxins
>   Polypeptides
>   Leukotrienes
> Diffuse mucosal disease
>   Celiac sprue
>   Tropical sprue
> Congenital ion transport defects
>
> Osmotic diarrhea
> Exudative or inflammatory diarrhea
>   Invasive diarrheas
>   Ulcerative colitis
>
> Motility disorders
>   Hypermotility as in thyrotoxicosis
>   Hypomotility encourages bacterial
>   overgrowth

NOTE: More than one mechanism may contribute to diarrhea in any one patient.

or protozoa such as *Giardia* or *Cyclospora,* whereas diarrheal illnesses with predominant large-bowel involvement are due to invasive organisms such as *Shigella.* Organisms that infect the colon may, in the early stages, produce a small-bowel type of diarrhea (watery diarrhea).

Once it is determined whether the small bowel or large bowel is predominantly involved, it is then useful to determine the underlying mechanism of the acute diarrhea. This may be secretory, osmotic, exudative, or inflammatory or be due to a disorder of motility (Table 12-3). More than one mechanism may contribute to diarrhea in a single patient.

SECRETORY DIARRHEA

Secretory diarrhea may be a result of one of the following:

1. The action of bacterial toxins, gut peptides such as vasoactive intestinal polypeptide, 5-hydroxy-

tryptamine (in patients with the carcinoid syndrome), inflammatory cell mediators, some laxatives, or bile acids on intestinal cell cyclic nucleotides, calcium, or protein kinases
2. Diffuse mucosal disease (e.g., celiac and tropical sprue, resulting in the loss of the absorptive villus cells and, therefore, net secretion)
3. Rare congenital ion transport defects (e.g., Cl^-/HCO_3^-, which causes congenital chloridorrhea and alkalosis, and Na^+/H^+ exchange defects, which result in high sodium concentrations in the stool and metabolic acidosis)

OSMOTIC DIARRHEA

Osmotic diarrhea is a result of fluid secreted into the intestinal lumen in response to poorly absorbed osmotically active intraluminal substances (e.g., intraluminal lactose in lactase-deficient individuals). Table 12-4 shows the distinguishing features between secretory and osmotic diarrhea.

EXUDATIVE OR INFLAMMATORY DIARRHEA

Inflammatory diarrhea, as in ulcerative colitis or bacillary dysentery, causes not only blood, mucus, and protein exudation, but also impaired water and electrolyte absorption. The result is diarrhea with blood and mucus.

MOTILITY DISORDERS

Changes in motility may play a role in the pathogenesis of diarrhea in some conditions. Hypermotility may be an important contributory cause of diarrhea in hyperthyroidism, whereas hypomotility allows bacterial overgrowth, which then causes deconjugation of bile salts and, therefore, secretory diarrhea.

OTHER FACTORS

Some organisms, such as enterotoxigenic *Escherichia coli* (ETEC), in addition to producing the secretogenic toxins also produce fimbrial colonization factor antigens. These factors facilitate

Table 12-4

Features of Secretory and Osmotic Diarrhea

	SECRETORY	**OSMOTIC**
Effect of fasting	Diarrhea persists	Decreases or stops
Volume	Usually >1 liter/24 h	Usually <1 liter/24 h
Osmotic gap*	<50	>125
Fecal Na$^+$	>90	70
pH	6	<5
Reducing substances	−	±

*$290 - 2 [Na^+ + K^+]$; 290 is stool osmolality as it passes through the rectum. This value is more accurate than measured stool osmolality, which changes rapidly at room temperature.

adherence of the bacteria to the ligand receptors on the enterocyte surface. The ability to adhere to the intestinal epithelial cells serves two functions. First, it prevents the organism from being propelled caudally by peristalsis and therefore eliminated from the host. Second, it allows elaboration of the toxin close to the intestinal epithelial cell where it can exert its deleterious effects. A different mechanism of adherence has been described for Enteropathogenic *E. coli* (EPEC). In these organisms localized adherence is brought about by a bundle-forming pilus.

Several other factors also govern whether individuals exposed to enteric pathogens develop diarrhea and/or vomiting. These include the number of organisms ingested (inoculum size, Table 12-5), the

Table 12-5

Inoculum Size Necessary to Produce Disease

Shigella 10^{1-2}
Salmonella 10^5
Escherichia coli 10^6-10^8
Vibrio cholerae 10^{2-6}
Campylobacter 10^{2-3}
Giardia 10^{1-2} cysts
Entamoeba histolytica 10^{1-2} cysts
Cryptosporidum 10^{1-3} cysts

virulence of the organism, and host factors such as gastric acidity, intestinal motility, secretory gamma-A globulin (IgA) and circulatory gamma-G globulin (IgG) and gamma-M globulin (IgM) levels. Of these host factors, intestinal motility is probably the most important.

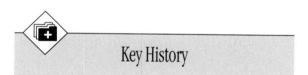

Key History

The history provides clues about the etiology of the diarrhea and which part of the bowel is predominantly involved. It also affords the opportunity to assess the severity of the diarrhea and the degree of intravascular volume depletion. Information regarding stool volume, frequency, character (color and consistency), presence of blood and mucus, tenesmus, and incontinence helps in determining whether abnormalities in the small intestine or the colon are primarily responsible for the diarrhea. The history also provides useful information about the underlying mechanism of the diarrhea (see Table 12-3).

History may be invaluable in pointing to the etiology. For example, patients may report a history of previous abdominal surgery (which may result in blind-loop syndrome); travel; recent food ingestion (its type and origin); contact with others

Table 12-6

Common Medications Which Can Cause Diarrhea

Antacids	Antidiabetic agents
Magnesium-containing	Metformin
H_2-receptor antagonists	Antihypertensives
Antiarrhythmic drugs	ACE inhibitors
Digoxin	Methyldopa
Quinidine	Hydralazine
Procainamide	Guanethidine
Antibiotics	Propranolol
Cephalosporins	Antiretrovirals
Clindamycin	Diuretics (especially the loop
Penicillins	diuretics)
Anticancer drugs	Prostaglandin analog
Azacitidine	Misoprostil
Actinomycin D	Laxatives
Cytosine arabinoside	Anthraquinones
Doxorubicin	Bisacodyl
5-Fluorouracil	Magnesium compounds
Methotrexate	Phenolphthalein
Antidepressants (especially the SSRIs)	Ricinoleic acid

Note: SSRIs, selective serotonin reuptake inhibitors; ACE, angiotensin-converting enzyme.

who have diarrhea; drinking potentially contaminated water (e.g., stream water); and sexual practices such as anal intercourse (associated with an increased risk for rectal herpes and gonorrhea). Diarrhea may be the presenting symptom in patients with AIDS.

The occupational history is also important. Day care workers are at increased risk for viral gastroenteritis, *Giardia,* and *Cryptosporidium* infections, whereas health care workers and nursing home residents may develop nosocomial enteric infections such as *Clostridium difficile, Salmonella,* and *Candida albicans.* It should be noted that nosocomial enteric infections may be followed by infections at other sites, particularly the urinary tract. In addition, a family history of diarrhea may provide clues to the rare multiple endocrine neoplasia syndromes and congenital transport defects.

A complete list of medications including over-the-counter medicines and herbs or health foods should be carefully documented since many medications can cause diarrhea (Table 12-6).

Finally, careful attention should be paid to patients' diets, particularly any recent dietary changes. Increased fiber intake, ingestion of milk or milk products, alcohol and seafood consumption, and foods that contain poorly absorbed sugar-alcohol may all be underlying causes or contributions to diarrhea.

Blood in the stool indicates that the mucosal lining of the gut has been eroded. Important noninfectious causes of blood in the stools include ulcerative colitis, Crohn's disease, ischemic bowel, diverticulitis, and radiation-induced mucosal damage.

Severe disease and, therefore, the need for clinical evaluation and possibly hospitalization are suggested by any of the following: persistent vomiting, profuse watery diarrhea or the passage of frequent blood and mucus stools, or marked or persistent abdominal pain or diarrhea for 48 h or longer. Excessive thirst, postural dizziness in the absence of autonomic neuropathy or medications, and a decrease in urine output are indicative of severe intravascular volume depletion.

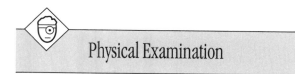

Physical Examination

Physical examination is not useful in identifying the cause of acute diarrhea. It is, however, useful in determining the degree of intravascular volume depletion (Table 12-7) and the severity of illness. High fever, abdominal tenderness, or distention indicates severe disease. Fever >101.3°F (38.5°C) is generally indicative of an invasive organism (see Table 12-1). A colonoscopy may be considered in the initial evaluation of patients with severe bloody diarrhea, particularly in immuno-

compromised patients or in those with any of the extraintestinal manifestations of inflammatory bowel disease, such as arthralgias, ankylosing spondylitis, erythema nodosum, pyoderma gangrenosum, iritis, uveitis, or cholangitis.

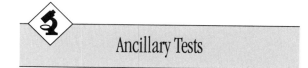

Ancillary Tests

The major reasons for attempting to find the cause of diarrhea are to identify those infectious agents for which treatment is available, to institute suitable control measures to contain the diarrhea, and to identify new organisms as a cause for diarrhea. Since acute diarrhea is self-limited in the majority of patients, mild illness requires no laboratory investigations. With more severe or protracted diarrhea, the etiology of infectious diarrhea may be deter-

Table 12-7

Assessment of Dehydration

SYMPTOMS AND SIGNS	MILD DEHYDRATION	MODERATE DEHYDRATION	SEVERE DEHYDRATION
General appearance	Thirsty, alert, irritable	Thirsty, restless, irritable, postural giddiness	Thirsty, restless, irritable, postural giddiness, peripheral cyanosis, wrinkled skin, muscle cramps
Pulse	Normal rate and volume	Rapid and decreased volume	Thready; may not be palpable
Systolic blood pressure	Normal	Normal	Low or unrecordable
Postural fall in systolic blood pressure	No	Present	If recordable, marked postural fall
Skin elasticity*	Normal	Decreased	Markedly decreased
Eyes	Normal	Sunken	Markedly sunken
Mucous membranes	Moist	Dry	Very dry
Urine volume	Normal	Diminished	Markedly diminished
Respiration	Normal	Increased†	Markedly increased†

*Not useful in malnourished or very obese individuals or the elderly.
†An indication of metabolic acidosis.

mined by a stool study—be it a smear (*Entamoeba histolytica*), culture (*Salmonella, Campylobacter*), electron microscopy (viruses), or an antigen (toxin). Appropriate stool examination must be carried out in the following situations:

1. Blood in the stool
2. High fever (>101.3°F, 38.5°C)
3. Severe abdominal pain
4. History of recent travel to an endemic area
5. Presence of an epidemic
6. Immunocompromised individual
7. Sickly appearance
8. History of tenesmus
9. History of antibiotic use

Stool Examination

It should be remembered that the etiologic agent is identified in only a minority of patients in an outpatient setting and in only 25 to 40 percent of hospitalized patients with severe diarrhea and repeated stool examinations. Fecal leukocytes, lactoferrin, and blood are useful in indicating that the diarrhea is inflammatory in origin (Table 12-8). Published studies report wide differences in the sensitivities (20 to 90 percent) and specificities (also 20 to 90 percent) for fecal leukocytes and blood as markers of an invasive organism in culture positive stools. The absence of fecal leukocytes suggests that the diarrhea may be due to a toxin, virus, or medication. Since stool cultures are expensive, to be cost-effective, the following guidelines are recommended:

1. Only stools from patients likely to have diarrhea secondary to an invasive organism are sent for culture.
2. The stool specimen must be fresh.
3. The mucus in the stool, if present, should be cultured rather than the stool itself. The likelihood of a positive yield is increased if the stool specimen has leukocytes present.
4. The laboratory should be alerted to the likely organism so that appropriate culture media and environment are used. For example, *Campy-*

Table 12-8

Investigations in Acute Diarrhea

Stool
    Leukocytes[*]
    Lactoferrin[†]
    Occult blood
    Ova and parasites[‡]
    Culture
    Detection of toxins
    Electron microscopy[§]
    pH
    Electrolytes
    Osmolality
    Alkalinization, to detect phenolphthalein-containing laxatives
Jejunal fluid
    Giardia
Blood tests
    Those useful in establishing a diagnosis
        Giardia antibody
        Peptide levels (e.g., VIP)
        Ameba, indirect hemagglutination
    Those useful in detecting the effects of acute diarrhea
        CBC, leukemoid reaction
        Electrolytes
        Renal function
Flexible sigmoidoscopy
Plain abdominal x-rays

[*]Detected by Wright's stain (1% methylene blue). A few white blood cells are normal.
[†]An indicator of inflammation.
[‡]In hospitalized patients after 3 days yield is close to zero.
[§]Primarily a research tool, most helpful in identifying viruses.
NOTE: VIP, vasoactive intestinal polypeptide; CBC, complete blood cell count.

lobacter require specially enriched media and a microaerophilic environment, whereas *Yersinia* require incubation at temperatures of 22 to 25°C (71.6°F to 77°F) and *Vibrio* require a thiosulfate-citrate-bile salts-sucrose (TCBS) agar, which inhibits growth of other organisms. The cytotoxin assay for *C. difficile* has a sensitivity of ~65 percent and specificity of 99 percent.

Stool Ova and Parasite Examination

Detection of ova and parasites in the stools is highly dependent on the skill of the examiner and on the freshness of the stool. Microscopic stool examination is the usual method for detecting *G. lamblia, E. hystolytica,* and *Cryptosporidium*. An acid-fast stain is required for *Cryptosporidium* detection. When stool examination is performed by an experienced examiner, the yield rate can be as high as 80 percent. Examination of serial fresh stool samples increases the yield. Barium, antacids, polyethylene-containing solutions, and previous antibiotic therapy can decrease parasite detection rates.

Measuring the stool's pH, sodium, and potassium concentrations and calculating the stool osmotic gap may help in distinguishing secretory from osmotic diarrhea (see Table 12-4). Serum electrolytes, glucose, blood urea nitrogen, and creatinine levels are required to assess metabolic status and renal function.

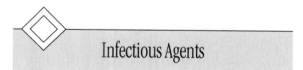

Infectious Agents

Viral Diarrheas

If all age groups are taken into consideration, viruses account for about one-third of all episodes of acute infectious gastroenteritis. Rotavirus, calcivirus, enteric adenovirus, Norwalk virus, and astrovirus multiply preferentially in the gastrointestinal tract and cause illness primarily in children and less often in adults.

Viruses are cytopathic to the absorptive villus cells, which then slough into the intestinal lumen. Villus cells are replaced by immature crypt cells that have poor absorptive function. This results in water, electrolyte, and nutrient malabsorption. Despite these functional abnormalities, the sodium-coupled glucose transport mechanism—the integrity of which is the basis for oral rehydration therapy

(ORT)—remains sufficiently intact to permit effective rehydration with glucose or starch-based electrolyte oral rehydration solutions.

The viruses responsible for gastroenteritis can be visualized by electron microscopy or detected by specific immunoassays, polymerase chain reactions, and nucleic acid probes—all research tools except for rotavirus antigen detection.

Generally the disease is abrupt in onset with vomiting a prominent symptom, especially in children. Diarrhea is usually mild and has the features of a small-bowel diarrhea (see Table 12-2). There may be associated crampy periumbilical pain, low-grade fever, headaches, and myalgias. The illness is short-lived, usually less than 48 h for the Norwalk virus and less than 5 days for rotavirus group B (the group usually responsible for diarrhea in adults). Abdominal examination may reveal hyperactive bowel sounds, generalized tenderness, particularly in the periumbilical region, with no evidence of peritonitis. Leukocytes are not found in the stool.

Bacterial Diarrhea

TOXIN-INDUCED DIARRHEA

A number of enteric bacteria produce an array of toxins (e.g., heat-stable toxins, heat-labile toxins, cytotoxins, and hemolysins). Some organisms, such as *Campylobacter, Shigella, Salmonella, C. difficle, Aeromonas,* and *Plesiomonas* are also invasive. The diarrhea may therefore be watery (from toxin production) or contain blood and mucus (from invasion).

ENTEROTOXIGENIC *ESCHERICHIA COLI* Enterotoxigenic *E. coli* (ETEC) is responsible for approximately 50 percent of all cases of traveler's diarrhea and, in developing countries, is a common cause of diarrhea in children. Both the organisms, heat-labile toxin (which resembles cholera toxin and acts by activation of adenyl cyclase) and heat-stable toxin (which activates guanylyl cyclase), result in net intestinal secretion of water and electrolytes.

There is nothing distinctive about the vomiting and diarrhea caused by ETEC. Disease severity can vary enormously. The illness may be mild and simply a nuisance or may be so severe as to result in prostration and severe dehydration. Fever is low grade, and stool leukocytes are absent.

CHOLERA   Both the classic and the El Tor biotypes of *V. cholerae* serotype 01 and the relatively new serogroup 0139 Bengal produce disease. While cholera is endemic in developing countries, it has been reported in the United States and Western Europe in individuals who have returned or eaten foods from countries where the disease is endemic. Most individuals who are exposed to the organism remain asymptomatic. The disease may be mild or severe. When severe, it is characterized by profuse and persistent vomiting and profuse, painless watery (secretory) diarrhea with more than 10 percent of body weight being lost in a matter of hours, severe electrolyte abnormalities, obtundation, and death. Fever is typically absent. The stool is watery and cloudy and has the appearance of water in which rice has been washed; hence the description of "rice-water" stools. Mucous flecks in the stools are characteristically present.

A rapid diagnosis can be made using dark-field or phase-contrast microscopy, which shows motile organisms. Stools should be plated directly onto a TCBS agar, which inhibits the growth of most other enteric organisms.

Restoration and maintenance of water and electrolyte balance are vital to survival and require aggressive ORT with glucose-electrolyte or starch polymer electrolyte solutions. Intravenous glucose-electrolyte solutions should be used if indicated. Concurrent antibiotic therapy for 2 days with either tetracycline, one of the macrolides, or trimethoprim-sulfamethoxazole decreases both diarrhea volume and duration. Tetracycline can be used for prophylaxis.

The killed vaccine, given intramuscularly, once thought to give protection, especially to travelers to endemic areas, is ineffective and is no longer recommended. Several live vaccines are currently being evaluated.

INFLAMMATORY DIARRHEA DUE TO INVASIVE ORGANISMS

Large-bowel-type diarrhea and systemic symptoms such as fever generally characterize the illness produced by these organisms.

SHIGELLA   *Shigella* organisms are highly pathogenic. Therefore, relatively few organisms are required to cause disease (see Table 12-5) and person-to-person disease transmission occurs easily. There are four *Shigella* subgroups (Table 12-9). Of these, group A *S. dysenteriae* causes the most severe illness and is associated with more complications than any one of the other subgroups. *S. sonnei* belongs to subgroup D, causes the mildest illness, and is the most prevalent species in the United States and in Britain.

All *Shigella* species are resistant to gastric acidity, the body's first line of defense against ingested pathogens. In the small intestine, the organism multiplies, releases enterotoxins (Shiga toxin and ShET-1 and -2) that cause watery (secretory) diarrhea, which frequently precedes the blood and

Table 12-9
Shigella Subgroups

Shigella sonnei	Most common in the United States
	Usually watery diarrhea
	Mild disease
S. flexneri	More severe disease
	Usually bloody diarrhea
S. boydii	Least common form
	Clinical features similar to *S. flexneri*
	Mainly found in the Indian subcontinent
S. dysenteriae	Severe blood and mucus diarrhea
	May result in prostration
	Can be fatal
	Multidrug resistant strains common in developing countries

mucus diarrhea. In the colon, the bacteria enter the colonocytes and possibly the M cells of mucosal lymphoid follicles by phagocytosis. Once within the cell they escape from the phagocytic vacuole and multiply. Spread from cell to cell occurs by bacteria-containing protrusions, which are endocytosed by adjacent cells generating, in the process, a severe inflammatory response. The Shiga toxin is enterotoxic, cytotoxic, and neurotoxic. Examples of other cytotoxin-producing bacteria are enterohemorrhagic *E. coli* (EHEC) 0157 and *C. difficile*.

With *S. sonnei* infection the illness is mild and is frequently associated with watery diarrhea without blood and mucus. In contrast, with the virulent *S. shiga*, blood and mucus diarrhea, fever, low abdominal colicky pain, tenesmus, vomiting, anorexia, and malaise are common. Complications are rare in adults and include toxic megacolon, intestinal obstruction, colonic perforation, bacteremia, leukemoid reaction, seizures, reactive arthritis, and the hemolytic-uremic syndrome. A diagnosis of shigellosis can be established by stool culture, or it can be more rapidly detected by finding the Shiga toxin in the stool. Rehydration and maintenance of water and electrolyte balance, as in all severe diarrheas, are of primary importance. Antibiotics shorten the duration of illness and reduce the incidence of the carrier state. Ampicillin (but not amoxicillin), trimethoprim-sulfamethoxazole, tetracycline, and ciprofloxacin are all effective.

***CAMPYLOBACTER* INFECTION**   Several *Campylobacter* species (*C. jejuni, C. coli, C. upsaliensis,* and *C. lari*) are pathogenic to humans. In the United States, *Campylobacter* infection is probably a more common cause of diarrhea than are *Shigella* and *Salmonella* combined.

The bacteria reach the human host from contaminated foods, but the pathogenesis of diarrhea has not been elucidated. As with other diarrheal illnesses, the disease can be mild, with only a few watery-semisolid stools, to severe bloody diarrhea, which is seen in 30 percent of all patients. The enteric illness caused by *Campylobacter* has been mistaken for acute appendicitis and ulcerative colitis. Complications include the hemolytic-

uremic syndrome, Reiter's syndrome, and Guillain-Barré syndrome.

Dark-field or phase-contrast microscopy shows darting organisms similar to *V. cholerae*. Micro-aerophilic conditions are required for growth in culture. It is not clear whether patients with *Campylobacter* benefit from antimicrobial therapy. The macrolides, quinolones, and tetracycline can be used.

ESCHERICHIA COLI   Enterohemorrhagic *E. coli* causes bloody diarrhea in the majority of cases. Transmission is by ingestion of contaminated foods, especially undercooked ground beef. Hemolytic-uremic syndrome and thrombotic thrombocytopenic purpura are known complications. Enteroinvasive *E. coli* (EIEC) is strikingly similar to *Shigella*, genetically, biochemically, and in the mode of presentation. Watery diarrhea is more common than is bloody diarrhea. In the United States, the disease is limited to rare, food-borne outbreaks. EPEC is primarily a disease of children and is extremely rare in industrialized countries.

PARASITIC DISEASES

G. lamblia and *Cryptosporidia* are the most common pathogenic intestinal parasites diagnosed in the United States. *Giardia* is transmitted by contaminated water and less frequently by contaminated foods. It tends to be more severe in hypochlorhydric individuals or those with secretory IgA deficiency.

Most of the individuals infected with *Giardia* remain asymptomatic or have a mild self-limited diarrheal illness. In acute giardiasis, watery diarrhea, crampy epigastric pain, nausea, vomiting, a characteristic "taste of rotten eggs in the mouth," bloating, flatulence, sulphurous burping, and fatigue are common. Symptoms generally persist for about a week and then either resolve or become chronic.

Diagnosis is established by identifying the cyst or the trophozoite form of the parasite in the stools, duodenal aspirate, or duodenal biopsy. Enzyme immunoassays and direct fluorescent antibody techniques to detect *Giardia* in stool have a sensitivity >95 percent and a specificity >95 percent. Metronidazole and furazolidone are effective in treating giardiasis. Medications not available in the United States that can be used for treatment include tinidazole and mepacrine.

HOSPITAL-ACQUIRED DIARRHEA

Hospital-acquired diarrhea is often thought to be secondary to *C. difficile* infection, especially in patients who have received or are currently receiving antibiotics, particularly clindamycin, the penicillins, or the cephalosporins. The diarrhea may occur several weeks after cessation of antibiotic therapy. Not all antibiotic-associated diarrheas are due to *C. difficile*. Antibiotics impair colonic fermentation of carbohydrates. This could result in an osmotic diarrhea. Some antibiotics such as erythromycin are prokinetic, binding to the motilin receptor and, therefore, resulting in diarrhea. Other potential causes of diarrhea in hospitalized patients include intolerance to nutrient supplements, tube feedings, a side effect of a medication, or the use of sorbitol- or mannitol-containing elixirs. Nevertheless, *C. difficile* remains the most common cause of diarrhea in hospitalized patients.

Traveler's Diarrhea

Of all Americans, 30 to 50 percent who travel to Africa, Southern Asia, the Middle East, and Latin America will develop diarrhea usually within the first few days of their arrival in the endemic area. The diarrhea, which may or may not be associated with vomiting, usually lasts from 1 to 5 days. A small percentage of travelers to high-risk areas may experience diarrhea only on their return home. Therefore, physicians in industrialized countries (low-risk areas) are faced with the challenge of advising travelers on preventive measures and treatment strategies should the traveler develop diarrhea. Recommendations for the prevention of infection in travelers are available on the Internet at www.cdc.gov.

Travelers should be advised to drink bottled beverages only, including water, or beverages that have been boiled. Water that has been filtered through an appropriate device or treated with a halogenated compound (e.g., chlorine) is also potable. Only fruits that are peeled by travelers should be eaten. Foods should be well cooked, and the core temperature of the food should reach over 70°C (158°F).

Prophylactic pharmacotherapy is generally not recommended because of the brief nature of the illness, the cost of antibiotics, the risk of side effects (some of them potentially fatal, e.g., Stevens-Johnson syndrome), the increased risk of promoting resistant organisms, and the risk, albeit small, of *C. difficile* diarrhea. Prophylactic antimicrobial therapy may be considered in the following circumstances: an insistent individual, an individual traveling to a high-risk area on an important business trip, immunocompromised individuals, and individuals with comorbid conditions such as inflammatory bowel disease, diabetes, and renal failure. Typically, prophylaxis should begin on the day of arrival in the endemic region and be continued for 2 days after the return home. Rarely should prophylactic treatment be continued beyond 3 weeks. The country visited and the season may determine the choice of prophylactic agent. Agents that may be used include bismuth subsalicylate, trimethoprim-sulfamethoxazole, doxycycline, azithromycin, and the quinolones (particularly ciprofloxacin).

Diarrhea in the Immunocompromised Host

Immunocompromised individuals are at risk of developing the same infections to which healthy individuals are susceptible. However, the clinical syndrome may be more severe, and organisms that rarely cause diarrhea in the normal host may do so in the immunocompromised host. These organisms include *Mycobacteria, Isospora belli, Cyclospora* species, *Microsporidium, Strongyloides stercolaris;* viruses such as astrovirus and picornavirus, cytomegalovirus, herpes simplex; and fungi such as histoplasmosis, coccidioidomycosis and *Candida albicans*. More than two pathogens may be detected in patients with diarrhea and AIDS. Patients with AIDS who have diarrhea without any obvious cause are said to have idiopathic AIDS enteropathy.

Neutropenic patients may develop typhilitis, an acute necrotizing colitis involving mainly the cecum. It is characterized by abdominal pain, mainly in the right lower quadrant, cecal edema and necrosis, and either watery or bloody diarrhea.

Patients with impaired cell-mediated immunity or on steroids are at particular risk of developing hyperinfection with *S. stercolaris*. This parasite can reside in human hosts for decades and cause few symptoms only to become a life-threatening illness when patients are given steroids.

Medications as a Cause of Diarrhea

Since a vast number of medications can cause diarrhea it is important to consider these as possibly causative in patients with diarrhea (see Table 12-6). Careful inquiry should be made concerning over-the-counter medications and herbal supplements, as well as health foods. Laxatives (in laxative abusers this history may be near impossible to obtain), antacids (especially magnesium-containing antacids), antineoplastic medications, antibiotics, antiarrhythmic agents, nonsteroidal anti-inflammatory drugs, antidepressants (especially the selective serotonin reuptake inhibitors), lithium, hypolipidemics, and antiretrovirals are most frequently implicated.

Idiopathic Inflammatory Bowel Disease

Ulcerative colitis and Crohn's disease are the two major idiopathic inflammatory bowel diseases. While the onset of idiopathic inflammatory disease is typically insidious, these diseases, particularly ulcerative colitis, may present as blood and mucus diarrhea, which, at least early in the course of the illness, is indistinguishable from that caused by invasive organisms. It is therefore important

that steroid therapy not be initiated until an infectious agent has been excluded with certainty.

Diarrhea in Runners

Gastrointestinal symptoms, including diarrhea, are common and occur in up to 25 percent of individuals who exercise vigorously, especially female marathon runners. Release of gut peptides (vasoactive intestinal polypeptide and gastrin) and mediators of inflammation have been implicated. No specific therapy has been found useful.

Awareness of this syndrome is important, not because it is common, but because in our health-conscious society it is likely that more and more individuals will be involved in vigorous exercise and will come to their primary care physician with abdominal symptoms including diarrhea.

Alcohol-Induced Diarrhea

It is important to ask patients with acute diarrhea about ingestion of alcohol, large quantities of which can cause diarrhea. Shortened transit time, decreased intestinal disaccharidase levels, reduced bile salts, and decreased sodium and water absorption have been implicated.

Emergence of New Diarrheal Syndromes and Pathogens

All physicians should be aware of the emergence of new diarrheal syndromes. One such syndrome is Brainerd diarrhea. This syndrome is named after the town of Brainerd, Minnesota, where it was first described. It is thought to be caused by either an infectious agent or a chemical toxin. Although a chronic illness, it can present as acute watery diarrhea that is explosive and is associated with urgency, fecal incontinence, mild abdominal cramps, and, later, mild weight loss. Nausea, vomiting, and fever are rare. Antimotility agents offer some relief.

ENTEROAGGREGATIVE *ESCHERICHIA COLI*

It is well known that ETEC, EPEC, EIEC, and EHEC cause diarrhea. Enteroaggregative *E. coli* (EAEC) is only now recognized as a pathogen not only in infants and children, in whom it is most often found, but also in adults. The illness is characterized by nausea, vomiting, diarrhea, and, less often, fever. It has been reported in adults from both developing and industrialized countries.

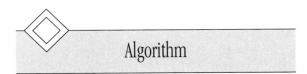

Algorithm

Figure 12-1 is an algorithm for the evaluation and treatment of acute diarrhea. Patients should be adequately rehydrated orally, unless there are specific indications for intravenous rehydration. The next step is to decide whether the diarrhea is due to an infection or to a noninfectious agent. If it is concluded that the diarrhea is due to an infection, a determination as to whether the diarrhea is inflammatory (i.e., blood and mucus) or noninflammatory (i.e., watery) should be made. If there are indicators of severe disease [>6 stools in 24 h, fever >101.3°F (38.5°C), or severe abdominal pain], the stools should be cultured and examined for ova and parasites. In immunocompromised individuals or in those with a possible nosocomial infection and bloody diarrhea, a sigmoidoscopy with rectal and colonic biopsies should be considered, in addition to examining the stools.

If patients have received antibiotics, *C. difficile* enterocolitis should be considered. If the stools are watery, for sporadic cases generally only rehydration is recommended.

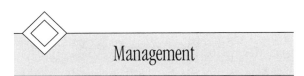

Management

The primary goal of acute diarrhea treatment in adults is to correct water and electrolyte deficits and maintain homeostasis. This is because acute diarrheal illness is short-lived irrespective of the etiology. In malnourished adults and children, adequate nutrient replacement during a bout of acute diarrhea is also important. Antimicrobial therapy is reserved for specific circumstances only.

Fluid and Electrolyte Replacement

Rehydration or maintenance of hydration by the oral route (ORT) with a glucose-electrolyte or a glucose-polymer-electrolyte solution is the therapy of choice. ORT has been used successfully in all age groups, worldwide, irrespective of the etiologic agent. The use of intravenous electrolyte solutions should be reserved for patients who are in hypovolemic shock, unable to drink adequate volumes of fluid (e.g., those with underlying swallowing problems or altered mental status, extremes of age, high-purging rates, and *severe* vomiting). It should be noted that ORT is often effective with high-purging rates and mild-to-moderate vomiting.

The World Health Organization (WHO) Oral Rehydration Solution (ORS) is composed of (in mM) sodium 90, potassium 20, chloride 80, bicarbonate 30, and glucose 111 with an osmolality of 330 mosm/kg; citrate can be substituted for bicarbonate. It is highly effective in repleting intravascular volume and correcting electrolyte abnormalities (hyponatremia, hypokalemia, hypochloremia, metabolic acidosis, and, less commonly, metabolic alkalosis—the latter of which reflects gastric acid losses) in adults, children, and infants, in industrialized as well as developing countries. It is equally effective as a maintenance oral fluid in patients with ongoing diarrhea and/or vomiting. Drinking adequate amounts of a solution made by adding ⅛ tsp salt and 1 level tsp sugar to 200 ml of water provides enough sodium and water to prevent dehydration and hyponatremia. Potassium should be supplemented with citrus juice.

Glucose-electrolyte solutions with low glucose and sodium concentrations and resultant hypotonicity are at least as effective as the WHO-ORS. The solution used by the International Study Group on reduced-osmolarity ORS used a solution with

Figure 12-1

Algorithm for Evaluation and Treatment of Acute Diarrhea

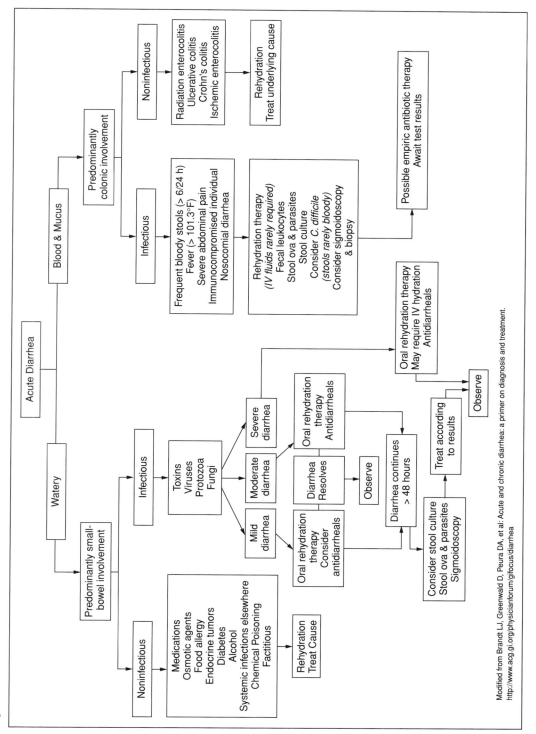

Modified from Brandt LJ, Greenwald D, Peura DA, et al: Acute and chronic diarrhea: a primer on diagnosis and treatment.
http://www.acg.gi.org/physicianforum/gifocus/diarrhea

the following composition (in mM): sodium 60, potassium 20, chloride 50, citrate 10, and glucose 84 with an osmolality of 224 mosm/kg. Adding excess water to rice, wheat, lentils, or potatoes and boiling results in the release of glucose polymers into the supernatant. Adding salt to the supernatant results in a solution that, if ingested in adequate volumes, effectively repletes intravascular volume, corrects electrolyte deficits, and provides more nutrients than a glucose-electrolyte solution. Commonly recommended fluids such as dilute tea, sodas, or Gatorade, to name but a few, should be avoided. They contain inadequate electrolytes and some are hypertonic and therefore have the potential to worsen diarrhea because of their osmotic effect. An ideal ORS should correct water and electrolyte deficits, replace ongoing losses, decrease purging rates, provide nutrients, have no side effects, and be inexpensive, easy to use, and widely available.

Food Restriction

Food restriction should not be recommended, particularly in children, because calorie and nitrogen deficits can occur rapidly in acute diarrhea due to decreased food intake, increased catabolism, and fecal nitrogen losses. Continued nutrition during acute diarrhea has been shown to improve gastrointestinal structure and function and, more importantly, clinical outcome.

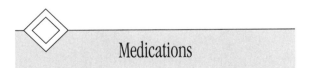

Medications

Adsorbents

Adsorbent drugs such as kaolin, pectin, and attapulgite are widely used for symptomatic relief of acute diarrhea. They have not been shown to alter the course of the illness but do increase the bulk of stools and, possibly, decrease the stool frequency.

Bismuth subsalicylate does reduce diarrhea because of the antidiarrheal effect of salicyclate. It also helps decrease vomiting.

Antimotility Agents

The opiate derivative lomotil (diphenoxylate plus atropine), an analog of meperidine and loperamide which is chemically related to haloperidol, is an antimotility agent that has an antisecretory effect as well. It is effective in reducing the duration and frequency of diarrhea. However, it should be used with caution, if at all, in patients with invasive diarrhea or inflammatory bowel disease for fear of precipitating a toxic megacolon. Its use should not take the place of ORT in any patient. Drugs such as zaldaride maleate and provir are currently being evaluated and may become the drugs of choice for symptomatic treatment of acute diarrhea because they have predominantly antisecretory effects with little or no antimotility action.

Antimicrobials

Antimicrobial therapy in general should not be used because it has little effect on the course of illness of most infectious causes of acute diarrhea, may prolong the carrier state, have potentially serious side effects, and expose patients to the risk of developing a *C. difficile*–induced diarrhea. Antimicrobials are useful in certain instances such as amebic dysentery, shigellosis, and *C. difficile*–induced diarrhea.

Antiemetics

Antihistamines with antiemetic activity (e.g., diphenhydramine and hydroxyzine) and the phenothiazines (e.g., prochlorperazine and promethazine) may be helpful in decreasing vomiting frequency. Drowsiness (which may interfere with ORT) and the more bothersome occasional extrapyramidal side effects, such as dystonia and oculogyric crisis with phenothiazines, should make one use these medicines with caution, especially in the elderly.

Biotherapeutic agents are microorganisms that are antagonistic to pathogenic microorganisms in vivo. These are not currently recommended either for treatment or prevention of acute diarrhea. Nevertheless, there are emerging data that bacteria such as *Lactobacillus casei* and *L. acidophilus* and the nonpathogenic yeast *Saccharomyces boulardii* may help decrease the incidence of antibiotic-associated diarrhea and prevent traveler's diarrhea. The results of carefully conducted double-blind clinical trials will help decide whether these agents should be used in routine clinical practice.

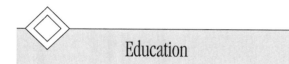

Education

Since the majority of cases of acute diarrhea are due to fecal contamination of drinking water and foods, ensuring a potable water supply, improving sanitation, and cooking foods at adequate temperatures are critical to interrupting the transmission of pathogens responsible for diarrhea. These measures have largely been achieved in industrialized countries. Hand-washing with soap and water and proper storage of foods can further reduce the incidence of these infections.

Although there is an abundance of data on the efficacy of ORT in acute diarrhea treatment, there continues to be a general reluctance by health care providers to accept and use this treatment modality. It should be recognized that ORT represents pharmacotherapy at its best. It is highly effective as a rehydrating agent, is cheap, easily administered, and when used correctly is virtually devoid of complications.

The public needs to be made aware of the ease with which an effective oral rehydration solution can be prepared at home for treating diarrhea of mild-to-moderate severity. Adding ⅛ tsp salt, 1 level tsp sugar to 200 ml of water provides

enough sodium and glucose to facilitate adequate water and sodium absorption to prevent dehydration and hyponatremia. Potassium should be supplemented with citrus juice.

Unfortunately the development of effective and safe vaccines against enteric pathogens has progressed slowly. Once effective vaccines become available, their use will constitute an important strategy in any intervention program.

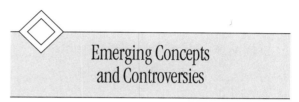

Emerging Concepts and Controversies

Oral rehydration therapy is now a well-established treatment modality for ensuring adequate hydration and electrolyte balance in patients with acute diarrhea. There is some discussion about whether a solution of one composition should be used for *rehydration* and another solution for *maintenance of hydration*. This is probably not an important issue because numerous studies have shown that a single glucose-electrolyte solution is effective for both purposes.

There are data indicating that oral rehydration solutions with lower glucose and sodium concentrations than the WHO-ORS may be more effective. Hypotonicity of these solutions is believed to be important in the improved efficacy of these solutions. Base precursors such as bicarbonate and citrate are probably not necessary for correcting the acidosis of mild-to-moderate diarrhea. Finally, the role of biotherapeutic agents in acute diarrhea treatment needs to be clarified.

Bibliography

Aranda-Michel J, Giannella RA: Acute diarrhea: A practical review. *Am J Med* 106:670, 1999.

Blacklow NR, Greenberg HB: Viral gastroenteritis. *N Engl J Med* 325:252, 1991.

Blaser MJ: How safe is our food? Lessons from an outbreak of salmonellosis. *N Engl J Med* 334:1324, 1996.

Caeiro JP, DuPont HL: Management of traveller's diarrhoea. *Drugs* 56:73, 1998.

Cody SH, Glynn MK, Farrar JA, et al: An outbreak of *Escherichia coli* 0157: H7 infection from unpasteurized commercial apple juice. *Ann Intern Med* 130:202, 1999.

Duggan C, Nurko S: "Feeding the gut." The scientific basis for continued enteral nutriton during acute diarrhea. *J Pediatr* 131:801, 1997.

DuPont HL: Guidelines on acute infectious diarrhea in adults. The Practice Parameters Committee of the American College of Gastroenterology. *Am J Gastroenterol* 92:1962, 1997.

Elmer G, Surawicz CM, McFarland LV: Biotherapeutic agents: A neglected modality for the treatment and prevention of selected intestinal and vaginal infections. *JAMA* 275:870, 1996.

Fine KD: Diarrhea, in Feldman M, Scharschmidt BF, Sleisenger MH (eds): *Gastrointestinal and Liver Disease,* 6th ed. Philadelphia, W.B. Saunders Co, 1998, p 128.

Grohmann GS, Glass RI, Pereira HG, et al: Enteric viruses and diarrhea in HIV-infected patients. *N Engl J Med* 329:14, 1993.

Guerrant RL, Steiner TS, Lima AAM, Bobak DA: How intestinal bacteria cause disease. *J Infect Dis* 179 (suppl 2):S331, 1999.

Herwaldt BL, Beach MJ, *Cyclospora* Working Group: The return of cyclospora in 1997: Another outbreak of cyclosporasis in North America associated with imported raspberries. *Ann Intern Med* 130:210, 1999.

International Study Group on Reduced-Osmolarity ORS Solution: Multi-centric evaluation of reduced osmolarity oral rehydration salt solution. *Lancet* 345:282, 1995.

Jones EM: Hospital acquired *Clostridium difficile* diarrhea. *Lancet* 349:1176, 1997.

Kotloff KL: Bacterial diarrheal pathogens. *Adv Pediatr Infect Dis* 14:219,1999.

Lebenthal E, Khin-Maung-U, Rolston DDK, et al: Thermophilic amylase-digested rice-electrolyte solution in the treatment of acute diarrhea in children. *Pediatrics* 95:198, 1995.

Lebenthal E, Khin-Maung U, Rolston DDK, et al: Safety and efficacy of a hydrolyzed rice-based oral rehydration solution in children. *J Am Coll Nutr* 14:299, 1995.

Lew EA, Poles MA, Dieterich DT: Diarrheal diseases associated with HIV infection. *Gastroenterol Clin North Am* 26:259, 1997.

Manabe YC, Vinetz JM, Moore RD, et al: *Clostridium difficile* colitis: An efficient clinical approach to diagnosis. *Ann Intern Med* 123:835, 1995.

McNeely W, DuPont HL, Matherson J, et al: Occult blood versus fecal leukocytes in the diagnosis of bacterial diarrhea. A study of US travelers to Mexico and Mexican children. *Am J Trop Med Hyg* 55:430, 1996.

Nataro JP, Steiner T, Guerrant RL: Enteroaggregative *Escherichia coli. Emerg Infect Dis* 4:251, 1998.

Passaro DJ, Parsonnet J: Advances in the prevention and management of traveler's diarrhea. *Curr Clin Top Infect Dis* 18:217, 1998.

Powell DW: Approach to the patient with diarrhea, in Yamada T, Alpers DH, Laine L, et al (eds): *Textbook of Gastroenterology,* 3rd ed. Philadephia, Lippincott Williams & Wilkins, 1999, p 858.

Rolston DDK: Treatment of acute watery infectious diarrhea in the tropics, in Rustgi VK (ed): *Gastrointestinal Infections in the Tropics.* Basel, Karger, 1990, p 224.

Schiller LR: Antidiarrhoeal pharmacology and therapeutics. *Aliment Pharmacol Ther* 9:87, 1995.

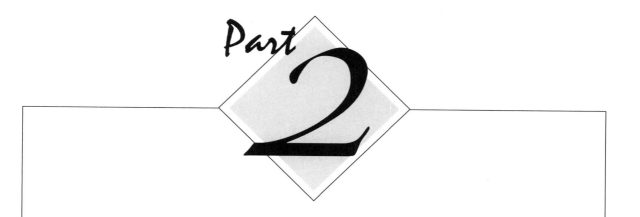

Lower GI Problems

Dordaneh Maleki

Chapter
13

Constipation

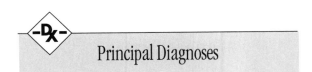

Incidence and Background

Epidemiology

Constipation is the most common digestive complaint in the United States, accounting for 2.5 million physician visits annually. It most commonly occurs in people 65 years old or older. In the United States alone, $400 million is spent annually on laxatives. A meta-analysis of 30 epidemiologic studies reported widely varying prevalence rates ranging from 1.4 to 16.9 percent depending on the definition of constipation. A population-based study of Olmstead county residents showed a prevalence rate of 11.0 percent for straining and 19.0 percent for the subjective complaint of constipation.

The prevalence of constipation increases in people 65 years old and older, with a small peak in young children. In addition, constipation is reported more in women and in nonwhite people than in white individuals. Epidemiologic studies have shown a geographical distribution. Constipation appears to be common in rural areas, cold temperatures, and low socioeconomic conditions.

Definition

Constipation is a symptom and, therefore, a subjective report of an individual's bowel function. Historically, *constipation* has been defined as the passage of less than three bowel movements per week. However, frequency alone is not a sufficient criterion; many constipated patients complain of excessive straining or discomfort on defecation. In addition, there is a discrepancy between what physicians and patients perceive as constipation. In view of the difficulty in defining *constipation*, an international committee has recommended an operational definition of chronic functional constipation (Table 13-1).

Table 13-1

Rome Criteria for Chronic Functional Constipation

> A. Patients not taking laxatives complain of 2 or more of the following for at least 12 months:
>   1. Straining with at least 25% of bowel movements
>   2. A feeling of incomplete evacuation with at least 25% of bowel movements
>   3. Hard or pellet stools with at least 25% of bowel movements
>   4. Stools less frequent than 3 per week.
>   **OR**
> B. Patient has fewer than 2 bowel movements per week on average for at least 12 months.

Principal Diagnoses

Based on the Rome criteria outlined in Table 13-1, constipation has been classified on the basis of stool frequency, consistency, and difficulty of defecation. With these recommendations, constipation has been categorized into two syndromes of "slow transit" and "rectosigmoid outlet delay."

The slow transit constipation syndrome may be caused by dietary habits, chronic diseases (Table 13-2), medications (Table 13-3), decreased mobility, and altered patterns of fluid intake. Rectosigmoid outlet delay refers to anorectal dysfunction. This syndrome is characterized by prolonged defecations (usually spending more than 10 min to complete a bowel movement) or by feelings of anal blockage (that is, often using manual maneuvers to aid in the passage of stool by placing fingers in or around the rectum or vagina). Rectosigmoid delay can also be caused by painful anorectal diseases such as anal fissures, perianal surgical procedures, trauma, or anorectal incoordination (dyschesia).

Table 13-2

Common Conditions Associated with Constipation in the Elderly Population

Metabolic conditions
   Diabetes mellitus
   Hypercalcemia
   Hypokalemia
   Heavy metal poisoning
   Hypothyroidism
   Hypomagnesemia
   Uremia
Mechanical obstruction
   Colon cancer
   External compression from malignant lesion
   Rectocele
   Strictures: diverticular or postischemic
   Postsurgical abnormalities
   Anal fissures
   Megacolon
Myopathies
   Scleroderma
   Amyloidosis
Neuropathies
   Spinal cord injury or tumor
   Cerebrovascular disease
   Parkinson's disease
   Multiple sclerosis
   Autonomic neuropathy
Miscellaneous conditions
   Depression
   Immobility
   Cardiac diseases

Table 13-3

Medications with a Side Effect of Constipation

Anticholinergic agents
Tricyclic antidepressants
Calcium channel blockers
Sympathomimetics
Antipsychotics
Diuretics
Antihistamines
Antiparkinsonian drugs
Opiates
Aluminum-containing antacids
Iron supplements
Bismuth
Calcium supplements
Nonsteroidal anti-inflammatory agents
Antidiarrheal medications

with outgoing, confident personalities had larger stools than did their introverted counterparts.

Constipation in children may involve psychological, as well as physiologic, factors and often results in fecal impaction. When clinically indicated, Hirschprung's disease should be excluded in this population. Some children withhold stool to gain attention, while others might have an aversion to defecation as a result of drafty houses or filthy plumbing.

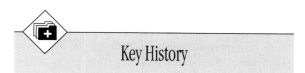

Key History

Many psychological conditions are associated with constipation, such as depression, anxiety, obsessive-compulsive neurosis, and psychological trauma as a result of sexual abuse. In the elderly population, dementia has also been reported to predispose to fecal impaction and fecal incontinence. In some adults, the inability to have a bowel movement due to social circumstances may cause constipation. One study found that after controlling for dietary fiber intake, the individuals

A careful history should evaluate patients' symptoms for the true presence of constipation based on the frequency (such as fewer than three bowel movements per week), consistency (lumpy or hard), and excessive straining as evidenced by prolonged defecation time or need to support the perineum or digitate the anorectum. A thorough diary of food and fluid intake, including the amount of dietary fiber, should be obtained from patients, as

Table 13-4
Indications for Gastroenterologist Referral

1. Recent onset of constipation associated with weight loss, abdominal pain, blood per rectum, heme-positive stool, or family history of colon cancer
2. Chronic constipation associated with a change in stool frequency or consistency, anemia, abdominal pain, or evidence of gastrointestinal bleeding
3. Failure to treat constipation with trial of diet, exercise, and bowel-training regimen
4. Constipation requiring high doses of laxative
5. New onset of fecal incontinence

well as a complete list of medications, including those that are over-the-counter and prescribed.

Attention to the medical conditions predisposing to constipation (see Table 13-2), including psychological issues, is important. In patients 50 years of age or older, any history of rectal bleeding or black stool or family history of colon cancer should prompt a colonoscopy to exclude malignancy (Table 13-4).

An effort should be made to distinguish between the two constipation syndromes of slow transit constipation and rectosigmoid delay. The history contains clues showing the amount of time spent on the toilet to have a bowel movement (usually more than 10 min), excessive straining, use of digits in or around the rectum or vagina to aid defecation, desire to defecate with inability to expel the stool, and history of sexual abuse.

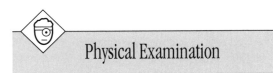

Physical Examination

Onset of constipation in persons 50 years of age and older warrants evaluation to exclude medical illness or mechanical obstruction due to colon can-

cer. Particular attention should be given to detection of masses in the rectum and abdomen. The rectal exam should also include the assessment of external anal sphincter tone, abnormal pelvic floor ballooning, and perineal descent during straining. A complete blood cell count, fasting blood glucose level, serum chemistry panel, and serum thyroid-stimulating hormone level should be done to exclude anemia, diabetes mellitus, hypokalemia, hypercalcemia, uremia, and hypothyroidism.

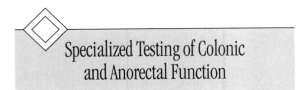

Specialized Testing of Colonic and Anorectal Function

For the small minority of patients who do not respond to dietary changes, mild laxative use, or bowel training, referral to a gastroenterologist is appropriate. Studies suggest that further evaluation of the physiologic function of the colon and anorectum help the physician to choose treatment.

Colonic transit time could be measured by a radiopaque marker, and the contractile activity of the colon can be measured by placing various pressure probes in the colon. The rectosigmoid outlet obstruction can be evaluated by anorectal manometry, balloon expulsion, and measurement of the anorectal angle. Anorectal manometry measures the pressures of the internal and external anal sphincter, while balloon expulsion and measurement of the anorectal angle evaluate the strength and coordination of the pelvic muscles. Defecography, a barium x-ray examination of the dynamics of defecation, is useful in evaluating the pelvic muscle coordination at defecation. Endorectal ultrasound evaluates anatomic integrity of the external and internal anal sphincter. Among patients with constipation who had thorough evaluation, including colonic transit time, colonoscopy, and anorectal function, a physiologic cause was found in only 50 percent of cases. Therefore, empiric treatment is often justified for constipation.

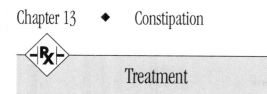

Treatment

The initial management of constipation is trial of nonpharmacologic measures. Patients should be informed about what is "normal" bowel movement. Ninety five percent of the population have at least three bowel movements per week. Patients should be educated about the gastrocolic reflex after meals and encouraged to have their bowel movements 30 min after meals. If possible, medications with a side effect of constipation should be discontinued. Treatment starts with a trial of increased fiber, fluid intake, and exercise. If there is no response within 2 to 3 weeks, the next step should be use of osmotic laxatives. If patients give a history of sigmoid outlet obstruction, then regular glycerin suppository or tap water enema is recommended. Stimulant laxatives are reserved for refractory cases because of their high side effect profile. Various agents used in the treatment of constipation and their most common side effects are listed in Table 13-5.

In the treatment of fecal impaction in the elderly, manual disimpaction is the first step. If the stool is beyond the reach of the examining finger, then oil retention or tap water enemas should be tried. Oral osmotic or stimulant laxatives should not be administered before rectal evacuation is achieved. Patients with fecal impaction should increase daily fluid intake to 1 to 2 liters a day and be on a regular enema schedule.

Exercise and Fiber

Dietary fiber is the first therapeutic measure. Most patients with constipation respond to a diet containing 20 or 30 g of dietary fiber and ample hydration (usually 8 to 10 glasses of noncarbonated fluid a day). Wheat bran is the best source of dietary fiber, but the side effect of bloating makes it less popular. Psyllium-containing fiber also causes abdominal gas and bloating since it is metabolized by colonic bacteria. Synthetic fiber products such as methylcellulose (Citrucel) and calcium polycarbophil (Fibercon tablets) are not digestible and hence produce less gas and discomfort than non-synthetic fiber. Introducing fiber in the diet should be done gradually, as a sudden increase may cause excess abdominal gas and discomfort. In addition, administration of fiber alone without increase of fluid intake may exacerbate constipation. The role of exercise in the pathogenesis of constipation is still not clear; however, increased physical activity has been recommended in patients with constipation.

Pharmacology

NONABSORBABLE DISACCHARIDES

Sorbitol, lactulose, and saline laxatives pass unchanged through the colon where they are broken down to smaller molecules, drawing fluid into the colonic lumen. These agents have minimal side effects and should be used as first-line agents. Sorbitol is as effective as lactulose but less expensive.

SALINE CATHARTICS

The most commonly used saline cathartics are the magnesium-containing products (e.g., Milk Of Magnesia). Their general mechanism of action is similar to the nonabsorbable disaccharides. The aluminum- and magnesium-containing products should be used with caution in patients with renal failure.

LUBRICANTS

Mineral oil taken orally lubricates the stool. In the elderly or those with impaired swallowing mechanism, there is a risk of aspiration and lipid pneumonia. In addition, long-term use of mineral oil can cause malabsorption of fat-soluble vitamins. Mineral oil may also cause fecal incontinence. In general, the use of these agents is not recommended. Topical ointment, sitz baths, and tucks pad can be beneficial to ease defecation.

Table 13-5

Medications Commonly Used for Constipation

Type	Generic Name	Dosage	Side Effects	Time to Onset of Action (h)
Fiber	Bran	1 cup/day	Bloating, iron, and Ca malabsorption	12–72
	Psyllium	1 tsp up to tid	Bloating, flatulence	
	Methylcellulose	1 tsp up to tid	Minimal bloating	
	Calcium polycarbophil	2–4 tablets qd	Bloating, flatulence	
Stool softener	Docusate sodium	100 mg bid	Ineffective for constipation	12–72
Hyperosmolar agents	Sorbitol	15–30 ml qd or bid	Transient abdominal pain, flatulence	24–48
	Lactulose	15–30 ml qd or bid	Same as sorbitol	24–48
	Polyethylene glycol	8–12 oz glass as needed	Fecal incontinence	0.5–1
Irritant	Glycerine suppository	Up to 2 daily	Rectal irritation	0.25–1
Stimulants	Bisacodyl	10 mg supp. 3 times/week	Incontinence, abdominal pain, hypokalemia, rectal burning with frequent use	0.25–1
	Anthraquinones	2 tablets qd to	Degeneration of enteric neurons, abdominal pain, dehydration, melanosis coli	8–12
	Senokot	4 tablets bid		
	Perdiem	1–2 tsp qd		
	Peri-colace	1–2 tsp qd		
	Phenolphthalein	1–3 tablets qd	Rash, malabsorption, dehydration	6–8
Saline Laxatives	Magnesium	15–30 ml qd or bid	Magnesium toxicity, abdominal pain, fecal incontinence	1–3
Enemas	Mineral oil retention	100–250 ml qd per rectum	Fecal incontinence, mechanical trauma	6–8
	Tap water	500 ml per rectum	Mucosal damage	5–15 min
	Phosphate	1 U per rectum		5–15 min
	Soapsuds	500 ml per rectum		5–15 min
Lubricants	Mineral oil	15–45 ml po qd	Lipid pneumonia, fat-soluble vitamin malabsorption, fecal incontinence, dehydration	6–8

bid=Twice a day; tid=three times a day.

STOOL SOFTENERS

Stool softeners have been shown to be useful only in cases where excessive straining is hazardous, such as in cardiac diseases or postoperative states; otherwise they have not been shown to be effective. Stool softeners may exacerbate fecal incontinence.

ORAL STIMULANTS

There are several over-the-counter oral stimulant preparations such as anthraquinones, phenolphthalein, castor oil, and bisacodyl. These agents act by changing the electrolyte concentration in the lumen of the colon and by producing propulsive activities. Prolonged and excessive use of stimulant laxatives can cause fat, calcium, and potassium malabsorption.

ENEMAS

Enemas evacuate the rectum and occasionally the rectosigmoid and descending colon. In the elderly, enemas should be administered by health care workers to avoid the risk of perforation. Phosphate and soapsuds may cause injury to the rectal mucosa. Rectal ischemia has been reported with long-term use of enema preparations.

PROKINETIC AGENTS

The role of prokinetic agents such as cisapride in the treatment of constipation is not clearly defined. The current studies show variable results. Cisapride (Propulsid) has been removed from the U.S. market, however, because of concerns regarding serious cardiac arrhythmias that may have developed in patients taking this agent.

OTHER PHARMACOLOGIC AGENTS

Antidepressants have been used in patients with "hypochondriacal" constipation, when reassurance and patient education fail. These agents should be used with caution since constipation is one of their side effects. Misoprostol can also be used for short-term treatment of intractable constipation; however, more long-term studies are needed.

Biofeedback Therapy

Patients with disordered defecation or rectosigmoid outlet delay syndrome (discussed earlier) may benefit from biofeedback therapy—training of the pelvic floor muscles used in defecation. The success rate of biofeedback therapy in the treatment of intractable constipation has been reported to be as high as 80 percent in some studies. Psychological counseling is helpful in combination with biofeedback, especially in those patients with an underlying psychological condition.

Surgical Treatment

In patients with intractable constipation who fail medical therapy, total or partial colectomy may be considered. The key to a successful surgery is careful selection of patients. Those with rectosigmoid outlet delay, as well as small-bowel and gastric dysmotility, should be excluded from consideration for total or partial colectomy for constipation. Patients with rectosigmoid delay syndromes should undergo biofeedback therapy before surgical removal of the large bowel. More studies are needed to show the long-term effectiveness of partial colectomy in the treatment of chronic constipation.

Patients who have significant anatomic defects associated with constipation are prime candidates for surgical therapy in the treatment of rectocele and rectal intussusceptions. During defecography, these patients should demonstrate preferential filling of the rectocele at defecation instead of expulsion of barium. In the case of rectal intussusceptions, there should be evidence of complete rectal outlet obstruction due to funnel-shaped plugging at the anal canal.

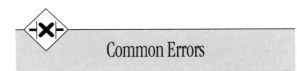

Patient Education

The most important part in the education of patients and health care workers is to correctly define constipation. Next, patients should be educated on the beneficial effects of dietary fiber, ample fluid intake, and physical exercise on regular bowel habits. Physicians should make a careful review of over-the-counter and herbal preparations, and patients should be educated about the use of over-the-counter "natural" laxatives. Many "natural" or herbal preparations contain laxatives such as senna alkaloids that are used in last steps of the recommended stepwise approach to treatment of constipation. Patients should be given a list of various food choices with corresponding fiber contents in order to help them match their dietary fiber intake to the recommended 20 to 30 g of fiber a day.

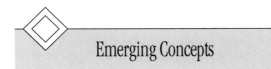

Common Errors

One of the most common errors made is in the diagnosis of constipation. It is important for physicians to use the correct definition of constipation and to distinguish between slow transit and sigmoid outlet obstruction syndromes. Another common error is the incorrect use of laxatives. It is important to start with laxatives that cause the least amount of side effects first (see "Pharmacology" and Table 13-5).

Emerging Concepts

New developments in the field of colorectal function are mainly in the areas of treatment and diagnosis of abnormal colonic motor and sensory function. New $5HT_4$ agonists are currently in the forefront of research for treatment of constipation.

Bibliography

Anti M, Pignataro G, Armuzzi A: Water supplementation enhances the effect of high-fiber diet on stool frequency and laxative consumption in adult patients with functional constipation. *Hepatogastroenterology* 45:727–732, 1998.

Badiali D, Corazziari E, Habib FI, et al: Effect of wheat bran in treatment of chronic nonorganic constipation: A double blinded controlled trial. *Dig Dis Sci* 40:349–356, 1995.

Camilleri M, Thompson WG, Fleshman JW, et al: Clinical management of intractable constipation. *Ann Intern Med* 121:520–528, 1994.

Corazziari E, Badiali D, Habib FI, et al: Small volume isosmotic polyethylene glycol electrolyte balanced solution (PMF-100) in treatment of chronic nonorganic constipation. *Dig Dis Sci* 41:1636–1642, 1996.

Farup PG, Hovdenak N, Wetterhus S: The symptomatic effect of cisapride in patients with irritable bowel syndrome and constipation. *Scand J Gastroenterol* 33:128–131, 1998.

Frame PS, Dolan P, Kohli R: Use of colchicine to treat severe constipation in developmentally disabled patients. *J Am Board Fam Med* 11:341–346, 1998.

Glia A, Gylin M, Gullberg K: Biofeedback retraining in patients with functional constipation and paradoxical puborectalis contraction: Comparison of anal manometry and sphincter electromyography for feedback 40:889–895, 1997.

Harari D, Gurwitz JH, Minaker KL: Constipation in the elderly. *J Am Geriatr Soc* 41:1130–1140, 1993.

Meza JP, Peggs JF, O'Brien JM: Constipation in the elderly patient. *J Fam Pract* 18:695; 698–699; 702–703, 1984.

Pemberton JH, Rath DM, Iistrup DM: Evaluation and surgical treatment of severe chronic constipation. *Ann Surg* 214:403–413, 1991.

Prather CM, Camilleri M, Zinsmeister AR, et al: Tegaserod accelerates orocecal transit in patients with constipation-predominant irritable bowel syndrome. *Gastroenterology* 118:463–468, 2000.

Romero Y, Evans JM, Fleming KC, et al: Constipation and fecal incontinence in the elderly population. *Mayo Clin Proc* 71:81–92, 1996.

Sandler RS, Jordan MC, Shelton BJ: Demographics and dietary determinants of constipation in the US population. *Am J Public Health* 80:185–189, 1990.

Schiller LR: Clinical pharmacology and use of laxatives and lavage solutions. *J Clin Gastroenterol* 28:11–18, 1999.

Soffer EE: Constipation: An approach to diagnosis, treatment referral. *Cleve Clin J Med* 66:41–46, 1999.

Sonnenberg A, Koch TR: Physician visits in the United States for constipation: 1958 to 1986. *Dig Dis Sci* 34:606–611, 1989.

Stark ME: Challenging problems presenting as constipation. *Am J Gastroenterol* 94:567–574, 1999.

Tedesco FJ, DiPiro JT, American College of Gastroenterology Committee on FDA-Related Matters: Laxative use in constipation. *Am J Gastroenterol* 80:303–309, 1985.

Thompson WG, Drossman DA, Funch-Jensen P, et al: Functional bowel disorders and functional abdominal pain, in Drossman DA (ed.): *The Functional Gastrointestinal Disorders: Diagnosis, Pathophysiology, and Treatment: A Multinational Consensus.* Boston: Little, Brown, 1994, pp 115–173.

Towers AL, Burgio KL, Locher JL, et al: Constipation in the elderly: Influence of dietary, psychological and physiological factors. *J Am Geriatr Soc* 42:701–706, 1994.

Wald A: Constipation in elderly patients: Pathogenesis and management. *Drugs Aging* 3:220–231, 1993.

Whitehead WE, Chaussade S, Corazziari E, et al: Report of an international workshop on management of constipation. *Gastroenterol Int* 4:99–113, 1991.

David S. Weinberg
Christine Laine

Colorectal Cancer Screening

Colorectal cancer (CRC) is one of the most common malignancies in the developed world and the second leading cause of cancer-related death in the United States. Approximately 1 of every 20 Americans will develop CRC during their lifetime. Nearly half of those who develop CRC will die as a direct result of their disease. These statistics are particularly tragic since appropriate disease screening has the potential to prevent death from CRC.

The "adenoma-carcinoma" sequence, the well-described progression from normal colonic mucosa to nonmalignant polyp (adenoma) to cancer, is a prototype for human carcinogenesis. The molecular abnormalities underlying this process require 5 to 10 years to occur. Screening for CRC exploits this large window of opportunity. Detection (and removal) of a polyp at any point before malignant transformation prevents CRC. The National Polyp Study best demonstrated the magnitude of this effect. This study reported up to a 90 percent reduction in CRC mortality rates for persons who underwent polypectomy compared to those who did not.

Despite the documented benefits of screening, clinicians and patients substantially underuse it for CRC. Participation in CRC screening lags behind screening for other malignancies such as breast and cervical cancer. Surveys suggest that fewer than 40 percent of the eligible population has ever completed a fecal occult blood test (FOBT) or flexible sigmoidoscopy, two current mainstays of CRC screening. Less than 10 percent of the average-risk population has completed both of these tests within the screening intervals recommended by most authorities.

Growing public awareness of CRC and its impact, increasing evidence that CRC screening is a cost-effective method to decrease mortality, wider promulgation of screening recommendations, and greater willingness by insurers to reimburse costs of CRC screening may improve CRC screening rates.

Who Gets Colorectal Cancer?

The age-specific incidence of CRC rises rapidly starting at age 40, with 90 percent of cases diagnosed in persons 50 years and older. Risk increases inexorably with age. Persons with familial CRC syndromes such as familial adenomatous polyposis (FAP) or hereditary nonpolyposis colon cancer (HNPCC) make up a small minority of all CRC cases, but CRC typically affects these persons early, often by the age of 40. Despite a common misconception that men are more likely than women to get CRC, this disease affects men and women equally. However, incidence curves for women lag around 5 years behind men until after menopause. No ethnic or religious group consuming a typical Western diet is spared from CRC. However, African Americans have a slightly increased risk of developing CRC than do other ethnic groups.

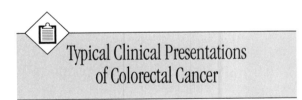

Typical Clinical Presentations of Colorectal Cancer

The progression from adenoma to carcinoma is generally slow. It is widely believed that 5 to 10 years must lapse before a small benign polyp progresses to cancer. While this slow growth allows a large window of opportunity for early detection, it also tends to limit any dramatic or characteristic symptoms. Four patterns of CRC-related symptoms are typically described.

The first results from obstruction of the bowel lumen by an enlarging mass, resulting in pain, distention, or, in the case of complete obstruction, nausea and vomiting. Because the colonic lumen is smallest in the transverse and left bowel, obstruction generally results from tumors in this location. Since a large mass is required to obstruct even here, the prognosis for these cases is generally poor.

A second presentation is bleeding, manifested as bright red blood per rectum for lower left-sided tumors, or occult blood for more proximal lesions. Because heavy bleeding from CRC is unusual, fecal occult blood testing is designed to detect minimal amounts of fecal blood loss. Abrupt discharge of large volumes of blood per rectum suggests other diagnoses. Gradual but continuing blood loss may be missed by FOBT, but may present as iron deficiency anemia.

The third category of symptoms are those stemming from local invasion, either into the bowel wall itself, resulting (as in rectal cancer) in tenesmus, or into adjacent organs such as the bladder, ureters, or surrounding soft tissues.

Finally, as with any malignancy, wasting secondary to colon cancer is well described. The basis for tumor-based cachexia from CRC is the topic of intense research. Not surprisingly, the prognosis of patients with wasting is usually grim.

Overall, when symptoms are associated with CRC they tend to suggest disease that is more advanced. As discussed below, detection of CRC at the asymptomatic stage results in improved clinical outcomes, lending support to the more aggressive use of CRC screening as the best way to minimize CRC-related morbidity and mortality.

Table 14-1

Factors that Increase or Decrease Risk for Colorectal Cancer

Increase risk
  Age
  Family history of polyps or cancer
  Personal history of polyps or cancer
  Inflammatory bowel disease
  Prior endometrial or ovarian cancers
  Diets high in fat or low in fruit and vegetables
  Ureterosigmoidostomy

Decrease Risk
  Long-term ingestion of aspirin or other NSAIDs
  Long-term ingestion of folate
  Regular exercise
  Hormone replacement therapy

NSAIDs, nonsteroidal anti-inflammatory drugs.

agent. Other nonsteroidal anti-inflammatory medications should theoretically reduce risk as well. The key appears to be duration of use rather than dose. For example, aspirin consumed at typical doses for cardioprotection reduces long-term CRC risk by 50 percent only after 20 or more years of regular use.

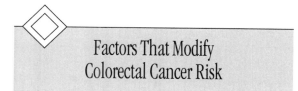

Factors That Modify Colorectal Cancer Risk

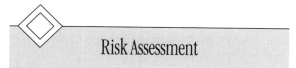

Risk Assessment

Many environmental and genetic risk factors for CRC have been identified (Table 14-1). On balance, most population studies suggest that diets high in fiber, fruits, and vegetables and low in fat reduce CRC risk. The value of various dietary supplements and vitamins is less certain. The most likely protective supplement is folic acid, while any advantage from consumption of other vitamins or minerals requires further evaluation.

In addition to dietary factors, regular, long-term consumption of aspirin is the best-defined protective

By definition, screening is intended for asymptomatic persons. The majority of signs and symptoms associated with CRC are nonspecific. However, the presence of symptoms such as weight loss or occult blood in stools should trigger a full diagnostic evaluation rather than the use of screening tests.

Family history is the key factor for CRC risk assessment. Approximately 5 percent of persons with CRC suffer from FAP or HNPCC. Early development of CRC in 80 (HNPCC) to 100 percent (FAP) of affected persons characterizes these autosomal dominant diseases. Other characteristics typical of FAP are the presence of hundreds to thousands of colonic polyps, as well as a propensity for polyp formation elsewhere in the GI tract. Hereditary nonpolyposis colon cancer is notable for proximal CRCs, few polyps, and strong association with extracolonic malignancy. Screening for persons known or suspected to have these syndromes is different than for persons of average risk. Early, periodic endoscopic evaluation is the standard of care for these persons. Referral to centers that are equipped to provide molecular diagnostics and genetic counseling should be considered for all patients with these diseases.

Far more common are patients with a less extensive family history of colon cancer, for instance, those with a single first-degree relative. "Familial" colon cancer represents about 25 percent of new colon cancer cases. Individual risk rises stepwise with increasing numbers of affected relatives. In general, a single first-degree relative with CRC increases personal risk by approximately threefold relative to the general population. It is also important to note that first-degree relatives of persons with adenomatous polyps exhibit approximately the same degree of cancer risk as first-degree relatives of persons with CRC. However, studies describing this risk were more likely to include persons with large or symptomatic polyps. Extrapolating this data to the more common scenario of risk assessment for patients with a first-degree relative with small polyps is difficult. Until studies that stratify risk by polyp size (or other factors) are available, it is reasonable to consider polyps greater than 1 cm in relatives to confer a risk similar to CRC.

Several diseases are associated with excess CRC risk. The most common is inflammatory bowel disease, where CRC risk parallels the extent and duration of colonic involvement. Previous endometrial or ovarian cancer predisposes women to colon cancer risk two to three times greater than average, but only if these gynecological cancers developed before age 50 to 60. Previous breast cancer appears to confer little or no increased risk of CRC.

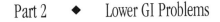

Screening Based on Risk Assessment

Most discussions of CRC screening assume that asymptomatic persons 50 years or older without family history of polyps or cancer are at average risk for CRC. It is much easier to identify persons at greater, rather than lesser, risk. Table 14-2 outlines the relative risk elevations for multiple scenarios of family history and prior personal history of polyps or CRC. There are no reliable data to assess individual risk reduction for persons who, for example, have consumed aspirin for extended periods of time.

It is important to emphasize the silent nature of most colon polyps and early colon cancers. By the time patients develop anemia, abdominal pain, change in bowel habits, weight loss, or visible blood in stools, they are more likely to have an advanced neoplasm. The aim of screening is to sort persons into high-risk versus low-risk categories. Once signs or symptoms have arisen, "screening" for colon cancer is no longer appropriate. Specific complaints warrant expedient evaluation, usually with endoscopy.

The most widely used method of CRC screening for average-risk persons in the United States is the combination of annual FOBT and flexible sigmoidoscopy (FS) every 3 to 5 years. Support for this approach is widespread, and advocates include the American Cancer Society, United States

Table 14-2

Relative Colorectal Cancer Risk Elevations Based on Family History

Average lifetime population risk is 2–5%
One first-degree relative affected = 2–3:1
One first- and one second-degree relative = 4:1
One affected relative under age 45 = 5:1
Two first-degree relatives = 8:1

Table 14-3

Screening Recommendations for Persons at High Risk*

FAP	Genetic counseling and, if appropriate, genetic testing; gene carriers and persons of indeterminate status should undergo FS starting annually at puberty.
HNPCC	Genetic counseling and, if appropriate, genetic testing; colonoscopic examinations performed starting at age 20 every 2 years until age 40 and then annually
Prior adenomatous	For persons with polyps greater than 1 cm or with multiple adenomatous polyps, colonic polyps colonoscopy should be repeated 3 years after the index procedure. Findings determine frequency of long-term screening. For persons with no polyps or 1 small polyp on index colonoscopy, repeat in 5 years.
Prior colorectal cancer	For persons undergoing curative resection, a preoperative colonoscopy to clear the colon of any other neoplasia. If colonoscopy is not possible, perform postoperative procedure within 6 months. If this evaluation or the preoperative study is normal, then follow-up in 3–5 years.

*FAP, familial adenomatous polyposis; FS, flexible sigmoidoscopy; HNPCC, heredity nonpolyposis colon cancer.

Preventive Health Services Task Force, and the World Health Organization. Some authorities have also advocated as acceptable substitutes, either double-contrast barium enema (BE) every 5 years or colonoscopy every 10 years. While polyp detection is greater with colonoscopy than it is with other screening methods, neither colonoscopy nor BE have been studied as screening mechanisms. At present, payers do not universally consider BE or colonoscopy as reimbursable substitutes for FOBT and FS.

Screening recommendations for persons at high risk due to family history of colon cancer or polyps advocate the combination of FOBT and FS starting at age 40 rather than at 50. However, there is near uniform agreement in clinical practice that colonoscopy is the screening test of choice for persons at moderately elevated risk (i.e., one or more first-degree relatives with cancer or polyps). Table 14-3 displays screening recommendations for persons at risk for FAP or HNPCC or with a history of polyps or cancer.

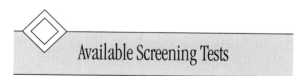

Available Screening Tests

Fecal Occult Blood Testing

Fecal occult blood testing is the most commonly used screening test. It is simple to employ, inexpensive, noninvasive, and acceptable to many patients. The best studied of several FOBT methods is the guaiac-impregnated slide test.

The pseudoperoxidase activity of hemoglobin is the basis for a true-positive FOBT result. However, there are many important causes of both false-positive and false-negative tests (Table 14-4). False-positive tests result most often from nonneoplastic sources of gastrointestinal bleeding or from various foods with peroxidase-like activity. Dietary restrictions as recommended by the manufacturer should be followed if possible. However, a positive FOBT result should be evaluated even if dietary restrictions have not been observed, since there is less likelihood of a false-positive result than there is of a true-positive result. Intermittently bleeding or nonbleeding polyps or cancers are the most frequent reason for false-negative tests. Bleeding from the gastrointestinal tract must generally be fivefold to tenfold greater than that of the normal physiologic blood loss for a positive test. It is important to emphasize that FOBT is a method to test the stool for blood, not for cancer.

Table 14-4

Causes of False-Positive and False-Negative Fecal Occult Blood Testing

> False Positive
>> Exogenous peroxidase activity (red meat, uncooked fruits, or vegetables)
>> Nonneoplastic sources of gastrointestinal blood loss
>> Oral or nasal blood loss
>> Medications (anticoagulants, NSAIDs?)
> False Negative
>> Nonbleeding neoplastic lesion at time of sampling
>> Vitamin C
>> Incorrect sampling or development
>> Prolonged slide storage
>> Degradation of hemoglobin by colonic bacteria

NSAIDs, nonsteroidal anti-inflammatory drugs.

TEST CHARACTERISTICS

Although it is of primary importance for population-based screening, the sensitivity of FOBT in the asymptomatic population is not clear. Estimates have been derived largely from studies of symptomatic persons with known polyps or colon cancer. These estimates range from 10 to 39 percent for polyps and 50 to 92 percent for malignancy. The specificity of FOBT in this setting is more than 95 percent.

The more clinically relevant positive predictive value (PPV) of FOBT is better described. The positive predictive value reflects the likelihood that persons with positive tests have the target disease (adenomatous polyp or CRC). The PPV for any test depends in part on the prevalence of the disease (colonic neoplasia) in the screened population. The PPV of FOBT in population-based screening has been found to be 2.5 to 50 percent for carcinomas and 16 to 40 percent for adenomas. This low PPV is virtually inevitable in the general population because most people do not have CRC.

Because of the limitations of FOBT, efforts have been made to develop other methods of detecting blood in stool, including tests based on the porphyrin-like moiety of hemoglobin (HemoQuant), as well as a human hemoglobin assay. While they may ultimately prove more useful than standard FOBT, they have not yet been the subjects of large-scale clinical testing.

TRIALS IN AVERAGE-RISK PERSONS

Four large prospective studies of FOBT have been completed. They document a reduction in CRC mortality rates of 15 to 33 percent, depending on whether FOBT was performed annually or every other year. Periodic FOBT use is likely to reduce CRC mortality for two reasons. First is the detection of neoplasia prior to the development of cancer. Many polyps, particularly those greater than 1 cm in diameter, bleed sufficiently for detection. The second reason for decreased CRC mortality is earlier cancer detection. Regular use of FOBT results in cancer detection at earlier stages, compared to detection stemming from symptom development. All major studies reveal that at least 70 percent of cancers in the "screened" group are confined to the bowel wall at diagnosis, compared to about 33 percent in persons with symptoms. As CRC survival closely parallels cancer stage at diagnosis, these findings are not surprising.

SUMMARY

The benefits of FOBT include low unit cost, noninvasive nature of the testing, patient self-administration, and relative ease of use. Conversely, the price paid for these advantages is limited sensitivity and specificity, low predictive value of positive and negative tests, and high cost of evaluation of false-positive tests. As described more fully below, models of CRC screening cost-effectiveness reveal that FOBT-based screening is not significantly different from more invasive screening tests, in great part because of the cost of evaluating many persons to identify one case of cancer. Also, FOBT screening involves a fair number of colonoscopies and the associated costs since positive tests require endoscopic evaluation.

Flexible Sigmoidoscopy

The relative inefficiency of FOBT as a screening tool has prompted the consideration of alternative methods for colon cancer screening. Current guidelines recommend annual FOBT plus periodic sigmoidoscopy beginning at age 50 years for screening of average-risk patients. Only 15 to 30 percent of eligible persons undergo such testing. Many patients view sigmoidoscopy as embarrassing and physically uncomfortable. Physicians' reluctance stems from several issues: the continued absence of any prospective data suggesting that sigmoidoscopy reduces colon cancer morbidity or mortality, confusion over screening guidelines, and concerns about cost and acceptability.

The effectiveness of sigmoidoscopy has not been sufficiently studied. The benefits of screening sigmoidoscopy theoretically could result from either of two mechanisms. The first would be the detection of polyps as nonmalignant precursors of colon cancer. The second would be if the risk of subsequent cancer could be predicted based on items such as polyp location, size, or histology, as detected at initial sigmoidoscopy. This knowledge could then be used to modify the intensity of subsequent screening. As discussed later, the significance of distal polyps found on sigmoidoscopy remains uncertain.

Increasing age appears to be the single greatest risk factor for polyp formation, correlating not only with the presence of polyps, but also their multiplicity, size, and degree of dysplasia. While approximately 40 percent of the adult population will develop a polyp at some point, only 5 to 6 percent of individuals develop colon cancer; therefore, few polyps progress to carcinoma. The average distribution of polyps throughout the colon is essential to the evaluation of sigmoidoscopy as a screening tool. However, this information is generally lacking, as studies in asymptomatic, randomly selected individuals are few. The distribution of polyps within the colon differs depending on the method of detection. There is uniform distribution of adenomas throughout the colon in autopsy studies, with large adenomas more frequently seen in the distal colon. The prevalence of polyps in persons from 50 to 70 years old is 25 to 50 percent at autopsy. In the few studies of colonoscopy in healthy populations older than 50 years, nearly 25 percent of all persons had adenomas, with the majority (greater than 70 percent) distal to the transverse colon.

Hyperplastic (nonadenomatous) polyps are frequent findings in the distal colon. They pose no significant risk to progress to colon cancer, nor do they serve as "sentinel" lesions for more dangerous proximal polyps. Polyps greater than 0.5 cm in diameter in the distal bowel are likely to be adenomas, whereas smaller polyps are more frequently hyperplastic. Based on limited evidence, it is estimated that the 60-cm flexible sigmoido-scope will reach sufficiently proximal in the colon to detect 50 to 60 percent of colon cancers in the average population.

Sigmoidoscopy has a very high sensitivity and specificity for distal colonic polyps, both 95 per-cent or greater. However, sigmoidoscopy produces frequent false-positive results if one considers the detection of polyps with no or little malignant potential as a false-positive test. As noted earlier, most polyps detected on routine examination will not progress to clinically significant neoplasia over time. At endoscopy, however, it is currently impos-sible to differentiate the fate of individual polyps. Because standard practice is to remove all polyps at the time of detection, it would be unethical to leave polyps in place for observation in some individuals. However, when the cost of sigmoi-doscopy-based screening programs are calcu-lated, consideration should be given to the number and cost of follow-up colonoscopies in persons very unlikely ever to develop CRC. It has been estimated that, for patients 50 to 59 years old, 2000 FSs must be done to prevent one colon can-cer death, whereas 1000 are necessary for the group 60 to 69 years of age.

To date, there have been no prospective, ran-domized trials evaluating the benefits of sigmoi-doscopy. Two early, uncontrolled, observational studies of rigid sigmoidoscopy suggested that sig-moidoscopy resulted in colon cancers detected at an earlier stage. However, critics of both of these nonrandomized studies have pointed out that, although cancer was detected earlier, there was no evidence of cancer prevention. Further, when age-adjusted colon cancer mortality rates were calcu-lated, they were equivalent in the screened groups to those expected in the general population.

However, two other case-control studies also using rigid sigmoidoscopy have appeared provid-ing more useful results. Selby et al. retrospectively studied 261 patient deaths from colon cancer that arose within 20 cm of the anus. When compared to controls, significantly fewer of the cases had undergone rigid sigmoidoscopy within the previ-ous 10 years. Exposure to sigmoidoscopy was associated with a 70 percent reduction in cancer mortality resulting from tumors within reach of the rigid endoscope. There was no change in mortality arising from tumors beyond the reach of the endoscope, suggesting that there were no sig-nificant biases between cases and controls. A sim-ilar but smaller study reported an 80 percent reduction in CRC mortality for those individuals who had a sigmoidoscopy compared with those persons not examined.

Despite that these latter studies were not ran-domized, prospective clinical trials, they provide important information regarding the role of sig-moidoscopic screening. If the benefits of FS screen-ing were limited only to that gathered through the performance of a single endoscopy, detection of colonic polyps and cancers would still be greatly improved relative to no screening or to FOBT alone. Because most positive sigmoidoscopic examinations are followed by evaluation of the remaining colon, prevention of colon cancer as a result of sigmoidoscopy would exceed the 50 per-cent predicted based on the percentage of poten-tial cancers accessible to the flexible endoscope. These small studies are provocative. The National Cancer Institute has initiated a large-scale pros-pective study of FS screening, but results will not be available for a number of years.

Combined Flexible Sigmoidoscopy Plus Fecal Occult Blood Testing

Intuitively, the combination of FOBT and FS is attractive. While the former is valuable to "survey" the colon in its entirety for blood loss, the latter adds a very sensitive and specific method to visu-alize the colorectal segments where polyps and cancers most commonly occur. Surprisingly, there are very few data to support such speculation. In the only controlled trial studying the benefits of the combination, there was a significant reduction in CRC mortality in the group submitting to both procedures periodically, rather than sigmoidos-copy alone. Other computer models in a hypo-thetical population of 100,000 eligible persons project a 62 percent reduction in CRC incidence compared to baseline for those participating in screening with both tests.

Colonoscopy

Complete visualization of the colon would seem to overcome the limitations of either FOBT or FS. For instance, in one trial of 210 persons with negative FOBT, colonoscopy detected two cancers and 13 polyps greater than 1 cm. Periodic examination of the whole colon by BE or colonoscopy has been advocated by some as the optimal mode of screening. Although such procedures would increase detection of colonic neoplasia, it would be in exchange for significantly higher cost and risk compared with FOBT or sigmoidoscopy. The risk of significant complication from colonoscopy is estimated at 2 per 1000 procedures, while the charge per procedure is generally $1000 or more. By comparison, sigmoidoscopy charges are approximately $150 with a significant complication rate of 0.5 per 1000 procedures.

A substantial advantage to colonoscopy is the interval between examinations. The high prevalence and slow growth rate of colonic polyps has prompted suggestions of screening strategies using a single colonoscopy at age 55 to 60. Cancer incidence rates increase markedly from approximately 50 per 100,000 at age 50 to 244 per 100,000 at age 65 and 415 per 100,000 by age 75. A negative examination at age 60 would not only screen for neoplasia, but also contribute important prognostic indications regarding a given individual's propensity for polyp formation.

One small study tested this hypothesis by performing an initial colonoscopy and then a follow-up procedure no less than 5 years later. It was hypothesized that persons free of polyps on initial colonoscopy would be less likely to have polyps on subsequent investigation. Instead, the polyp prevalence was higher than predicted on the subsequent colonoscopy, equal to the general population, suggesting either that polyps had been missed initially or that the appropriate interval for screening colonoscopy needed greater study. Given the natural history of polyps, presumably 7 to 10 years could elapse between examinations.

Others have argued that, if the cost of colonoscopy were decreased, it would be more cost-effective than any other screening procedure because of better colon visualization, the opportunity for concurrent polypectomy, and the savings from colon cancer averted by early removal of polyps. However, manpower concerns may limit the feasibility of widespread screening with colonoscopy. Colonoscopy is more difficult to learn and to perform than FS. Although nonphysician providers have been recruited to perform sigmoidoscopy, it is unlikely that nonphysicians could easily be trained to perform polypectomy. Who would perform all these procedures, and at what interval, would need to be determined.

Barium Enema

Single-contrast BE is an inadequate method to detect polyps in most cases. When single-contrast BE is performed, followed by colonoscopy, only 40 percent of polyps seen endoscopically were noted radiographically. Double-contrast (air and barium) techniques greatly improve the ability of BE to detect polyps. The accuracy of double-contrast BE in screening for polyps and cancers larger than 1 cm is 90 to 95 percent. Colonoscopy is more sensitive for polyps both smaller and larger than 1 cm. However, for the larger polyps there is a small difference between endoscopic and radiographic detection rates. As the great majority of cancers originate in these larger polyps, for screening purposes, these may represent equivalent sensitivities. The main limitation of BE is that biopsy or polypectomy cannot be performed. Thus, patients who require these interventions would need to undergo a second procedure. Given the widespread availability of BE, however, it is unlikely to disappear as a screening tool in the near future.

Many authorities have advocated BE as an alternative to FS in persons at average risk for colon cancer. Although less expensive and less risky than colonoscopy, concerns regarding manpower and quality control with BE are the same as for colonoscopy. Barium enema also has a small associated risk of radiation exposure.

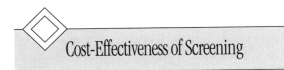

Cost-Effectiveness of Screening

It is unlikely that there will ever be a clinical trial directly comparing the various modes of CRC screening for clinical effectiveness or cost-effectiveness. In lieu of such trials, researchers have constructed several computer models. The most obvious drawback of modeling is the possibility for error in the various assumptions about, for example, the natural history of colon polyps or cancer, the screening tests themselves, or compliance with testing.

Allowing for these potential shortcomings, these models suggest that broad-based CRC screening would be expensive. Screening 60 million average-risk Americans older than 50 years with FOBT and FS is estimated to cost $3 billion annually, not including the cost of follow-up colonoscopies. Despite this impressive figure, CRC screening by any standard technique is cost-effective. All screening modalities would cost less than $20,000 per year of life saved. This figure compares favorably to the cost-effectiveness of other cancer screening strategies, such as mammography. It is valuable to recognize that the direct costs of colon cancer therapy were estimated to be over $4 billion. Any calculation of the overall cost of CRC needs to consider associated costs ranging from screening through therapy. While each screening modality is essentially equally cost-effective, it is valuable to recognize that the basis for cost savings varies with each modality. Fecal occult blood testing is the single least expensive test. It prevents the fewest cancers and therefore has the greatest associated treatment costs. Colonoscopy on the other extreme is the most expensive test, but also prevents the greatest number of cancers.

Ultimately, decisions about cost-effectiveness are societal ones. At present, most screening programs emphasize the immediate costs of testing, neglecting to consider more intermediate concerns.

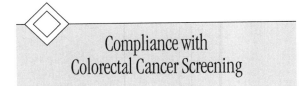

Compliance with Colorectal Cancer Screening

Most studies of compliance with CRC screening report only FOBT, presumably because of its greater dissemination and ease of use compared to other tests. The 1993 Behavioral Risk Factor Surveillance Study reported that less than 30 percent of persons 50 years or older had ever been screened using FOBT. Despite growing interest in screening, the 1997 update of this study reported that less than 20 percent of eligible persons had completed a screening FOBT in the previous year.

Compliance with CRC screening seriously lags behind screening rates described for other common malignancies, including breast, cervical, or prostate cancer. Patient factors linked to high rates of compliance with FOBT include knowledge about CRC, high educational level, having friends or relatives with the disease, and belief in the importance of preventive care. Women are generally more likely to participate in CRC screening than are men.

Reasons patients most frequently cited for noncompliance with FOBT include lack of symptoms, the unpleasant and embarrassing nature of the test, operational difficulty with the testing procedure, and fear about test results. Barriers to screening for physicians include misperceptions that comorbidity precludes the effectiveness of screening, concerns about screening effectiveness, and low reimbursement. Most studies suggest that physicians do not recommend FOBT frequently enough. There is little known about factors that increase use of other screening modalities, particularly colonoscopy or BE.

Interventions to Encourage Colorectal Cancer Screening

Interventions to increase CRC screening have met with only modest success. There has been increasing interest by public figures in promulgating the benefits of CRC screening. Broad public education has been effective in changing health behaviors, including breast cancer screening and smoking cessation. To date, community education programs stressing the role of FOBT in CRC screening have been less effective than programs targeting individual patients. Methods that emphasize patient education in combination with physician recommendation tend to be more successful.

The most effective techniques have provided written CRC educational material to patients in advance of clinician visits. One of the most effective methods to increase patient participation in any health-related behavior is the strong endorsement of a trusted clinician. The most common reason women give for not undergoing screening for breast or cervical cancer is that it is not recommended or offered by their physicians. Personal reminders from physicians to their patients increase CRC screening. Providing patients with FOBT cards improves compliance compared to various techniques where patients are responsible for obtaining cards. Aggressive use of patient-targeted education has resulted in improved CRC screening. Given baseline screening rates of approximately 20 percent, such results are encouraging.

Two Common Problems in Colorectal Cancer Screening

Myths about Fecal Occult Blood Testing

While much effort has been expended to identify patient- and physician-based reasons for under-

utilization of FOBT-based CRC screening, little attention has been devoted to understanding those forces driving the follow-up of positive tests. Only 40 percent of FOBT-positive patients undergo appropriate evaluation, meaning either colonoscopy or a combination of FS and BE. In the majority of cases, misconceptions about the use or interpretation of FOBT undermined physician intent to arrange appropriate evaluation. The most common physician reasons for not following up with patients who have positive FOBTs are listed in Table 14-5. While a full discussion is beyond the scope of this chapter, it is safe to conclude that the moderate reduction in colon cancer rates afforded by regular use of FOBT are substantially undermined if persons with positive tests do not undergo complete evaluation.

The Appropriate Management of a Distal Polyp Detected on Flexible Sigmoidoscopy

Screening FS identifies distal colonic adenomas in approximately 10 percent of patients. In addition,

Table 14-5

Top 10 Reasons Why Fecal Occult Blood Testing (+) Patients Do Not Undergo Complete Colonic Examination (Flexible Sigmoidoscopy Plus Barium Enema or Colonoscopy)

1. Follow up recommended, but not CCE
2. Patient had some evaluation already, but not CCE
3. Medical history suggested another reason for FOBT(+)
4. No family history
5. Normal hemoglobin
6. Age greater than 75 years
7. Fewer than 3 FOBT (+) results
8. Concurrent use of medications that could increase FOBT (+) rate
9. Nonadherence to diet
10. FOBT(+), but patient never contacted

CCE, complete colonic evaluation; FOBT, fecal occult blood testing.

a similar proportion has hyperplastic polyps. Differentiation based on endoscopic appearance between the two histologic types can be challenging. The weight of current evidence suggests that distal hyperplastic polyps confer no risk for more dangerous proximal neoplasia. For many clinicians, the decision to proceed with a colonoscopy in persons with polyps identified by FS is based on the existence of adenomatous polyps. Hence, the ability to perform biopsies at the time of screening FS is crucial in the identification of patients who require more extensive evaluation.

A far more controversial topic is whether any distal adenomatous polyp requires subsequent total colonic evaluation. Opinions range from advocating colonoscopy for all patients with adenomatous polyps no matter what, to suggesting that only patients with polyps larger than 1 cm undergo colonoscopy. While it is generally agreed that adenomatous polyps larger than 1 cm predict the presence of significant proximal neoplasia more adequately than polyps less than 1 cm, other important factors deserve consideration. Most important are polyp number and histologic type, specifically the presence of a villous component. Many authorities suggest that if any of three criteria—size (1 cm or greater), polyp number (>1), or histology (villous or tubulovillous component)—is satisfied, then colonoscopy is warranted. While the authors favor this approach, it is admittedly conservative, and most experts recommend colonoscopy if polyps are detected.

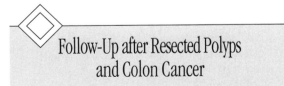

Follow-Up after Resected Polyps and Colon Cancer

Appropriate follow-up of persons who have had adenomatous polyps removed endoscopically is not clearly defined. The risk of recurrent polyps, while small, is real, suggesting that surveillance should be performed using testing that visualizes the entire bowel (i.e., BE or colonoscopy) rather than using FOBT. As there are no reported studies of postpolypectomy surveillance using BE, only data specific to colonoscopy can be used.

The chance of detecting a significant polyp (greater than 1 cm, villous histology, or dysplasia) is slightly more than 3 percent during colonoscopies performed 3 years after index colonoscopy. Because this rate does not differ substantially from follow-up colonoscopy at 1 year, most authorities recommend a 3-year interval. However, it is likely that factors that modify risk, for example, size or number of polyps, are important. Persons with a single, small (less than 1 cm), tubular adenoma that was removed have a subsequent risk of colon cancer one-half that of the general population, while persons with multiple adenomas suffer risk elevations more than five times greater than average.

Clearly, no definitive recommendations about screening intervals can be made. Until better data are available, the majority of persons who have had small polyps removed can be followed with colonoscopy at 3-year (or greater) intervals. Those with more worrisome initial examinations would benefit from more frequent examinations, at least until subsequent examinations show the colon to be free of polyps.

At present, there is unfortunately little evidence supporting aggressive endoscopic, radiographic, or laboratory follow-up of patients who have undergone colon cancer resection with curative intent. Such evaluation is unlikely to hasten detection of recurrent disease. However, it is important to note that persons with prior CRC are at elevated risk for other colon polyps or metachronous CRCs. Consequently, it is imperative that the colon be cleared of all other neoplasia either before surgical resection of the cancer or, if this is not possible, within 1 year after resection. If the preoperative examination is normal, then the follow-up schedule should revert to the recommendations noted earlier, with the next colonoscopy planned for 3 years post-resection.

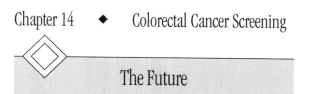

The Future

The future of colon cancer screening is easily described: genetic testing to predict overall susceptibility to colon cancer used in conjunction with a rapid office-based rectal biopsy performed by a primary care physician to survey the effect of environmental exposure on the colonic mucosa.

While awaiting the development of such technology, much effort has been focused on identification of biomarkers more predictive than stool blood. A number of candidate oncogenes, growth factors, mucins, and other proteins have been proposed. Issues around sensitivity, specificity, and cost have conspired to prevent the widespread use of any to date.

At present and for the foreseeable future, variants of FOBT using new reagents may be the most effective for colon cancer screening. The role of virtual colonoscopy presently is unclear.

Issues of cost and patient acceptability will still need to be addressed if this new diagnostic method is found to have clinical utility comparable to present techniques. No test, new or old, will have substantial effect to reduce colon cancer unless screening for the disease is more widely adapted.

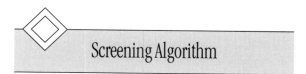

Screening Algorithm

A suggested algorithm for CRC screening is displayed in Figure 14-1. The key decision point is the initial assessment of colon cancer risk. The majority of patients seen in the primary care setting will clearly be at average risk for colon cancer. Physicians should encourage patients to have periodic, but continuous, FSs and FOBTs. Some patients may opt for BE or colonoscopy, espe-

Figure 14-1

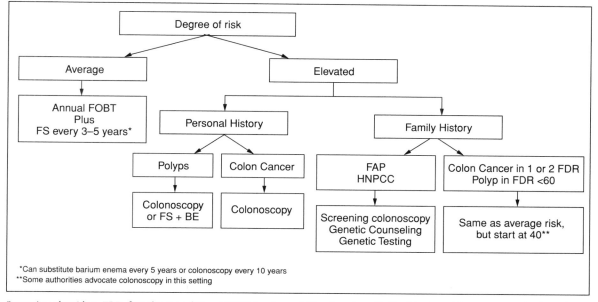

Screening algorithm. FDR, first-degree relative; FOBT, fecal occult blood testing; FS, flexible sigmoidoscopy; HNPCC, hereditary nonpolyposis colon cancer; BE, barium enema.

cially if third-party payers are willing to cover the greater immediate expense.

Patients at more elevated risk require more individualized screening programs. Colon cancer screening when appropriately used can prevent both CRC and its associated mortality. Increasing patient and physician involvement in adequate CRC screening programs remains a formidable challenge.

Bibliography

Allison JE, Tekawa IS, Ransom LJ, et al: A comparison of fecal occult-blood tests for colorectal-cancer screening. *N Engl J Med* 334:155–159, 1996.

Atkin WS, Morson DM, Cuzick J: Long-term risk of colorectal cancer after excision of rectosigmoid adenomas. *N Engl J Med* 326:658–662, 1992.

Burke W, Petersen G, Lynch P, et al: Recommendations for follow-up care of individuals with an inherited predisposition to cancer. I. Hereditary nonpolyposis colon cancer. Cancer Genetics Studies Consortium. *JAMA* 277:915–919, 1997.

Burt RW: Screening of patients with a positive family history of colorectal cancer. *Gastrointest Endosc Clin N Am* 7:65–79, 1997.

Cho KR, Vogelstein B: Genetic alterations in the adenoma-carcinoma sequence. *Cancer* 70(6 Suppl): 1727–1731, 1992.

Giovannucci E, Egan KM, Hunter DJ, et al: Aspirin and the risk of colorectal cancer in women. *N Engl J Med* 333:609–614, 1995.

Giovannucci E, Stampfer MJ, Colditz GA, et al: Multivitamin use, folate, and colon cancer in women in the Nurses' Health Study. *Ann Intern Med* 129:517–524, 1998.

Levin TR, Palitz A, Grossman S, et al: Predicting advanced proximal colonic neoplasia with screening sigmoidoscopy. *JAMA* 281:1611–1617, 1999.

Hardcastle JD, Chamberlain JO, Robinson MHE, et al: Randomized controlled trial of fecal occult blood screening for colorectal cancer. *Lancet* 348:1472–1477, 1996.

Kronborg O, Fenger C, Olsen J, et al: Randomized study of screening for colorectal cancer with fecal occult blood test. *Lancet* 348:1467–1471, 1996.

Mandel JS, Bond JH, Church TR, et al: Reducing mortality from colorectal cancer by screening for occult blood. *N Eng J Med* 328:1365–1371, 1993.

Selby JV, Friedman GD, Quesenberry CP, et al: A case-control study of screening sigmoidoscopy and mortality from colorectal cancer. *N Engl J Med* 326: 653–657, 1992.

Wagner JL, Tunis S, Brown M, et al: Cost-effectiveness of colorectal cancer screening in average-risk adults, in Young GP, Rozen P, Levin B (eds): *Prevention and Early Detection of Colorectal Cancer*. Philadelphia, Saunders, 1996, pp 321–357.

Winawer SJ, Fletcher RH, Miller L, et al: Colorectal cancer screening: Clinical guidelines and rationale. *Gastroenterology* 112:594–642, 1997.

Winawer SJ, Stewart ET, Zauber AG, et al: A comparison of colonoscopy and double-contrast barium enema for surveillance after polypectomy. *N Engl J Med* 342:1766–1772, 2000.

Winawer SJ, Zauber AG, Ho MN, et al: Prevention of colorectal cancer by colonoscopic polypectomy. The National Polyp Study Workgroup. *N Engl J Med* 329:1977–1981, 1993.

James W. Fleshman

Chapter

15

Anal Pain

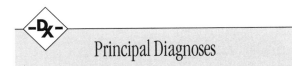

How Common is Anorectal Pain?

Anorectal pain is the most common reason why patients seek care from colorectal surgeons, and it is also a frequent problem seen in primary care practice. The symptom of anal pain can be caused by either benign or malignant disease. When patients are seen in the office complaining of anal pain, the problem is usually easily diagnosed with a superficial exam and the most common cause is an anal fissure. When patients are seen in hospitals, however, anal pain usually occurs in patients being treated for other problems such as total joint replacement or bone marrow transplant and diagnosis is often a more serious problem.

The management of anal pain is dictated by the diagnosis and by other problems that patients may have. In young healthy individuals with anal fissure, treatment may be as simple as raising their fiber intake. In individuals who are HIV-positive or elderly persons immunocompromised from diabetes or steroids, the pain may represent something completely different and will need to be managed in a more aggressive manner. This chapter will define those circumstances in which a more aggressive approach is required and yet set the background for the simple treatment of anal pain in the office setting.

Principal Diagnoses

Anal pain is commonly caused by the following conditions: anal fissure, thrombosed external hemorrhoids, perianal and perirectal abscess, infectious proctitis, levator syndrome and pelvic floor abnormality, Crohn's disease, and anal cancer. While the character of the pain may not be the same in each of these conditions, patients still present with chief complaints of anal pain and each of these conditions is a possibility and must be considered.

Anal Fissure

An anal fissure is a split in the anoderm at the dentate line. Of these patients, 80 percent will have a single midline anterior fissure. However, 18 percent may present with a posterior fissure and 2 percent with an anterior/posterior fissure.

Thrombosed External Hemorrhoids

External hemorrhoids occur in the superficial venous plexus under the anoderm in one of three quadrants. Thrombosis in these hemorrhoids causes anal pain. Typically, external hemorrhoids produce anal pain with thrombosis, but internal hemorrhoids do not.

Perianal and Perirectal Abscess

Inflammation and obstruction of anal glands at the level of the dentate line will occasionally cause an abscess to form in the base of one or more of the glands. The glands can then enlarge, and the infection dissects in many different directions, resulting in an anal abscess. Typically, abscesses arising from glands located in the anterior half of the anal canal will track to the perineum in a radial fashion and involve varying amounts of the internal and external anal sphincter in their course. Glands in the posterior half of the anal canal cause abscesses that usually appear in the posterior midline and extend first to the postanal space and then dissect laterally toward the ischial rectal fascia on either side of the anal canal. This will sometimes result in a fistula or abscess that can extend as far forward as the perineal body. It is difficult to detect these abscesses on a superficial exam; frequently patients will require an exam under anesthesia to make the diagnosis.

Infectious Proctitis

The most common anal infections seen by primary care physicians are gonorrhea and condyloma (veneral warts); the most common infections seen by colorectal surgeons are herpes, condyloma, and cytomegalovirus. Most patients with infectious proctitis are either immunocompromised or sexually active. Herpes zoster or shingles can also occur in the rectal area and is not necessarily related to sexual activity or immunocompromise. Any of these infections will cause pain in certain circumstances. Herpes and cytomegalovirus are more commonly associated with pain than is condyloma; however, large condyloma may cause pain.

Levator Syndrome and Pelvic Floor Abnormality

Spasm of the muscle in the pelvic floor can be a source of pain even for healthy individuals. As the patients overuse the pelvic floor muscle, muscle fatigue occurs, spasm occurs, and a symptom of aching anal or low pelvic pain is reported.

Crohn's Disease

Crohn's disease causes anal fissuring, ulceration, and/or abscess formation in approximately 20 percent of patients affected by the disease.

Anal Cancer

A squamous cell cancer of the anus causes pain. The cancer occurs in patients with a history of urogenital human papillomavirus (HPV) infection.

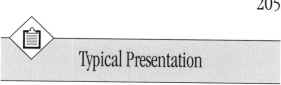

Typical Presentation

Anal Fissure

A number of symptoms are normally present when patients complain of anal pain due to an anal fissure. Patients may complain of pain with bowel movements, especially during hard bowel movements or after an episode of diarrhea. Additional symptoms include anal spasm for 2 to 4 h after bowel movement, bright red blood per rectum with a bowel movement or during wiping, and anal itching.

Thrombosed External Hemorrhoids

Symptoms of external hemorrhoids include a palpable lump, straining during a hard bowel movement, or diarrhea. Symptoms may be worsened by prolonged sitting or heavy lifting.

Perianal and Perirectal Abscess

The key symptom of an abscess is constant anal pain. The exceptions to this rule are:

1. Mass with pointing or fluctuance on the perianal skin. The one exception of this is the intersphincteric abscesses that cause anal pain with no external findings and the only finding is a bulge extending into the anal canal on palpation.
2. Anal abscesses may be silent in immunosuppressed patients.

Anal Infection

Gonorrhea is often asymptomatic but may present with anal pain or discharge. Condylomas cause pain if they are extremely large; the warts are most commonly in a butterfly pattern distributed on all sides of the anal canal. Cytomegalovirus is typically found in immunocompromised patients as a large deep anal ulcer in an atypical location from those where anal fissures are usually seen. In herpes zoster, ulcer-like lesions have an erythematous base and usually follow a dermatome. Patients have a history of varicella zoster or chickenpox. Herpes simplex (genital herpes) usually is associated with perineal or genital distribution as well as anal lesions.

Levator Syndrome and Pelvic Floor Abnormality

The pain caused by pelvic floor abnormalities is typically chronic in nature and associated with straining and squatting. Patients generally complain of pain at night and wake up in the morning feeling improved. There may be a history of anal incontinence or constipation as a source of overuse.

Crohn's Disease

The ulcers of Crohn's disease contrast with those of ideopathic ulcer disease by occupying atypical positions around the anal canal (rather than being located anteriorly or posteriorly). They are often associated with tags and weeping mucositis. When present, fissures generally arise from the base of the ulcer and extend out into the perianal skin.

Anal Cancer

Anal cancer is most often present with pain or a mass in the rectum associated with a lesion palpable on digital rectal exam. An atypical or chronic ulcer may be also seen. Patients will have a history of HPV 16, 18, or 21.

Anal Incontinence

The pain associated with anal incontinence usually is due to excoriation of the perianal skin or deep muscle pain due to overuse.

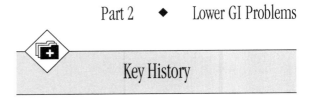

Key History

Pain

Anal pain may be reported as constant or intermittent or associated with bowel movements. It is important to distinguish whether this pain is internal or external. Patients should be questioned as to the nature of the pain. A tearing type of pain is common for anal fissures. A dull ache is more common with pelvic floor abnormality or anal cancer. Severe muscle spasm is most commonly identified with levator syndrome, and pressure-like pain is usually present with anal incontinence or anal cancer.

Bleeding

Bleeding associated with pain should be characterized. Bright red blood per rectum is typical of anal ulcers as opposed to dark venous type bleeding from proctitis or diverticular disease. The presence of blood mixed with or in the stool suggests a source higher in the gastrointestinal tract. Blood on the stool suggests surface bleeding. Bright red blood on toilet paper indicates less volume of bleeding than does blood dripping into the toilet; the latter usually indicates a large volume of bleeding.

Bowel Patterns

Bowel pattern is relevant to the development, as well as the management, of the anal pain. Hard bowel movements will generally need to be softened; diarrhea will need to be stopped; constipation will need to be relieved; and an irritable bowel syndrome should be regulated.

Associated Diseases

Associated diseases may affect both the diagnostic process and the therapeutic measures needed. Diabetes in patients with a potential abscess indicates an increased likelihood of a larger abscess or development of complications. In immunocompromised individuals or patients undergoing chemotherapy for cancer in the remote past, anal pain may be a harbinger of disastrous events such as gangrene and sepsis. Individuals with Crohn's disease who have anal pain should be examined carefully to detect fistulas, abscesses, or other complications.

Condition: Specific History

ANAL FISSURE

Anal fissures result in a tearing, knifelike sensation in a specific area of the anal canal. This is intermittent and usually after bowel movement. A 2- to 4-h period of intense anal spasm sometimes follows.

THROMBOSED EXTERNAL HEMORRHOIDS

Thrombosed external hemorrhoids result in a constant localized external pain associated with a palpable lump under the skin.

PERIANAL AND PERIRECTAL ABSCESS

Perianal and perirectal abscesses result in a constant sharp pain that may be increased during bowel movement and that may not resolve after the bowel movement.

INFECTION

Herpes generally causes irritation, especially with wiping. The pain follows a dermatome. Condylomas are painful only when the lesions become large, in which case the pain is in a butterfly pattern, interferes with hygiene, and causes rubbing and bleeding. Cytomegalovirus results in a bleeding, painful ulcer. The individuals normally have significant underlying immunosuppression.

LEVATOR SYNDROME

Patients with levator syndrome usually report a dull ache with increased pain on sitting, especially during long car trips or airplane rides. Straining to have a bowel movement generally will cause the pain to worsen.

CROHN'S DISEASE

Patients with Crohn's disease usually only have pain where there is an abscess or where an acute fissure is irritated by diarrhea. The typical Crohn's ulcer with a large skin tag and weeping moisture does not usually cause pain.

Anal Incontinence

Anal incontinence typically causes anal pain with wiping, burning with seepage, and poor hygiene. Table 15-1 categorizes the anal pain in relation to etiology and is useful as a quick reference.

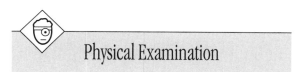

Physical Examination

When examining the anal canal, clinicians should look for several specific findings. First, the anoderm, which is skin without hair follicles, should be intact. The perianal skin where there may be hair is typically slightly thicker and should have no evidence of erythema or other lesion. Any discoloration such as hyperpigmentation or a raised lesion should be noted.

The anal canal can be everted partially by using a thumb placed on either side of the anal canal to exert gentle traction to evert the dentate line, at least in the lateral positions. Any mucositis or disease of the anoderm should be noted within the short anal canal.

Discharge per anum indicates ongoing inflammation, though a small amount of mucus is normal. The presence of stool or fresh blood on the skin is an indicator of either poor hygiene or prolapsing internal hemorrhoids. Any lumps, bumps, or divits should be noted and documented accordingly.

Table 15-1

Etiology of Anal Pain

Dx	Pain				Bleeding			Mass	Bowel Pattern	
	Sharp	Dull	Constant	Intermittent	Wipe	On Stool	In Stool		Constipation	Diarrhea
Fissure	+	–	–	+	+	+	–	–	+	+
Hemorrhoid	+	–	+	–	–	+	–	+	+	+
Abscess	+	–	+	–	–	–	–	+	–	–
Infection	+	–	+	–	+	+	–	–	–	+
Levator	+	+	–	+	–	–	–	–	±	±
Crohn's	+	–	–	+	+	+	–	±	–	+
Anal cancer	+	+	+	+	±	±	–	+	–	–
Incontinence	+	–	–	–	+	–	–	–	–	–

Anal Fissure

An anal fissure is the acute manifestation of tearing of the anoderm, typically located anteriorly and/or posteriorly in the midline. An ulcer will form with heaped rolled edges, exposed muscle, internal anal papilla, and an external skin tag over time. There is usually a band of hypertrophied internal anal sphincter. This is easily palpated on all sides, just outside the opening of the anal canal.

Thrombosed External Hemorrhoids

The external thrombosed hemorrhoid may vary from the size of a small pea to a large grape with overlying smooth intact skin in one of the three typical quadrants: right anterior, right posterior, and left lateral positions. It is the skin eroding over the thrombosed hemorrhoid that causes the pain and that may also be responsible for eventual gangrene of these hemorrhoid complexes. Sometimes it is possible to evacuate the clot through the erosion.

Incarcerated strangulated thrombosed internal hemorrhoids generally present with a rosette of red and black lumps of mucosa caught by the tight ring of the internal sphincter. These are typically associated with a pressure-like pain rather than with the sharp searing pain of a thrombosed external hemorrhoid. Strangulated, thrombosed hemorrhoids are an indication for surgery.

Perirectal and Perianal Abscess

As mentioned earlier, abscesses typically occur in the anterior/posterior midlines and track to the ischiorectal fossa, perineal body, or gluteal cleft. A small perianal abscess generally manifests as a tender lump with overlying erythema within 1 to 2 cm of the anal canal. An ischiorectal fossa abscess, in contrast, causes a large swelling of the inner aspect of either buttock with overlying induration, erythema, and fluctuance; these findings typically indicate a deeper abscess with a longer tract.

An intersphincteric abscess usually has no external findings. Patients complain of constant severe pain and, on digital rectal exam, the pain should be localized to an area of fluctuance under the mucosa and internal sphincter between the internal and external sphincters within the anal canal. This requires the examination to be performed under anesthesia for definitive diagnosis and treatment.

Anal Infection

Herpes manifests itself as erythematous punched-out lesions with a white ring in most circumstances. The ulcers are painful to touch and will typically follow a dermatome if they are due to zoster. Condyloma acuminatum results in raised white vegetation on the perineal and perianal skin. Unfortunately, these lesions may encroach on the anal mucosa due to receptive intercourse or long-standing disease. They will appear both on the anoderm at the dentate line as well as eventually on the mucosa.

Cytomegalovirus in immunocompromised patients is usually a large ulcerated area anywhere around the anal canal. The ulcers typically bleed and have a corrugated base.

Levator Syndrome

Patients with levator syndrome typically have normal anatomy and normal function of the anal canal. Occasionally, however, point tenderness over a muscle in the area of the puborectalis at the upper end of the anal canal or over a lateral portion of the levator ani muscle can be identified. With strong point pressure during the digital rectal exam, clinicians can regenerate patients' complaint and tenderness will sometimes lessen with a short period of massage.

Crohn's Disease

Rectal mucosal ulceration and mucosal granularity with friability, easy bleeding, and loss of vascular pattern are typical of anorectal Crohn's disease. Anal Crohn's disease may be seen in isolation from any intestinal disease. The anal fissures are usually in an atypical position and are accompanied by large edematous elephant-ear skin tags. Fistulas may arise from the base of the ulcers and extend out under superficial skin to abscesses in the subcutaneous fat around the anal canal. The most severe form of anal Crohn's disease is the "watering pot perineum," which is due to undermining anal fistulas arising from several anal ulcers within the anal canal, resulting in chronic weeping openings throughout the skin area.

Anal Cancer

Smooth white superficial change in the anoderm or the perianal skin is a mild form of anal cancer called Bowen's disease. This is an intraepithelial squamous cancer that should be biopsied for definitive diagnosis.

A typical anal cancer is a firm nodule or a hard ulcer that is sometimes less painful than the physical findings would otherwise indicate. Unfortunately, anal cancer sometimes appears serendipitously in a hemorrhoid specimen after excision. Squamous cell cancers are also found in large anal condylomas in HIV-positive patients.

Anal Incontinence

The anal skin in patients with anal incontinence typically has deep rugae with pseudoepithelial changes on the skin due to chronic wetness and bathing in mucus with a high pH. Prolapsing internal hemorrhoids may also cause this. Typical findings are a thin perianal body with an obvious defect in the anal sphincter. However, the sphincter injury may be more subtle and be identified only with transrectal ultrasound or anal physiologic testing such as manometry and electromyography. A patulous anus in elderly females with large amounts of excoriation may also indicate occult rectal prolapse.

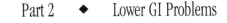

Ancillary Tests

If the cause of anal pain cannot be identified on observation or culture in the office setting, it is important to proceed with examination under anesthesia. This allows examination of the anal canal and surrounding tissues without causing patients pain . Endoscopy is necessary to inspect inside the anal canal and the rectal mucosa, but endoscopy is usually not possible in patients with severe anal pain, unless local or regional anesthesia is used.

A good anoscope with a light source to look at the anal transition zone, dentate line, and anal mucosa is probably the most useful piece of equipment for the practicing colorectal surgeon or primary care physician. Colonoscopy or complete evaluation of the entire colon with a flexible scope is indicated in patients with blood in the stool coming from above the rectum. If an inflamed mucosa is identified in the anal canal, colonoscopy may also be useful to identify colitis. In patients in whom infection is suspected, a white blood cell count may be useful. A white blood cell count will also aid in identifying patients who are immunosuppressed or neutropenic.

A viral culture of the anal ulcer or perianal lesions may lead to a diagnosis of herpes. Other sexually transmitted diseases have specific culture requirements that should be considered before obtaining specimens. Cytomegalovirus generally requires a biopsy to identify nuclear inclusion bodies in the tissue at the base of the ulcer. Therefore, an examination under anesthesia is necessary.

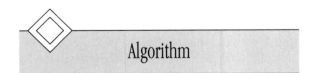

Algorithm

A simple algorithm is sometimes useful for making the diagnosis of anal pain (Figure 15-1).

Figure 15-1

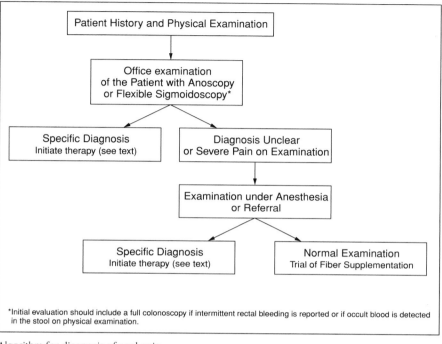

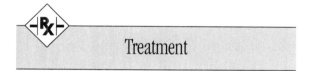

*Initial evaluation should include a full colonoscopy if intermittent rectal bleeding is reported or if occult blood is detected in the stool on physical examination.

Algorithm for diagnosis of anal pain.

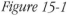

Treatment

Anal Fissure

The majority of patients with an anal fissure will respond to stool softeners with an increase in dietary fiber. A suppository with hydrocortisone and an antibiotic such as neomycin may also be useful. Substances that reduce the tone of the internal anal sphincter by stimulating the nitric oxide receptors in the autonomic internal sphincter have been shown to be effective in reducing the pain related to the anal fissure and initiating the healing process. A typical regimen is 0.5 g of nitroglycerin ointment (0.2%) 3 times a day applied to the perianal skin.

Another method of relaxing the internal anal sphincter is the use of botulinum toxin. The dose of toxin can be injected every 6 months to keep the sphincter relaxed. However, the most effective long-lasting method of treatment of the anal fissure is a lateral internal anal sphincterotomy. The distal third of the anal internal sphincter is divided in the midlateral position. Typically, this is the hypertrophied band that is palpable during anoscopy with an open-sided anoscope under local anesthesia. The sphincterotomy results in immediate relief of anal pain and spasm and results in rapid healing of the fissure over a 2- or 3-day period. Unfortunately, sphincterotomy may be associated with varying degrees of incontinence of gas and mucus or liquid. Care must be taken to limit the amount of sphincter divided, and patients must be warned of these potential side effects before undertaking sphincterotomy.

Thrombosed External Hemorrhoid

The initial treatment of patients with thrombosed external hemorrhoids includes bulk-forming agents such as psyllium, tub soaks 3 times a day to relax the internal anal sphincter, and local anesthetic ointments as needed for local relief. If the hemorrhoid has developed skin necrosis, a local excision of the skin clot and ligation of the vessel can be performed in the office. If the clot has begun to erode and there is no gangrene present, enucleation of the clot through the ulcer is often possible and provides immediate relief. However, the chance of recurrence is high. Antibiotics are essential if there is evidence of cellulitis or gangrene.

An examination under anesthesia and excisional hemorrhoidectomy are usually necessary to treat incarcerated, strangulated, fourth-degree hemorrhoids with necrosis or gangrene present on skin or mucosa. An operation to evaluate the anal canal is also essential in immunocompromised patients if there is any suspicion of ongoing bacterial infection due to thrombosis combined with gangrene.

Perianal and Perirectal Abscess

For small perianal abscesses with fluctuance and an obvious pointing site over a perianal cavity, it is possible to perform incision and draining in the office with a local anesthetic over the surface of the fluctuant cavity. The same applies to a large abscess in the ischiorectal fossa with an obvious site of potential spontaneous drainage.

However, if there is any evidence of necrosis or impending gangrene, patients should undergo examination under anesthesia. A large abscess draining pus from the anus but no clear site to drain requires examination under anesthesia as does a suspected intersphincteric abscess. Patients who drain spontaneously and with a continuously draining fistula will also require inspection in the operating room to identify the internal opening that persists as a draining source to the fistula.

Almost one-half of patients with a perirectal or perianal abscess will go on to develop a fistula tract in the future. An immediate fistulotomy at the time of abscess drainage is sometimes recommended if an obvious internal opening is present. However, this is not essential in the treatment of every abscess.

Anal Infection

Anal herpes responds to oral acyclovir 500 mg twice daily for 10 days in most circumstances. Local therapy with acyclovir ointment will take some of the symptoms away but is not considered definitive therapy. Large anal condyloma accumulatum will require examination under anesthesia and excision and coagulation in the operating room. Small recurrent warts or small, single, isolated condyloma can be treated in the office with trichloroacetic acid. Immiquimod ointment is also a reasonable treatment, but ointment should be applied for at least a month before evaluating results. Immiquimod usually causes an erythematous response within the anoderm and perianal skin. The ointment should be completely removed the following morning after placement overnight. Also the hands and fingers should be completely cleared of the ointment to avoid injury to the patient's skin.

Cytomegalovirus should be treated with oral acyclovir, especially in immunocompromised patients. However, most immunocompromised patients with cytomegalovirus are already on antivirals and the addition of acyclovir may provide no additional benefit. In such cases, palliative treatment for symptomatic relief includes fiber, tub soaks, and local anesthetics.

Levator Syndrome

Normally, the addition of a fiber, cessation of aggravating behaviors such as straining or lifting, avoiding unsupported cushion seats, and a nonsteroidal anti-inflammatory drug will relieve the levator syndrome. Nonsteroidal anti-inflammatory drugs are useful in reducing inflammation and pain. Occasionally nitroglycerin ointment 0.2% may be required to relieve the associated internal sphincter spasm. Patients should avoid inner-tube-type cushions that provide no support of the anal canal. Individuals should decide whether furniture at home or work provides adequate support.

Crohn's Disease

If Crohn's disease is suspected as the source for fissures and anal pain, patients require colonoscopy and may require surgical procedures. These patients usually require a multidisciplinary approach as the treatment is sometimes complicated. A conservative nonsurgical approach is usually pursued first to preserve the sphincter and anal tissue. Occasionally a lateral internal sphincterotomy is performed if the fissure is determined to be a true idiopathic anal fissure. Anal abscesses in Crohn's disease are normally treated with drainage, placement of soft setons, and preservation of the anal sphincter as much as possible. In the most extreme case, consideration can be given to use of a diverting colostomy.

The medical therapy for anal Crohn's disease is metronidazole orally and immunosuppressants. New forms of immunosuppression include anti-tumor necrosis factor alpha and 6-mercaptopurine or azathioprine. Prednisone may be useful for severe disease.

Anal Cancer

If anal cancer is suspected, patients should undergo an examination and biopsy under anesthesia. The treatment of Bowen's disease (intra-epidermal squamous cell carcinoma) is wide local excision and reconstruction with either skin flaps or grafting. True invasive anal squamous cell cancer is best treated by a combined chemoradiation protocol using 5-fluorouracil and mitomycin C in combination with external beam radiation ther-

apy, a treatment that has resulted in 90+ percent complete response of the tumor and a high cure rate. These treatments have eliminated the need for abdominal perineal resection and colostomy in almost all cases.

Squamous cell cancers at the anal verge outside the anal canal on the skin of the inner buttock are treated by local excision with adequate margins. The results of this technique are similar to excision of other squamous cell cancers in other portions of the anatomy.

Anal Incontinence

The symptoms caused by prolapse of internal hemorrhoidal mucosa and seepage of mucus onto the anal canal can easily be treated with increased fiber and internal elastic ligation of hemorrhoids. More severe hemorrhoidal prolapse should be treated with excisional hemorrhoidectomy using current techniques. Anal incontinence due to sphincter injury should be treated with repair of the sphincter muscle (if it is not responsive to a bowel routine with antidiarrheals, increased bulk fiber, and a bowel regimen with glycerin suppositories). Anal manometry and transrectal ultrasound in conjunction with pudendal nerve terminal motor latency determination will give a clear anatomic and physiologic view of the anal sphincter and its potential for use after a surgical repair. Results from anal sphincter reconstruction using an anterior overlapping muscle repair have been excellent. As the patient becomes older, the results are somewhat less consistent but certainly deserve consideration if there is an obvious sphincter defect. Biofeedback for anal incontinence is only effective if there is a functioning muscle. Biofeedback using sensory muscle retraining results in an improved minimal sensory volume and coordinated squeeze efforts. The muscle contraction may improve, but there has never been a correlation between increased squeeze pressure and an increase in muscle bulk. The treatment of anal incontinence is a complex issue and deserves a lengthy discussion on its own.

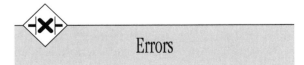

Patient Education

Dietary recommendations for many anal problems are focused on softening stool. High-fiber diets are appropriate for this purpose. The American Dietetic Association recommends 25 to 35 g of fiber daily, which is above the 10 to 15 g daily intake of fiber by most Americans. Vegetables high in fiber include broccoli, green peas, green beans, and other forms of peas and beans. Lettuce and bread have inadequate amounts of fiber to be considered high-fiber foods. Most flake cereals have a low-fiber content also. Only those cereals with psyllium or unprocessed bran should be considered high in fiber. Several fiber supplements are available. Psyllium is an inert insoluble fiber. Methylcellulose is partially soluble and yields stool softening but not bulking. Methylcellulose is also inert and does not result in long-term damage to the colonic mucosa or muscle. Fibercon is an inert but low-volume pill providing one-half gram of dietary fiber per pill. Psyllium should be administered in 3- to 6-g doses; methylcellulose in 3- to 6-g doses. Patients have varying tolerances and preferences to each of these compounds.

Patients should be educated on transmittable diseases including herpes, cytomegalovirus, and HPV. Good hand-washing, frequent follow-up, and use of condoms in sexual encounters should be recommended to prevent transmission of infection.

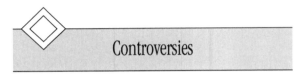

Errors

The major error when evaluating patients with anal pain is to forget to examine the anal canal and thus miss an abscess. The ultimate outcome of an undetected abscess can be Fournier's gangrene in patients with diabetes, HIV, or other immunosup-

pressions. The simple anal evaluation for detection is a sure means of avoiding this complication.

Another potential major mistake is to forego the digital rectal exam and miss a possible anal cancer. Similarly, rectal bleeding in persons at risk for colorectal cancer should never be attributed to hemorrhoids without first conducting a full colon examination to exclude a neoplasm.

A major misconception is that hemorrhoids cause all forms of anal pain. As mentioned earlier, hemorrhoids only cause pain if thrombosis is present and necrosis or ulceration has begun of the overlying skin. The assumption that anal pain is due to hemorrhoidal disease has led to morbidity or even mortality in many high-risk patients with immunosuppression and Fournier's gangrene.

Controversies

Anal Fissure

Lateral internal anal sphincterotomy is successful in 98 percent of patients in terms of resolution of anal pain, but up to 30 percent of patients undergoing this procedure develop anal incontinence. While this may be mild, it is often significant in its effect on the quality of life. Thus, nonsurgical management is being used with increased frequency. Nonsurgical management with nitroglycerin and botulinum toxin results in a higher recurrence rate of the fissure than does surgery, but the initial success rate is extremely high. The author's personal preference is to try conservative therapy first, inform patients of the risk of lateral internal sphincterotomy, and offer surgical treatment if other therapies have failed.

Colonoscopy to Evaluate Rectal Bleeding

Bright red blood per rectum usually implies a rectosigmoid source of bleeding. Colonoscopy may not be required in low-risk patients. *Low-risk patients,* however, refers only to individuals with no family history of rectal or colon cancer and an age under 40 years old. Colonoscopy is definitely indicated in patients over the age of 50 and in those over 40 with a positive family history for colorectal cancer, history of anal cancer, or mucosal abnormalities seen on anoscopy or proctoscopic exam. The yield for colonoscopy in the age group between 40 and 50 without other risk factors is relatively low and the need for colonoscopy in the group is somewhat controversial. However, most experts recommend colonoscopy for such patients.

Excision of Thrombosed External Hemorrhoids

The residual skin tag resulting after resolution of the thrombosis from an external hemorrhoid is present in most patients. The thrombosis resolves in 2 weeks spontaneously. Unfortunately, the skin tags sometimes cause symptoms due to poor hygiene or simply the feeling of the presence of tissue. If patients are extremely anxious and desire definitive therapy and an excision is performed, the usual recovery period is also 2 weeks. However, because pain resolution occurs spontaneously or with excision within 2 weeks, the need for excision is controversial. Most patients can be talked out of an excisional hemorrhoidectomy and encouraged to undergo tub soaks and conservative therapy and allow spontaneous resolution to occur.

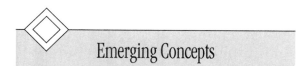

Emerging Concepts

Circular Stapled Hemorrhoidectomy for Internal Large Third-Degree Hemorrhoids

The use of a circular stapled hemorrhoid technique is being evaluated in Europe and the United States. This is a relatively painless procedure re-

sulting in resuspension of the anal canal and hemorrhoidal tissues within the distal rectum and removal of any prolapsing distal rectal mucosa. This technique may need long-term follow-up to evaluate recurrence data before becoming an established method in the armamentarium of colorectal surgeons.

Botulinum Toxin for Anal Fissure

The major side effect of nitroglycerin in the treatment of anal fissures and ulcers is the development of headaches. This side effect can be reduced by proper application techniques with patients in the left lateral decubitus position and the use of gloves to protect the skin of the digit. However, there are other products that may eventually allow the same success without the nitroglycerin-related side effects. These products include myphetopine and other similar calcium-channel-blocking drugs applied to the anal canal. Botulinum toxin, as mentioned earlier, is also effective. Currently a single injection is required every 6 months. The drug may be modified in the future to achieve a longer lasting effect.

Bibliography

ASCRS Standards Practice Task Force: Practice parameters for the management of anal fissure. *Dis Colon Rectum* 35:206–208, 1992.

Fleshman JW: Fissure-in-ano and anal stenosis, in Beck DA, Wexner SD (eds): *Fundamentals of Anorectal Surgery.* London, WB Saunders, Ltd., 1998, pp 209–224.

Fleshner PR: Anal fissure in Crohn's disease. *Semin Colon Rectal Surg* 8:36–39, 1997.

Hananel N, Gordon PH: Re-examination of clinical manifestations and response to treatment of fissure-in-ano. *Dis Colon Rectum* 40:229–233, 1997.

Jensen SL: Treatment of first episodes of acute anal fissure: Prospective randomized study of lidocaine ointment versus hydrocortisone ointment or warm sitz baths plus bran. *Br Med J* 292:1167–1169, 1986.

Jost WH, Schimrigk K: Botulinum toxin in therapy of anal fissure. *Lancet* 345:188–189, 1995.

Miles AJG: Pathophysiology of anoreceptive intercourse, in Allen-Mersh TG, Gottesman L (eds): *Anorectal Disease in AIDS*. London, Edward Arnold, 1991, pp 28–41.

Milsom JW: Hemorrhoidal disease, in Beck DE, Wexner SD (eds): *Fundamentals of Anorectal Surgery*. New York, McGraw-Hill, 1992, pp 192–214.

Saler ME, Gottesman L: Anal and rectal ulcer, in Allen-Mersh TG, Gottesman L (eds): *Anorectal Disease in AIDS*. London, Edward Arnold, 1991, pp 103–129.

Schouten WR, Briel JW, Auwerda JJA: Relationships between anal pressure and anodermal blood flow. The vascular pathogenesis of anal fissures. *Dis Colon Rectum* 37:664–669, 1994.

Stahl TJ: Anorectal physiologic testing in anal fissure disease. *Semin Colon Rectal Surg* 8:6–12, 1997.

Stein BI: Nitroglycerin and other nonoperative therapies for anal fissure. *Semin Colon Rectal Surg* 8:13–16, 1997.

Whalen TV, Lieutenant MC, Kovalcik PJ, et al: Tuberculosis anal ulcer. *Dis Colon Rectum* 23:54–55, 1980.

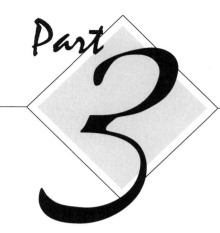

Part 3

Hepatic and Biliary Problems

Saeed Zamani
Steven K. Herrine

Chapter

16

Viral Hepatitis

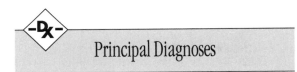

Incidence and Background

Viral hepatitis is the most common cause of chronic liver disease, cirrhosis, and hepatocellular carcinoma in the United States. Each year, some 200,000 to 700,000 new cases of acute viral hepatitis occur in the United States. Although the death rate from acute hepatitis is low, many patients with some types of viral hepatitis become chronically infected, with a large percentage progressing to significant liver disease. The Centers for Disease Control and Prevention (CDC) estimate that approximately 5 million Americans are chronically infected by hepatitis viruses.

Principal Diagnoses

Overview of the Hepatotropic Viruses

HEPATITIS A

Hepatitis A virus (HAV) is a ribonucleic acid (RNA) virus typically transmitted person to person via the fecal–oral route. Because mollusks filter large volumes of water, concentrating both bacteria and viruses, a common vehicle for source outbreaks has been raw or partially cooked shellfish. The reported incidence of acute HAV infection in the United States is 9.1 per 100,000, although infection rates tend to rise and fall sharply every 7 to 10 years. The seroprevalence of HAV in the United States is 38 percent, with rates from 11 percent in children under the age of 5 years to 74 percent in adults 50 years old and older.

HEPATITIS B

Hepatitis B virus (HBV) is a partially double-stranded deoxyribonucleic acid (DNA) virus. Transmission of HBV is primarily parenteral and sexual.

During the past decade, the annual reported incidence of hepatitis B in the United States has been 40 cases per 100,000 persons. Chronic HBV infection has an estimated global prevalence of more than 300 million carriers, or approximately 5 percent of the world's population. According to World Health Organization statistics, hepatitis B-induced cirrhosis and liver cancer is the ninth most common cause of death worldwide, accounting for more than 1 million fatalities each year. Of the more than 1 million Americans with chronic HBV infection, an estimated 15 to 25 percent will die of associated complications.

HEPATITIS C

Hepatitis C virus (HCV) is a single-stranded RNA virus that undergoes significant genetic changes during replication. These changes may explain the ability of HCV to evade the host's immune surveillance and cause chronic infection. It is transmitted via the parenteral route, with the majority of new infections occurring as a result of intravenous drug use.

The worldwide seroprevalence of HCV infection, based on antibody to HCV, is estimated to be 1 percent. It is currently estimated that 3.9 million people in the United States, or 1.8 percent of the population, are infected with HCV. The current incidence of acute infection in the United States is estimated at 28,000 cases per year, a nearly tenfold decrease over the last decade.

Since universal blood product testing was instituted in 1992, transmission by means of blood transfusion has become rare. Injection drug use, however, whether current or remote, has emerged as the most common cause of HCV infection. Although approximately 20 percent of infected individuals deny any known risk factors for HCV infection, the majority of this population have participated in some high-risk behaviors such as past drug use, history of sexually transmitted disease, body piercing, tattoos, intranasal cocaine use, or a prison stay.

HEPATITIS D

Hepatitis D virus (HDV) is an incomplete RNA virus that requires the presence of chronic HBV infection to replicate. Its mode of transmission is identical to that of HBV.

HEPATITIS E

Hepatitis E virus (HEV) is an RNA virus, similar in natural history and mode of transmission to HAV. Unlike HAV, however, HEV is rarely seen in the United States, with the disease occurring most commonly in the developing nations of Asia, Africa, and the Indian subcontinent. Epidemics typically occur after the rainy season and are spread by drinking water.

Clinical Syndromes

ACUTE VIRAL HEPATITIS

Early manifestations of acute viral hepatitis include fatigue, malaise, anorexia, nausea, vomiting, and right upper quadrant abdominal discomfort. Less common symptoms include fever, headache, arthralgias, myalgia, and diarrhea. Although patients can present with dark urine, light-colored stool, and scleral icterus, anicteric infections are three times more likely than are icteric infections for all forms of hepatitis virus infections. Tenderness and mild hepatomegaly are present in 85 percent of patients, while a minority of patients may have splenomegaly and posterior cervical lymphadenopathy.

Hepatitis A virus is an acute self-limited disease. The clinical spectrum of disease ranges from asymptomatic infection to fulminant hepatitis, as described later. Acute HBV infection can present with extrahepatic findings such as arthralgias and rashes. Less commonly, immune complex deposition can result in angioneurotic edema or systemic vasculitis. Acute HCV infection is rarely seen in practice since the vast majority of patients experience no clinical symptoms. Among persons identified as HCV positive through routine screen-ing, as many as 90 percent do not recall an episode suggesting the onset of acute illness. The HDV infection presents in a similar fashion to acute HBV when transmitted as a coinfection with HBV. However, if HDV is transmitted as a superinfection in patients with preexistent chronic HBV, the syndrome is generally more severe. Acute HEV, like HAV, is a generally a self-limited infection, except when seen in pregnant women, in whom fulminant hepatitis develops with high frequency.

FULMINANT HEPATIC FAILURE

The most profound complication of acute viral hepatitis infection is fulminant hepatic failure, defined as the onset of encephalopathy or coagulopathy within 6 weeks of the development of jaundice. Although fulminant hepatic failure is an infrequent form of acute viral hepatitis, occurring in less than 1 percent of patients, the prognosis is poor in the absence of liver transplantation. Fulminant hepatitis is infrequent in HAV and rare in HCV. Hepatitis B virus is responsible for 70 percent of fulminant hepatitis, but only 1 percent of cases of hepatitis B has a fulminant presentation. Fulminant hepatitis can occur in 10 to 20 percent of pregnant women infected with HEV.

CHRONIC VIRAL HEPATITIS

Chronic hepatitis is defined as the presence of elevated serum transaminases for longer than 6 months. In practice, however, the exact onset of abnormal liver blood tests is usually unknown. In such cases, clinical impression must be used to differentiate acute, self-limited hepatitis from chronic hepatitis.

No chronic carriers of HAV or HEV have ever been identified. Chronic HBV, however, occurs in approximately 5 percent of HBV-infected adults, although the incidence of chronic infection is much higher in the pediatric population. In contrast, approximately 85 percent of patients infected with HCV develop chronic infection.

Most patients with mild chronic hepatitis are asymptomatic, although a sizable percentage may note fatigue, depression, nausea, anorexia, abdominal discomfort, or difficulty with concentration. Once patients develop cirrhosis of the liver, they are at risk for complications of portal hypertension such as variceal hemorrhage, ascites, and hepatic encephalopathy. Important extrahepatic manifestations of chronic viral hepatitis include essential mixed cryoglobulinemia, membranoproliferative glomerulonephritis, and porphyria cutanea tarda.

END-STAGE LIVER DISEASE

Of patients with chronic hepatitis B and active viral replication, 15 to 20 percent develop cirrhosis within 5 years. It is estimated that at least 20 percent of patients with chronic HCV will develop cirrhosis within 20 years of infection. Of those with cirrhosis, approximately 1.5 percent per year will develop decompensated liver disease, manifested by portal hypertension, coagulopathy, encephalopathy, or hepatocellular carcinoma. The risk of developing cirrhosis is enhanced by the regular use of alcohol. Because of the large population of chronically exposed individuals and the frequency of chronicity of infection, HCV is the leading indication for adults with liver transplantation in the United States. While nearly all recipients will remain viremic with HCV following transplantation, their liver disease is usually mild and slowly progressive. Five-year survival in these patients is similar to patients transplanted for other disease.

HEPATOCELLULAR CARCINOMA

Chronic HBV infection is the leading cause of hepatocellular carcinoma throughout the world, accounting for 75 to 90 percent of the world's cases. The actual risk in individual patients depends on the activity of the infection, age of acquisition, duration of infection, and the presence or absence of cirrhosis. The rate of progression from chronic HCV to hepatocellular carcinoma is estimated at 0.2 to 0.7 percent per year. Screening for the development of hepatocellular carcinoma in patients with chronic HBV and in those with HCV-related cirrhosis may allow early detection and improvement in outcome.

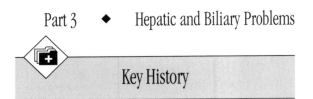

Key History

History in patients with hepatitis is focused on identification of risk factors that might predict the type of hepatitis. Identification of risk factors is also useful in the prevention of hepatitis in intimate contacts and the general population.

Risk Factors for Hepatitis A Virus

Risk factors associated with the acquisition of hepatitis A in the United States include personal contacts with an infected person, attendance in a day care center, travel to developing nations, food- and waterborne disease outbreaks, and injection drug use. In 40 to 50 percent of cases, the source of infection is not known (Figure 16-1). Native Americans and Latinos are at higher risk than other populations in the United States.

Risk Factors for Hepatitis B Virus

Percutaneous and mucous membrane exposure to infected bodily fluids (serum, semen, and saliva) and vertical transmissions from mother to child are the major sources of HBV infection. Although HBV viral antigens can be detected in breast milk, breast-feeding is not believed to be an important mode of transmission. Health care workers exposed to blood products have a higher prevalence of infection than does the general population. Immigrants from endemic areas such as Alaska, Asia, and the Pacific Islands are at high risk of exposure. Injection drug use and sexual practices such as receptive anal intercourse or heterosexual promiscuity also increase the risk of HBV infection.

Risk Factors for Hepatitis C Virus

Transmission patterns of HCV have changed in recent years. Prior to the discovery of HCV, there was a strong correlation found between hepatitis

Figure 16-1

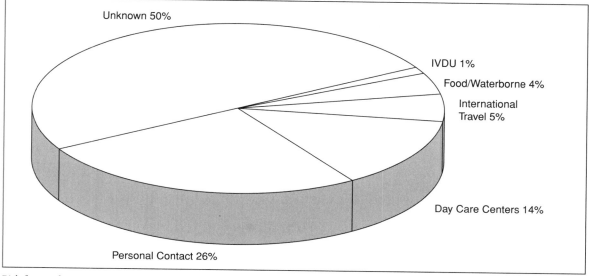

Risk factors for acute hepatitis A virus in the United States.

and a recent history of blood transfusion. Because transfused blood is now screened for the presence of HCV, injection drug use, sexual and household exposure, promiscuous sexual behavior, and low socioeconomic status have now become the most important risk factors (Figure 16-2). Estimates of the prevalence of HCV antibodies in patients requiring hemodialysis range from 15 to 48 percent in North America.

Most experts agree that sexual transmission of HCV occurs, but a growing consensus view such transmission as inefficient and relatively uncommon. Although early population-based reports on the risk factors for HCV mention household contact, documented cases of such transmission in the United States are absent. The currently accepted estimate of vertical transmission is around 6 percent. The prevalence of HCV in clinical and laboratory health care workers is variously estimated at 1.0 to 2.0 percent, some four times higher than in the volunteer donor population, but the same as the general population.

Risk Factors for Hepatitis D and E Viruses

The risk factors for HDV are identical to those for HBV. Because HDV can infect only those patients also infected with HBV, any decompensation in patients with previously stable HBV should prompt an evaluation for HDV infection. Hepatitis E virus is spread via the fecal–oral route in a similar fashion to HAV. Consideration of HEV infection should be given only to those patients from endemic areas as described earlier.

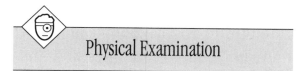

Physical Examination

Although anicteric viral hepatitis is more common than icteric infections, jaundice is an important finding, suggesting hepatocellular necrosis or biliary obstruction. Jaundice, usually detectable with

Figure 16-2

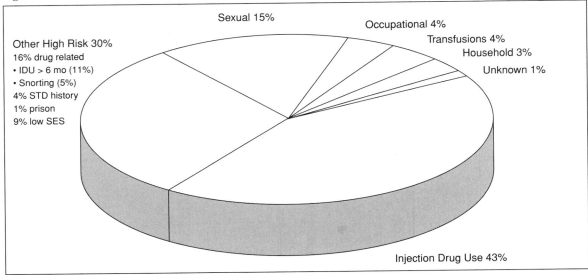

Risk factors for acute hepatitis C virus in the United States.

serum bilirubin above 3 mg/dl, is most noticeable in the sclerae and sublingual area. Abdominal tenderness and tender hepatomegaly are present in 85 percent of patients with acute viral hepatitis. The skin may be excoriated from the pruritus that often accompanies cholestasis. In disease that has advanced to cirrhosis, the left lobe of the liver may be nodular and enlarged, with associated splenomegaly. Abdominal wall collateral vessels, umbilical hernia, and ascites may be present. Other stigmata of chronic liver disease, such as spider telangiectasia, palmar erythema, gynecomastia, and testicular atrophy, can be seen.

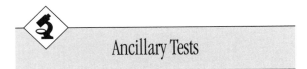

Ancillary Tests

Routine Blood Tests

In acute viral hepatitis, the rise in serum alanine aminotransferase (ALT) is typically greater than the increase in serum aspartate aminotransferase (AST), often exceeding 1000 IU/dl. Serum aminotransferase elevations usually precede changes in serum bilirubin and alkaline phosphatase. These elevations tend not to persist beyond 6 months and almost always return to normal within a year.

Persistently elevated serum ALT is the hallmark of chronic viral hepatitis. Even slight persistent abnormalities (i.e., a few points above the upper limit of normal) in serum aminotransferases should prompt a serologic evaluation for viral hepatitis. Approximately 30 percent of chronically infected patients have persistently normal ALT levels and, in some others, the ALT may be intermittently elevated. In chronic HCV, ALT levels do not correlate with the histologic extent of the liver disease.

Serologic Evaluation

HEPATITIS A VIRUS

The presence of immunoglobulin M (IgM) anti-HAV in serum collected during acute or convalescent period of the disease (>5 days following exposure) confirms a diagnosis of hepatitis A. In most patients, IgM anti-HAV then slowly declines becoming undetectable 3 to 6 months after infection. Infected individuals also will produce immunoglobulin G (IgG) anti-HAV during the convalescent phase. This marker, detectable in serum for the life of patients, is protective against reinfection (Figure 16-3).

HEPATITIS B VIRUS

Hepatitis B surface antigen (HBsAg), anti-HB core IgM, and HBV DNA are the first serum markers of acute HBV, becoming detectable within 6 weeks after infection and before the onset of clinical symptoms or biochemical abnormalities. These tests remain positive throughout the prodromal phase and during the early clinical phase of the illness.

In chronic infection, HBsAg and HBV DNA remain positive for at least 6 months. Anti-HB core IgG persists indefinitely as a marker of previous exposure. With time, there may a spontaneous loss of HBV DNA and Hepatitis B surface antigen (HBsAg). The latter, HBsAg, is a marker of active replication and infection (Figure 16-4).

HEPATITIS C VIRUS

Antibodies to HCV detected by the enzyme-linked immunoassay (EIA) are the primary screening tool for the diagnosis of hepatitis C. Supplementary testing for infection with HCV should always be performed on asymptomatic individuals from low-risk settings who are anti-HCV positive. Individuals in high-risk groups with positive EIA results do not usually require supplementary testing to confirm the diagnosis. For those with biochemical or clinical signs of liver disease, a positive EIA finding will be sufficient to make the diagnosis.

Viral RNA detection is accomplished by amplification methods such as polymerase chain reaction (PCR) or signal amplification methods such as branched-chain DNA (bDNA) assay. Quantification of viral RNA is useful in assessing the effectiveness of antiviral therapy. Hepatitis C now is classified as six major genotypes and many subtypes. Differentiation of these genotypes can be accomplished by direct sequencing. Genotyping allows the clinician to predict responsiveness to interferon therapy and, in some cases, to shorten the recommended course of therapy.

Figure 16-3

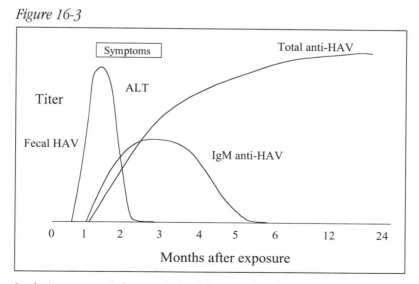

Serologic parameters in hepatitis A virus infection. Adapted from American Gastroenterological Association, Bethesda, Maryland. Used with permission.

Figure 16-4

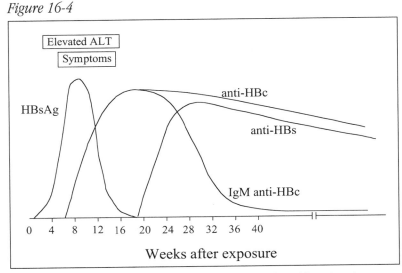

Serologic parameters in acute hepatis B virus infection. Adapted from American Gastroenterological Association, Bethesda, Maryland. Used with permission.

Imaging

Although most patients with hepatitis have normal liver ultrasound examinations, the technique is useful for detecting changes of cirrhosis, portal hypertension, and intraparenchymal masses. On ultrasound examination acute hepatitis may result in a diffusely hypoechoic liver with increased echogenicity to the periportal regions. Homogeneous coarsened echotexture with high periportal echogenicity can be seen in patients with chronic hepatitis. When the suspicion of hepatocellular carcinoma is high, computed tomography with intravenous contrast and magnetic resonance imaging with gadolinium are more sensitive and specific than ultrasonography.

Liver Biopsy

Liver biopsy is a safe and well-tolerated outpatient procedure. Under local anesthesia, a core of liver tissue is excised via transabdominal puncture, either with or without ultrasound guidance. In the setting of viral hepatitis, a random core is representative of the entire parenchyma. Liver biopsy can provide information about the severity of disease and is usually indicated to stage chronic hepatitis, especially if treatment is considered. The finding of periportal or bridging fibrosis in chronic hepatitis makes treatment more imperative since the rate of progression relates best to the degree of inflammation and scarring. In uncomplicated acute hepatitis, however, liver biopsy is seldom indicated unless the etiology of the illness is unclear.

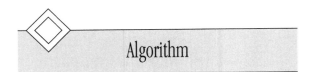

Algorithm

Please see algorithm for evaluation of abnormal liver function tests (Figure 19-1, page 277).

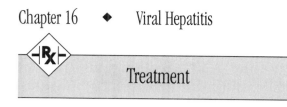

Treatment

Prevention

HEPATITIS A VIRUS

Prevention of HAV infection requires attention to public and personal health measures. Strict adherence to hand-washing in hospitals and in day care or institutional settings is important in preventing person-to-person spread. Travelers to endemic areas should be advised to avoid drinking water or beverages with ice from sources of unknown purity. Similarly, raw vegetables and uncooked shellfish may also harbor infection.

HEPATITIS B AND C VIRUSES

Improved screening measures of blood products, changes in sexual practice in response to the HIV epidemic, and changing practices in injection drug users have contributed to a declining incidence of hepatitis B and C infections in the United States. Epidemiologic studies suggest that the most important factor in the decline of incidence in acute HBV and HCV is a decrease in transmission from shared intravenous needles (Figure 16-5). Current U.S. Public Health Service recommendations advise that although HCV can be transmitted from persons with chronic disease to their steady sexual partner, the risk for transmission is low despite long-term, ongoing sexual activity. Infected persons should be informed of the potential risk for sexual transmission to assist in decision-making about precautions. Persons with multiple sex partners should adopt safer sex practices, including reducing the number of sex partners and using barriers (e.g., latex condoms) to prevent contact with bodily fluids. There is no evidence to advise against pregnancy in woman with chronic HCV nor has there been a documented case of HCV transmission by breast-feeding.

Figure 16-5

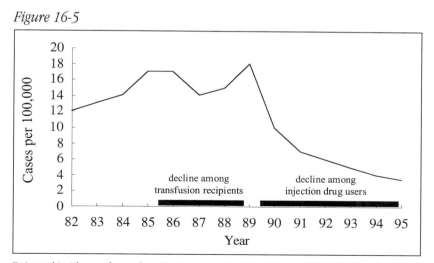

Estimated incidence of acute hepatitis C virus in the United States, 1982–1995. Data from Alter MJ: Epidemiology of hepatitis C. *Hepatology* 26 (Suppl 1): 62S–65S, 1997.

Table 16-1

Recommendations of the Advisory Committee on Immunization Practices of the Centers of Disease Control:
Groups Requiring Anti-Hepatitis A Virus Vaccination

> Persons traveling to or working in countries with high or intermediate rates of disease
> Children living in communities with high rates of disease or periodic outbreaks
> Children and young adults living in communities with intermediate rates of disease
> Individuals who engage in high-risk behaviors, such as the following:
>> Homosexual activities
>> Illegal drug use
> Patients with chronic liver disease
> Individuals with occupational risk of disease, such as primate handlers

Prophylaxis of Exposed Individuals

Passive immunization is recommended for household contacts of index cases and travelers to endemic areas. Household contacts of HAV-infected individuals should be given pooled human immune serum immunoglobulin (ISIg), unless there is a well-documented history of hepatitis A in the past. Contacts outside the home (at work or school) do not require passive immunoprophylaxis. The administration of ISIg before the exposure will prevent HAV infection in 85 to 95 percent of exposed individuals. Administration within 1 to 2 weeks of exposure will prevent or attenuate infection, and administration beyond 2 weeks after exposure is ineffective. The duration of protection appears to be dose-related, with the 0.02 ml/kg dose providing protection for approximately 3 months.

Passive immunoprophylaxis in HBV is used in four situations: (a) neonates born to HBsAg-positive mothers, (b) needlestick exposure, (c) sexual exposure, and (d) liver transplantation in HbsAg-positive patients. Immunoprophylaxis is recommended for all infants born to HBsAg-positive mothers.

There have been no studies of ISIg for the prevention of HCV infection. It seems unlikely that ISIg would contain sufficient neutralizing antibodies to be effective and is therefore not recommended.

Vaccination

HEPATITIS A VIRUS

The availability of hepatitis A vaccines provides a powerful tool to lower disease incidence and potentially eliminate infection by increasing the immunity of high-risk individuals. Table 16-1 outlines the list of those at risk in whom vaccination should be recommended. In the face of community outbreaks, vaccination is recommended for food service workers and health care providers.

The U.S. Food and Drug Administration (FDA) has licensed two formalin-inactivated hepatitis A vaccines, Havrix and VAQTA. Both are highly effective in adults and children. The most common adverse events are pain, tenderness, and warmth at the site of injection. The safety of vaccinations during pregnancy is unknown. Special precautions need not be taken for the immuno-compromised, as the vaccines are inactivated.

HEPATITIS B VIRUS

Effective vaccines against HBV have been available since the early 1980s. In 1988, the CDC recommended screening all pregnant women in the United States for HBV infection. In 1991, universal childhood vaccination against HBV infection was recommended. In 1994, the CDC expanded their recommendations to include all

11- and 12-year-olds who had not previously been vaccinated and all children less than 11 years of age of ethnic groups at high risk for HBV infection. More than 95 percent of healthy infants, children, and young adults who receive three intramuscular doses of vaccine develop protective serum titers of anti-HBs.

HEPATITIS C VIRUS

Vaccine development for HCV has been hampered by the same difficulties encountered in the vaccine development against HIV infection due to variability and mutability in strains of the virus. Regardless of other treatment considerations, all patients with hepatitis C should be vaccinated against hepatitis A and hepatitis B as these infections may cause significant morbidity and mortality when superimposed on preexisting liver disease.

Antiviral Therapy

Type 1 interferons have been available for the treatment of both chronic hepatitis B and C viruses for more than 10 years. These recombinant compounds are injected subcutaneously for 6 to 18 months in patients with chronic viral hepatitis. Side effects include flulike symptoms, fatigue, irritability, depression, thyroid abnormalities, and bone marrow suppression. Response rates range from 10 to 40 percent depending on the virus being treated and the length of therapy. Because of the complexities of patient and drug regimen choice, as well as the potential toxicity of the interferons, this therapy is generally administered by specialists in gastroenterology and hepatology. Newer therapies for chronic hepatitis B include nucleoside analogs such as lamivudine and adefovir, which can be taken orally with minimal adverse reactions. In hepatitis C, the nucleoside analog ribavirin, when used in combination with interferon, increases response rates by reducing posttreatment relapse.

Liver Transplantation

Despite improved prevention, detection, and treatment, end-stage liver disease will develop in a subset of patients with chronic hepatitis. It is generally agreed that patients with chronic liver disease qualify for liver transplantation if their chance of 1-year survival is less than 90 percent. Nationwide uniform listing criteria are based upon the type of liver disease (hepatocellular or cholestatic) and the Child-Pugh-Turcotte score (Table 16-2). Variceal hemorrhage, the development of ascites, or spontaneous bacterial peritonitis, hepatic encephalopathy, and worsening hepatocellular synthetic function should prompt consultation with

Table 16-2
Child-Pugh-Turcotte Score

	POINTS		
	1	2	3
Encephalopathy	None	1,2	3,4
Ascites	Absent	Slight	Moderate or controlled by diuretics
Bilirubin (mg/dl)	1–2	2–3	>3
Albumin (g/dl)	>3.5	2.8–3.5	<2.8
INR	<1.7	1.8–2.3	>2.3

INR, international normalized ratio.

a transplant center. A history of at least 6 months of alcohol abstinence is generally required for those patients with a history of alcohol-related liver disease before they will be considered for transplantation.

In the past, hepatitis B has been a controversial indication for liver transplantation because the high rate of recurrent infection has limited survival to only 40 to 50 percent after 3 years. Effective prophylaxis can be now be achieved, and most transplant hepatologists now recommend that patients with liver failure due to acute or chronic hepatitis B be considered candidates for liver transplantation, irrespective of their initial viral replication status.

Approximately 20 percent of hepatitis C patients develop cirrhosis during the first 2 decades of disease, although in rare cases, cirrhosis can develop within the first 2 years. The risk of developing cirrhosis appears to accelerate in patients over the age of 50 to 55 years and in the presence of alcohol intake. Chronic hepatitis C, accompanied by cirrhosis and hepatic failure, is the leading indication for liver transplantation in adults in the United States, accounting for 30 to 50 percent of cases at most transplant centers. While nearly all recipients will remain positive for HCV RNA following transplantation, liver disease usually is mild and only slowly progressive. Five-year survival in these patients is similar to recipients who receive transplants for other diseases.

Patient Education

Clinicians can help patients prevent the acquisition of viral hepatitis by way of education during different stages of their lives. Reinforcement of the recommended vaccination schedules may be the single most effective strategy. Young adults who have not received HBV vaccination should do so before commencing sexual activities. Travelers to endemic areas should have native or vaccine-

induced HAV antibodies. Users of intravenous drugs should be encouraged not to share needles, to sterilize injection instruments, or to enroll in needle exchange programs.

Patients who have chronic viral hepatitis should minimize or abstain from alcohol consumption. Consultation with specialists should be encouraged, as the agents available for therapy of chronic viral hepatitis are constantly improving. Transmission risk should be minimized by discouraging blood and organ donation, sharing of toothbrushes and razors, and using barrier methods with new sexual partners.

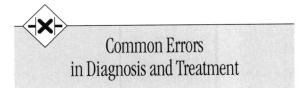

Common Errors in Diagnosis and Treatment

The two common errors in the diagnosis and treatment of viral hepatitis are the lack of recognition of chronic viral hepatitis and undue delay in referring patients for liver transplantation.

Diagnosis

Any elevation in ALT, no matter how slight, should be investigated. Although fatty liver, drug effects, and alcohol can account for some of these laboratory abnormalities, a high index of suspicion for chronic viral hepatitis must be maintained at all times. A careful history may reveal the presence of risk factors or previously recognized elevated transaminases. The finding of anti-HCV or HBsAg in the presence of increased serum aminotransaminases is highly suggestive of chronic hepatitis and should prompt consultation with a specialist.

Referral

Patients with cirrhosis who develop decompensation, manifested by variceal bleeding, the development of ascites, hepatic encephalopathy, or early synthetic dysfunction (elevated prothrombin time and decreased serum albumin), should be referred to a transplant center for evaluation. The lack of organ donors has led to progressively longer waiting times than previously for potential recipients. Early recognition and prompt evaluation of progressive liver disease will lead to improved outcomes at the time of transplantation.

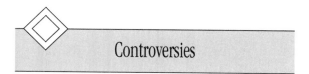

Controversies

Persistently Normal Liver Tests

The frequency of persistently normal ALT levels in patients who have chronic hepatitis C is unclear, but it may be as high as 25 percent. Data from a number of studies suggest that patients with chronic HCV infection who have persistently normal ALT levels are more likely to have minimal or mild liver disease. However, the extent of liver injury cannot be assumed without a liver biopsy, since a small number of patients may have advanced disease even with normal ALT levels. The treatment of this population has led to low response rates and is not recommended outside of controlled clinical trials.

HIV Coinfection

As the survival of HIV-infected patients improves, the need to consider treating chronic hepatitis virus infections in HIV-infected patients becomes necessary. Interferon therapy in patients with chronic HBV infection has been disappointing, with response rates only one-quarter of those seen in non-HIV-infected patients. Lamivudine, a nucleoside analog that inhibits reverse transcriptase in both HIV and HBV, may benefit this group. Early trials of interferon use in patients coinfected with HCV and HIV have led to acceptable response

rates in those with minimally damaged immune systems. Although few liver transplants have been performed in patients with HIV infection, more are sure to follow, allowing more data on graft function, immunocompetence, and survival.

Bibliography

Alter MJ, Mast EE: The epidemiology of viral hepatitis in the United States. *Gasteroenterol Clin North Am* 23: 437–455, 1994.

Alter MJ, Kruszon-Moran D, Nainan OV, et al: The prevalence of hepatitis C virus infection in the United States, 1988 through 1994. *N Engl J Med* 34: 556–562, 1999.

Anonymous: National Institutes of Health consensus development conference panel statement. Management of hepatitis C. *Hepatology* 26:2S–10S, 1997.

Bukh J, Miller RH, Purcell RH: Genetic heterogeneity of hepatitis C virus: Quasispecies and genotypes. *Semin Liver Dis* 15:41–63, 1995.

Carithers RL, Emerson SS: Therapy of hepatitis C: Meta-analysis of interferon alfa-2b trials. *Hepatology* 26: 83S–88S, 1997.

Centers for Disease Control and Prevention: Risk of acquiring hepatitis C for health care workers and recommendations for prophylaxis and follow-up after occupational exposure. Hepatitis surveillance Report No. 56. Atlanta, 1995.

Dienstag JL, Perrilo RP, Schiff ER, et al: A preliminary trial of lamivudine for chronic hepatitis B infection. *N Engl J Med* 333:1657–1661, 1995.

Dodson SF, Issa S, Bonham A: Liver transplantation for chronic viral hepatitis. *Surg Clin North Am* 79: 131–145, 1999.

Gumber SC, Chopra S: Hepatitis C: A multifaceted disease. Review of extrahepatic manifestations. *Ann Intern Med* 123:615–620, 1995.

Herrine SK, Weinberg DS: Epidemiology of hepatitis C viral infection. *Infect Med* 16:111–117, 1999.

Lai C-L, Chien R-N, Leung NWY, et al: A one year trial of lamivudine for chronic hepatitis B. *N Engl J Med* 339:61–68, 1998.

Lee WM: Management of acute liver failure. *Semin Liver Dis* 16:369–378, 1996.

Lemon SM, Thomas DL: Vaccines to prevent viral hepatitis. *N Engl J Med* 336:96–204, 1997.

Lucey MR, Brown KA, Everson GT, et al: Minimal criteria for placement of adults on the liver transplant
waiting list. *Transplantation* 66:956–962, 1998.

McHutchinson JG, Gordon SC, Schiff ER, et al: Interferon alfa-2b alone or in combination with ribavirin
as initial treatment for chronic hepatitis C. *N Engl
J Med* 21:1485–1492, 1998.

Poynard T, Leroy V, Thevenot T, et al: Meta-analysis of
interferon randomized trials in the treatment of viral
hepatitis C: Effects of dose and duration. *Hepatology*
24:778–789, 1996.

Sharara AI, Hunt CM, Hamilton JD: Hepatitis C. *Ann
Intern Med* 125:658–668, 1996.

Soriano V, Garcia-Samaniego J, Bravo R, et al: Inter-
feron-alpha for the treatment of chronic hepatitis C
in patients infected with human immunodeficiency
virus. *Clin Infect Dis* 23:585–590, 1996.

Stehman-Breen C, Willson R, Alpers CE, et al: Hepatitis
C virus-associated glomerulonephritis. *Curr Opin
Nephrol Hypertens* 4:287–294, 1995.

Tong MJ, el-Farra NS, Reikes AR, et al: Clinical outcomes after transfusion-associated hepatitis C. *N Engl
J Med* 332:1463–1466, 1995.

Wejstal R, Widell A, Mansson A, et al: Mother-to-infant
transmission of hepatitis C virus. *Ann Intern Med*
117:887–890, 1992.

Cheryl A. Cox
Stephen J. Bickston

Chapter

17

Right Upper Quadrant Pain: Gallbladder Disease and Its Complications

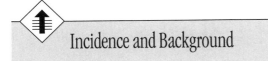

Incidence and Background

Right upper quadrant pain is a common problem that accounts for many elective and emergency room visits. Although the list of causes is extensive, one of the most common is cholelithiasis (gallstones) and its associated complications. Gallstone disease represents the most frequent and costly cause of hospital admissions due to gastrointestinal disease, and cholecystectomies are the most common elective abdominal operations performed in the United States. Gallbladder disease costs Americans an estimated $4.5 billion annually. A large multiethnic population-based study looking at the prevalence of gallstone disease in the United States found that the highest prevalence was in Mexican-American women (26.7 percent) and the lowest in non-Hispanic black men (5.3 percent). Women had about double the prevalence of men in the same ethnic group. Data from other countries estimate the prevalence to range from 5.9 to 21.9 percent. There is wide variability between certain subpopulations, with a prevalence of 70 percent among the Pima Indian women of Arizona and 5.2 percent among the Sudanese population of sub-Saharan Africa. African-Americans have a lower prevalence than whites.

The majority of gallstones are asymptomatic. When patients seek medical attention, it is most often for symptoms of uncomplicated biliary colic.

Acute cholecystitis and gallstone pancreatitis are more serious complications of gallstone disease.

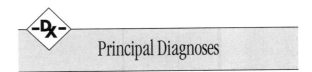

Principal Diagnoses

Types of Gallstones

There are three main types of gallstones categorized on the basis of composition. The first, and most common, are completely or primarily composed of cholesterol. They are referred to as cholesterol stones. The supersaturation of bile with cholesterol is the initial event in the formation of cholesterol stones. This is followed by the formation of submicroscopic crystals or amorphous particles that can condense to form gallstones. Finally, gallbladder hypomotility and biliary stasis also act to promote the formation of gallstones.

The second type of gallstones is a black pigment stone. Patients with cirrhosis and chronic hemolytic states are more likely to form black pigment stones. These stones are composed of calcium bilirubinate or complexes of calcium, copper, and mucin glycoproteins.

Brown pigment stones are the third type. They are composed of calcium salts of unconjugated bilirubin with variable amounts of cholesterol and protein. They may be caused by the action of anaerobic bacterial enzymes, although this has not been proved.

Risk Factors for Developing Gallstones

Several risk factors have been associated with the development of gallstones. The old saying, "fat, female, forty, and fertile" is often evoked in association with those most at risk for gallstone formation. Women have a two- to threefold increase in the prevalence of gallstones. This is felt to be associated with estrogen secretion, as the prevalence between men and women becomes essentially equal after the fifth decade of life. Obesity, as well as rapid weight loss, both greatly increase the risk of developing gallstones. The risk of developing gallstones after gastric bypass surgery is approximately 30 percent. Although hypercholesterolemia does not seem to be a risk factor for gallstone formation, high serum triglyceride levels have been positively associated with an increased incidence of gallstone disease. Certain drugs, such as estrogens and oral contraceptives, clofibrate, octreotide, and ceftriaxone, have also been associated with increased lithogenesis. Diabetics may be prone to gallstone formation although it is difficult to distinguish whether this is due to the diabetes or attendant obesity and hypertriglyceridemia.

◇
Complications of Gallstone Disease

Symptomatic Cholelithiasis

Most patients diagnosed with gallstones will remain asymptomatic for life. When symptoms occur, they are most often biliary colic and not more serious complications (Figure 17-1). According to the 1992 National Institutes of Health Consensus Conference report, 10 percent of patients develop symptoms during the first 5 years after diagnosis and 20 percent develop symptoms after 20 years. Approximately 30 percent of patients experiencing a first attack of biliary colic will have no further attacks over the following 2 years.

A landmark study by Gracie and Ransohoff at the University of Michigan suggested that the annual rate of developing symptoms once cholelithiasis has been diagnosed is 2 percent per year for the first 5 years with decreases over time. The annual rate of developing a serious complication of biliary disease requiring urgent surgical intervention is only about 1 percent.

As noted, biliary colic is the most common initial presentation of gallstone disease (see later). It is caused by the intermittent obstruction of the cystic duct by one or more gallstones without associated inflammation of the gallbladder. The pain is of visceral origin and therefore is usually poorly localized. Most often the pain is in the epigastric region or right upper quadrant, although it may also manifest in the left upper quadrant or is referred to the right subscapular or shoulder region. Studies of the pain of biliary colic found that about one-third of patients described it as maximal at onset, one-third noted a peak after 10 to 60 min, and the remainder reported the maximal pain intensity after several hours.

The quality of the pain was the same for most patients. Most patients (90 percent) described a steady, continuous pain that did not vary in intensity. A small percentage had a steady severe pain with short, intermittent exacerbation. Only 2 percent of patients had pain-free intervals and thus true colic. Typical intervals between attacks can be weeks to years.

Acute Cholecystitis

Acute cholecystitis is the most common and clinically important complication of gallstone disease. It occurs when a gallstone becomes impacted in the cystic duct and causes obstruction of the duct. The result is biliary stasis and inflammatory changes in the gallbladder mucosa. Enteric bacteria have been cultured from the gallbladder bile in only about one-half of patients with acute cholecystitis. Thus, infection is not felt to play a significant role in the development of the disease.

Chronic Cholecystitis

Chronic cholecystitis is a misnomer in that it implies a state of chronic inflammation, which may not be present in a given patient. Chronic cholecystitis usually presents as recurrent episodes of biliary colic. It may be associated with a scarred, shrunken gallbladder, but significant pathologic changes seen in the gallbladder have little correlation with the frequency and severity of biliary colic in these patients. Long-standing cholelithiasis and chronic cholecystitis may lead to the development of gallbladder malignancy.

Choledocholithiasis

When a gallstone either forms in the common bile duct (CBD) or migrates to the CBD from the gallbladder, it is referred to as choledocholithiasis. Of those with symptomatic cholelithiasis, 15 to 20 percent also have stones in the biliary ducts. This complication can lead to cholangitis and biliary pancreatitis.

Patients suspected of having choledocholithiasis can be grouped into categories based on their risk of having the condition (Table 17-1). Low-risk patients have no history of choledocholithiasis, normal liver function tests (LFTs), and no ultrasonographic evidence of biliary duct dilation. Bile duct stones will be found in only 2 to 3 percent of these patients. Intermediate-risk patients have moderate elevations in their LFTs, moderate dilation of the CBD (8- to 10-mm diameter) on ultrasonography, and/or a history of cholangitis or biliary pancreatitis, suggesting the passage of a previous stone. The likelihood of a CBD stone in this group is 20 to 40 percent. High-risk patients have cholangitis or recent acute pancreatitis and

Table 17-1

Categories of Risk for Patients with Choledocholithiasis

RISK	CHARACTERISTICS
Low	No history of choledocholithiasis
	Normal LFTs
	No evidence of common bile duct dilation
Intermediate	With or without history of pancreatitis/cholangitis
	Elevated LFTs
	Moderate dilation of common bile duct
High	Cholangitis or biliary pancreatitis
	Elevated LFTs, jaundice, alkaline phosphatase >2X normal
	Significant common bile duct dilation (10 mm)

LFTs, liver (hepatic) function tests.

jaundice and an alkaline phosphatase higher than twice that of normal patients as well as evidence of significant CBD dilation (>10 mm diameter). Choledocholithiasis will be found in 50 to 80 percent of these patients.

Cholangitis

Episodes of cholangitis are the most serious and life-threatening complications of gallstone disease. When obstruction occurs, biliary pressure increases and bile flow is diminished. This can allow for the seeding of bile with bacteria and result in infection of the biliary tree (cholangitis). Cholangitis occurs in 6 to 9 percent of patients admitted with gallstone disease. Its severity is highly variable and reported mortality rates range from 13 to 88 percent. Complete obstruction of the duct can lead to frank pus in the biliary system, septicemia, and intrahepatic abscess formation unless treated promptly. Intravenous fluids, antibiotics, and biliary decompression are the mainstays of therapy.

Gallstone Pancreatitis

Gallstones are responsible for 30 to 75 percent of all cases of acute pancreatitis. In 1901, Opie postulated that a gallstone becoming impacted in the ampulla of Vater causing biliary obstruction was the initiating event leading to acute biliary pancreatitis. This concept is still embraced today, although the exact mechanism of the development of gallstone pancreatitis is unknown. The leading theories are that either it is a result of obstruction to the flow of pancreatic enzymes or the reflux of bile or duodenal contents into the pancreatic duct, with either leading to inflammation of the pancreas. It is often difficult to document gallstones as a cause of pancreatitis because the majority of patients will have passed their stone by the time of presentation. Stool screening has shown stones in the feces of more than 90 percent of patients with gallstone pancreatitis. Careful screening of bile aspirate in patients thought to have idiopathic pancreatitis has shown over half to have microlithiasis. In patients with typical features of gallstone pancreatitis, but no stones on diagnostic studies, gallstone pancreatitis should be considered the default diagnosis. It is likely that stones too small to be documented may be the underlying cause in many patients diagnosed with idiopathic pancreatitis. Newer methods of detecting common duct stones and microlithiasis, such as endoscopic ultrasonography (EUS), may help clarify the cause of pancreatitis in these patients.

Mirizzi's Syndrome

Mirizzi's syndrome is an unusual complication of gallstone disease in which a gallstone becomes impacted in the cystic duct. This in turn compresses the CBD, leading to obstruction. Symptoms are similar to those seen from other causes of CBD obstruction.

Postcholecystectomy Syndrome

Postcholecystectomy syndrome refers to pain and abdominal symptoms that occur months or years after cholecystectomy. Often the complaints are of atypical pain and nonpain symptoms such as dyspepsia, bloating, and flatulence. Irritable bowel syndrome and acid dyspeptic disease commonly coexist with gallbladder disease and their symptoms persist after surgery. Patients with severe pain, jaundice, emesis, or fever will most likely have an identifiable source, such as choledocholithiasis, bile leak, or abscess and should be carefully evaluated.

Malignancy

Primary malignancy of the biliary system is fairly rare. A small focus of adenocarcinoma is found in 1 to 2 percent of surgically removed gallbladders and is usually associated with chronic cholecystitis. Other gallbladder malignancies include squamous cell carcinoma, cystadenocarcinoma, and adenoacanthoma. The overall prognosis for patients with malignant gallbladder disease is dismal, with only a 5 percent survival rate at 5 years. The exception is when gallbladder cancer is truly found incidentally. In those cases, surgery is usually curative. Other malignancies that may produce right upper quadrant pain include adenocarcinoma (90 percent) and squamous cell carcinoma (10 percent) of the extrahepatic bile ducts, adenocarcinoma of the ampulla, and various pancreatic tumors.

Motility Disorders

Like other digestive organs, the gallbladder is subject to disorders of muscle contraction. The most common of these is poor emptying or hypomotility. Complications from gallbladder hypomotility generally show up as two very different conditions.

The first is the well-recognized entity of acute acalculous cholecystitis. It is typically seen in critically ill patients who are hospitalized for another serious illness or injury, elderly patients, and as a complication of AIDS. Although the precise pathophysiology is unknown, biliary stasis and gallbladder hypomotility are presumed to play a significant role.

The other condition is acalculous gallbladder pain, which is predominantly seen in middle-aged women. The term is worded to describe the symptoms without presuming a specific pathology. These patients pose a diagnostic problem in that they have typical symptoms of biliary pain but no stones can be found. They frequently pass from doctor to doctor and undergo a variety of unrevealing investigations and treatments. The cause of acalculous gallbladder pain is unknown. Both increased and decreased contraction of the gallbladder has been suggested. Several studies have been done using cholecystokinin (CCK) cholescintigraphy, which showed that a majority of these patients had poor gallbladder emptying. In this group of patients, cholecystectomy relieved or improved their symptoms in 67 to 95 percent of cases. Changes consistent with chronic cholecystitis were found in 47 to 83 percent of the resected specimens. Although the placebo effect of surgery must be taken into account, these studies would suggest that cholecystectomy was a cost-effective treatment for patients with typical biliary pain and evidence of decreased gallbladder emptying.

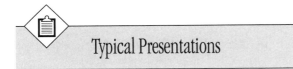

Typical Presentations

The term *biliary colic* is misleading. The pain is more often steady as opposed to intermittent, gradually increasing over a few minutes and then reaching a plateau for 1 to 3 h before diminishing. Rarely, the pain may have a sudden onset and cease more abruptly. The pain is often nocturnal and commonly occurs 1 to 2 h after eating a meal. About one-half of patients experience nausea and diaphoresis. Emesis is also common, although not usually protracted.

Atypical pain and nonpain symptoms are common among patients presenting for evaluation of gallbladder disease. The most typical nonpain complaints are bloating, fatty food intolerance,

dyspepsia, and flatulence. These are probably not related to the gallstones directly, as they are equally as frequent in patients without gallstones. The relation of fatty foods to gallbladder disease is also unclear. Many patients who complain of symptoms after fatty foods actually have conditions such as irritable bowel syndrome, reflux disease, or non-ulcerative dyspepsia. When cholecystectomy is done for these symptoms alone, the results are not as favorable as when the surgery is done for "classic" biliary pain. Only about one-half of patients with nonpain complaints will get relief with surgery.

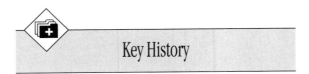

Key History

The objectives when taking histories of patients with suspected symptomatic cholelithiasis include accurately diagnosing biliary colic, excluding the presence of complications of gallstone disease, and identifying patients at special risk if a complication should arise.

Diagnosis of Biliary Colic

A thorough history of the timing and nature of the pain is the most important step in the diagnosis of biliary colic. When history leads to suspicion of gallstones as the source of pain, an ultrasonographic examination of the right upper quadrant usually confirms the diagnosis. This is often the only imaging study needed. Laboratory studies in patients with uncomplicated cholelithiasis are usually normal.

Diagnosing the Complications of Gallstone Disease

An important aspect in evaluating patients with right upper quadrant pain is recognizing the complications of gallstone disease. Again, the timing and nature of the pain are important. Patients with unrelenting pain for more than 6 h are likely to have more than uncomplicated biliary colic, especially when associated with fever. This presentation should lead one to suspect acute cholecystitis. The history of jaundice may suggest choledocholithiasis, cholangitis, or malignancy.

Patients with gallstone pancreatitis will typically report acute onset of pain, which may localize to the epigastric area, right or left upper quadrant, or, rarely, the lower abdomen. They may appear mildly ill or toxic depending on the severity of the disease process. The typical pain is maximal in about 10 to 20 min and, unlike biliary colic, lasts days as opposed to hours. Although one might expect it to occur after a fatty meal and gallbladder contraction, this is not the case. Often, the pain will start at night and cause awakening. Vomiting may also be a prominent feature in gallstone pancreatitis.

Diagnosis of Acute Acalculous Cholecystitis

In the intensive care unit setting, it can be difficult to make the diagnosis of acute acalculous cholecystitis. Ultrasound will show that many of these patients have distended gallbladders due to prolonged fasting. To make the diagnosis in a septic patient, all other sources of infection, such as line sepsis, pneumonia, and pleural effusions, need to be excluded. Then one can empirically place a cholecystostomy tube. If patients improve, the diagnosis is consistent with acalculous cholecystitis.

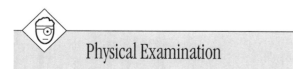

Physical Examination

After a careful history is obtained, a thorough physical examination is the next step in making the correct diagnosis. However, the variable loca-

tion and intensity of the pain in symptomatic gallstone disease can make assessment difficult. Half of patients will have tenderness in the right upper quadrant. One-third will have pain in the epigastrium, although this is also a common finding in patients with essential dyspepsia. Murphy's sign, an abrupt arrest of inspiration as the gallbladder moves downward and against the examiner's hand, which is placed in the right subcostal area, is present in about one-third of patients with gallbladder inflammation. Fullness in the right upper quadrant can only be appreciated in about 15 percent of patients. Rarely, hyperesthesia is noted in the upper abdomen or right infrascapular region.

Jaundice must make the examiner suspicious of biliary obstruction and when associated with pain and fever is considered cholangitis until proven otherwise. Scleral icterus may also be present due to biliary obstruction.

Most patients with pancreatitis have upper abdominal tenderness to varying degrees. Extravasation of pancreatic fluid can cause ecchymotic discoloration in one or both flanks (the Grey Turner's sign) or the periumbilical region (Cullen's sign). In severe cases, third-space fluid losses may lead to tachycardia and hypotension.

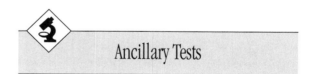

Ancillary Tests

Sonography

GALLSTONES

Ultrasound imaging of the gallbladder has been the main diagnostic test for cholelithiasis since the early 1980s. It has the advantages of being fast, simple, noninvasive, and safe. It is widely available, and portable units make it possible to evaluate critically ill patients at the bedside. Sonographic findings consistent with gallstones include mobile echogenic objects within the lumen of the

Figure 17-1

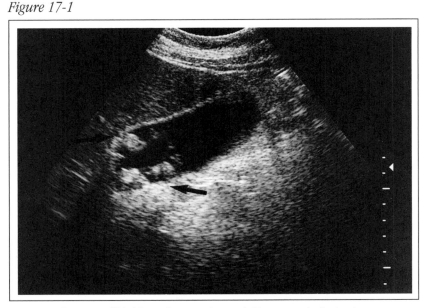

Sonogram showing gallbladder with stones (arrows). Note acoustic shadowing.

gallbladder that produce an acoustic shadow (Figure 17-1). Sludge is usually seen as layering echogenic material without acoustic shadowing. Generally, the stones can be seen in the most dependent portion of the gallbladder. These finding are best seen in the distended gallbladder, so ideally patients should have been fasted for at least 8 h.

Sonography has an overall sensitivity of greater than 95 percent for the detection of stones in the gallbladder that are larger than 2 mm in diameter. Its specificity is generally 95 percent or better when stones are seen with an accompanying acoustic shadow.

CHOLECYSTITIS

In addition to detecting the presence or absence of stones in the gallbladder, sonography can be very useful in diagnosing acute cholecystitis. Fluid seen around the gallbladder in the absence of ascites and thickening of the gallbladder wall to more than 4 mm are nonspecific indications of acute cholecystitis. These findings can also be helpful in diagnosing acalculous cholecystitis in the proper setting. When the sonographer elicits focal tenderness under the transducer while examining the gallbladder, it is known as a "sonographic Murphy's sign." This is a more specific finding of acute cholecystitis.

While an excellent study for the detection of cholelithiasis, sonography does have some limitations. Scarring and contraction of the gallbladder around stones can make it difficult to visualize. Ultrasound examination is also not useful in the detection of CBD stones. Gas in the lumen of the duodenum often obscures visualization of portions of the CBD, particularly in patients with ileus. As such, sonography can only detect these stones in about 50 percent of cases. Often stones in the bile duct will cause dilation of the duct above the point of obstruction. If ductal dilation is present, sonography has a sensitivity of 75 percent in detecting stones in the CBD. In a nondilated duct, the sensitivity falls to 35 percent.

Cholescintigraphy

For patients with suspected acute cholecystitis, cholescintigraphy can be a useful adjuvant to ultrasonography (Figure 17-2). It can be performed on an emergency basis without the requirement of an overnight fast. Patients are given a radionuclide (e.g., hydroxy iminodiacetic acid) intravenously, which is rapidly taken up by the liver and excreted into the bile. In patients without biliary tract disease, serial scans reveal that the radionuclide can be seen in the gallbladder, CBD, and small bowel in 30 to 60 min. The test is "positive" and acute cholecystitis indicated when the gallbladder is not seen, but contrast is excreted into the CBD or small bowel. Pericholecystic hepatic uptake is also a useful secondary sign of acute cholecystitis.

Generally, the sensitivity and specificity of cholescintigraphy is 95 and 90 percent, respectively, for the diagnosis of cholecystitis. However, false positives can be seen in critically ill patients. Significant delays in gallbladder visualization may be noted in these patients and those with chronic cholecystitis, intrinsic liver disease, or choledo-cholithiasis. To reduce the false-positive rate by one-half, intravenous morphine sulfate may be given to decrease the time required to get contrast uptake into the gallbladder. Morphine acts to increase the pressure within the sphincter of Oddi and leads to the preferential flow of bile into the gallbladder, unless there is cystic duct obstruction.

Scintigraphy can also be used to evaluate gallbladder motility. Cholecystokinin is a potent stimulant for gallbladder contraction. By measuring radioactivity before and after intravenous administrations of CCK, an estimate can be made of the gallbladder "ejection fraction." Normal subjects have an average ejection fraction of >75 percent. Although definitions of normal vary among institutions and practitioners, most agree that a value below 35 percent is definitely abnormal.

Oral Cholecystography

Used more frequently in the past, this imaging modality has now been largely replaced by sonography. To perform this test, patients take a single

Figure 17-2

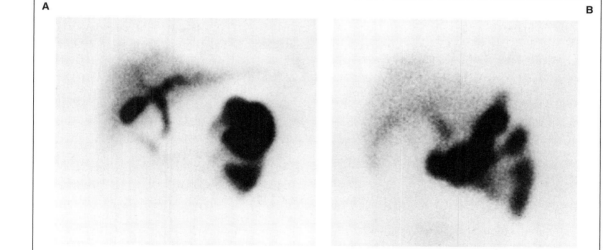

A. Cholescintigram showing radionuclide in the liver, gallbladder and bile duct. **B**. Delayed image showing emptied gallbladder with increased radionuclide in small bowel.

dose of oral contrast agent, which is secreted into the bile, much like intravenous pyelogram dye is secreted into urine. As bile is concentrated in the gallbladder, the iodine in the contrast material opacifies the lumen of the gallbladder and can be seen on a plain radiograph. Stones appear as mobile filling defects in the opacified gallbladder. This process usually takes about 12 h. About 25 percent of the patients will require a second dose of contrast and a repeat radiograph, and in 33 percent of these patients the gallbladder may still not opacify. "Nonvisualization" of the gallbladder can indicate multiple causes such as choledocholithiasis, malabsorption, or impaired secretion of the contrast, or intrinsic liver disease.

Today, the greatest use of oral cholecystography is to establish the patency of the cystic duct prior to attempts at medical dissolution therapy or lithotripsy. Occasionally, oral cholecystography can detect stones that cannot be seen on sonography due to scarring and contraction of the gallbladder. Because oral cholecystography may take up to 48 h to complete in some patients, it is a poor test for acute cholecystitis or other acute complications of cholelithiasis.

Computed Tomography and Magnetic Resonance Imaging

The role of computed tomography and conventional abdominal magnetic resonance imaging in the evaluation of the biliary tree is limited. Their main use is in the detection of complications of biliary disease, such as pericholecystic fluid, evidence of perforation, abscess formation, and occasionally evidence of malignancy.

Endoscopic Retrograde Cholangiopancreatography

Endoscopic retrograde cholangiopancreatography (ERCP) is used as both a diagnostic and therapeutic tool in the evaluation and treatment of choledocholithiasis and its attendant complications (Figure 17-3). It has a sensitivity and specificity of 95 percent and is now the preferred study for the detection of CBD stones.

Magnetic Resonance Cholangiopancreatography

Magnetic resonance cholangiopancreatography (MRCP) is rapidly emerging as an important tool in the diagnosis and management of biliary disease. Newer equipment and techniques have allowed for the production of images similar in appearance to those obtained by invasive studies such as ERCP. The basic principle of MRCP is that bile and pancreatic secretions have high signal intensity on heavily weighted T2-sequences and will appear white, whereas other body tissues will appear gray to black (see Figure 17-4). There are many attractive advantages to MRCP. The test only takes about 10 to 30 min to complete, it is noninvasive, and has virtually no contraindications. It can also offer cross-sectional magnetic resonance imaging, magnetic resonance angiography, and perfusion imaging as an all-in-one package.

Magnetic resonance cholangiopancreatography is particularly useful in detecting choledocholithiasis with a sensitivity reported in early studies of 71 percent and a large study reporting 100 percent. Its specificity ranges from 89 to 100 percent. Stones as small as 3 mm can be seen on MRCP.

Occasionally, surgical alterations and congenital anomalies of the upper gastrointestinal tract make ERCP difficult. In cases where ERCP is contraindicated or unsuccessful, MRCP can be a valuable option and is less expensive.

Its main limitations are a lack of availability and that therapy cannot be performed as part of the procedure. The image spatial resolution is inferior as compared to conventional radiographic cholangiography, and MRCP is currently unable to access small ducts. Placement of patients in a magnetic resonance scanner can cause claustrophobia in those prone to the disorder. Previous

Figure 17-3

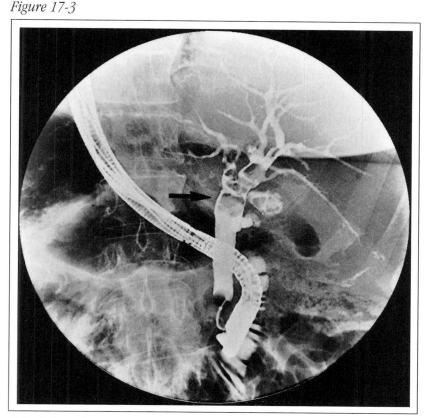

ERCP: Balloon cholangiogram shows stones in the gallbladder and bile ducts (arrow).

difficulties with metal clips, motion artifacts, gas in the intestine, and intraductal gas and debris have been largely overcome by using a variety of troubleshooting techniques.

Blood Tests

Laboratory studies would be expected to be normal in patients with uncomplicated biliary colic. Patients with acute cholecystitis may present with mild leukocytosis and elevated alkaline phosphatase, and bilirubin elevations in the range of 2 to 4 mg/dl. Elevations in bilirubin greater than this should lead the clinician to suspect biliary duct stones.

Slightly elevated amylase levels may be noted with acute cholecystitis even in the absence of pancreatitis. Higher amylase levels are associated with obstructing stones and pancreatic inflammation. If a stone causes obstruction and is then spontaneously passed, a transient "spike" in transaminases may be observed.

Cholangitis may be indicated by elevations in bilirubin, often exceeding 2 mg/dl. However, a level greater than 3 mg/dl raises the likelihood of parenchymal liver disease in addition to obstructive disease. Elevations in alkaline phosphatase and leukocytosis also suggest cholangitis. Blood cultures will be positive in the majority of patients with cholangitis.

Figure 17-4

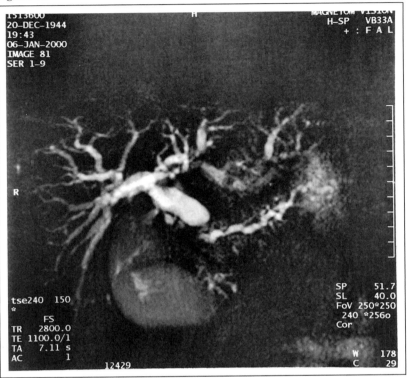

MRCP demonstrating dilated bile ducts without stones.

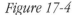

Algorithms

Algorithms for the evaluation and treatment of gallbladder disease are found in Figures 17-5 and 17-6.

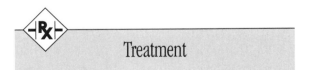

Treatment

Cholecystectomy

Surgical removal of the gallbladder, via open surgery or by laparoscopy, is the most definitive treatment of gallbladder disease irrespective of the pathology (Figure 17-7). The first reported cholecystectomy was performed in 1882. Removal of the gallbladder relieves the biliary symptoms for 90 to 95 percent of patients. It is less effective for the relief of symptoms such as dyspepsia, vague abdominal pain, bloating, and flatulence. In the last four decades, the overall mortality has declined to 1.5 percent and to only 0.5 percent in patients having elective surgery for biliary colic. Some common complications include bleeding, infection, bile duct injuries, and acute pancreatitis. The main contraindications to cholecystectomy include cardiac and pulmonary compromise that preclude the use of general anesthesia.

Since the introduction of laparoscopic cholecystectomy in 1988, the rate of cholecystectomies

Figure 17-5

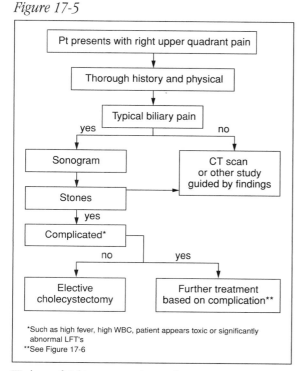

Work up of right upper quadrant pain.

performed in the United States has risen dramatically. This may, in part, be due to the surgical treatment of patients who previously would be treated medically. Patients who were hesitant to have open surgery for cosmetic or other reasons may be more willing to undergo laparoscopic surgery. It is important for the primary care physician to be familiar with the indications and contraindications for cholecystectomy. The most common indication for cholecystectomy is to relieve pain and prevent complications related to gallstones. Uncomplicated biliary colic is not an emergency. However, patients with recurrent attacks of biliary colic should be offered elective cholecystectomy.

Laparoscopic cholecystectomy has become the mainstay of therapy for the treatment of symptomatic cholelithiasis. Its wide acceptance has come about in part due to its shorter hospital stays, faster returns to work, and more desirable cosmetic results, though its mortality is not measurably lower than that of open surgery. This procedure involves making a small umbilical incision through which an instrument is introduced to establish a pneumoperitoneum. Three other small incisions are then made through which instruments are used

Figure 17-6

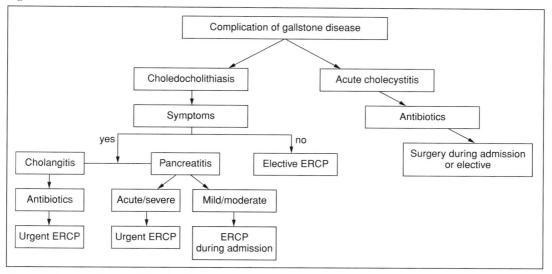

Treatment for complicated gallbladder disease.

Figure 17-7

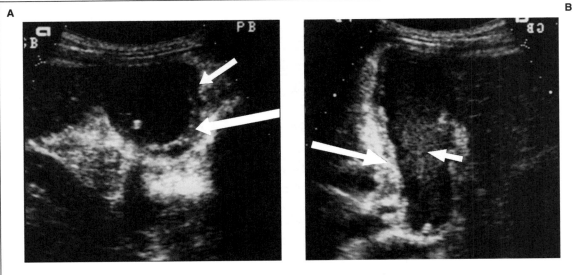

Complications of Gallstone Disease

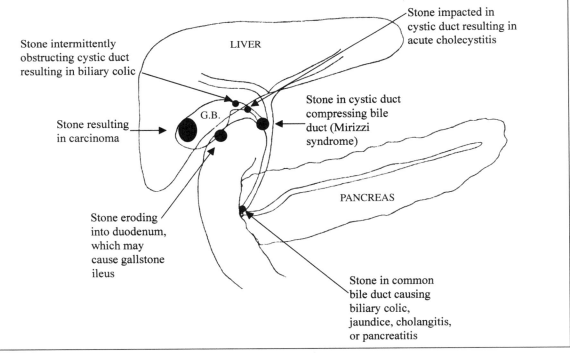

Stone intermittently
obstructing cystic duct
resulting in biliary colic

Stone impacted in
cystic duct resulting in
acute cholecystitis

LIVER

Stone in cystic duct
compressing bile
duct (Mirizzi
syndrome)

Stone resulting
in carcinoma

G.B.

PANCREAS

Stone eroding
into duodenum,
which may
cause gallstone
ileus

Stone in common
bile duct causing
biliary colic,
jaundice, cholangitis,
or pancreatitis

Complications of gallstone disease, CBD, common bile duct. **A**. Acute cholecystitis with gallbladder wall thickening (long arrow) and pericholecystic fluid (short arrow). **B**. Acute cholecystitis with loss of normal gallbladder wall architecture (long arrow). Sludge can be seen in the lumen of the gallbladder (short arrow).

to perform the procedure. As in an open chole-cystectomy, the cystic duct and artery are identified and divided. The gallbladder is then dissected from the liver bed and brought out through one of the incisions. In cases where unexpected complications arise, a laparoscopic cholecystectomy can be converted to an open cholecystectomy. The conversion rate is approximately 3.5 to 5 percent.

The risks of laparoscopic cholecystectomy are similar to the open method, although the risk of biliary injury is higher, especially in the hands of a less experienced surgeon. The risk of biliary injury is also high in patients with acute cholecystitis and inflammation around the gallbladder. This has led some to argue that it may be better to reserve surgery until after resolution of the acute phase. Male sex, recurrent pain attacks, stones >2 cm by ultrasound, thickened gallbladder wall or contracted gallbladder, and dilation of the CBD are all predictors of increased surgical difficulty. Also, because carbon dioxide is the gas of choice for establishing the pneumoperitoneum, patients with preexisting obstructive lung disease may retain carbon dioxide.

Percutaneous Cholecystostomy

Percutaneous cholecystostomy is used to decompress the gallbladder in patients with acute cholecystitis or acalculous cholecystitis who are too acutely ill to undergo cholecystectomy. Using ultrasound guidance, or a combination of ultrasound and fluoroscopic guidance, the gallbladder is punctured and bile aspirated. A guidewire is then introduced into the gallbladder and used to place a pigtail drainage catheter. Complication rates for this procedure approach 10 percent, largely due to the bias for more critically ill patients.

Medical Management

For patients with complications of gallstone disease, such as acute cholecystitis, choledocholithiasis, or cholangitis, immediate surgery may not always be the best option. Inflammation can make dissection of the gallbladder difficult in either a laparoscopic or an open case. Often, patients are hospitalized and treated with supportive intravenous fluids and electrolytes while they are allowed a brief period to "cool off."

Antibiotics are usually withheld in straightforward, uncomplicated cases. However, if patients are febrile to >102°F (38.39°C), have marked leukocytosis, or generally appear toxic, antibiotics should be given. A single agent that covers gram-negative organisms is sufficient for milder cases. For severely ill patients, broader coverage should be chosen. Surgical treatment is usually offered after the acute episode, either during the same admission or shortly thereafter.

In recent years, both open and laparoscopic cholecystectomies have become safe and easy for patients. The rapid recovery time and good cosmetic results of laparoscopic cholecystectomy have made it the treatment of choice for gallstone disease. However, some patients with gallstones do not wish to undergo surgery for a variety of reasons. Although rarely used today, dissolution therapy and extracorporeal shock-wave lithotripsy can provide alternatives to surgery for these patients.

DISSOLUTION THERAPY

Ursodeoxycholic acid (Actigall), which works by decreasing biliary cholesterol secretion, has become the agent of choice for gallstone dissolution. The goal of this therapy is to reverse the supersaturation of bile with cholesterol and thereby make the surrounding medium more capable of solubilizing the stone. This also acts to prevent the formation of new stones.

Several factors in addition to the degree of bile saturation influence the rate at which stones dissolve. Kinetic factors, such as the stirring of the bile and the surface and volume ratio of the stones, also play a key role in determining the efficacy of dissolution therapy. Therefore, patient selection is very important in determining who is likely to benefit from dissolution therapy. For example, patients with multiple small stones and normal gallbladder motility would be predicted to respond better to dissolution therapy than patients with single large stones and hypoactive gallbladders.

Oral bile salt dissolution therapy is rarely appropriate for patients with complications of gallstone disease. To be a candidate for dissolution therapy, episodes of biliary colic should be mild and infrequent. The cystic duct must be patent to allow unsaturated bile to fill and empty from the gallbladder. This can best be documented by oral cholecystography.

Oral bile acids are effective in treating only cholesterol stones. Plain films of the abdomen can be used to exclude calcium-containing stones. Stones that are hypodense or isodense to bile on computed tomography and that float when patients are turned upright during oral cholecystography are more likely to respond to dissolution therapy.

Patients with gallstones up to 10 mm in size are candidates for oral dissolution therapy, although the efficacy decreases with stones larger than 5 mm. The number of stones is not a significant factor as long as they occupy less than one-half the volume of the gallbladder.

Oral bile acid therapy with ursodeoxycholic acid is safe and has virtually no side effects. It can achieve complete dissolution of stones in 20 to 70 percent of cases, depending on patient selection, dosage, and treatment time. Treatment is usually continued for 6 months and then reassessment occurs. If no improvement is noted at that time, therapy is discontinued. If only partial dissolution is noted, treatment can be continued for a total of 2 years, after which time it is unlikely complete resolution will be achieved. This may be due to stone composition or structure that is unfavorable for complete dissolution. At this point, therapy should be discontinued. The overall gallstone recurrence rate after dissolution of the stones by oral bile acid therapy is 50 percent in 5 years, with most stones redeveloping in the first 2 years after treatment. Patients who have recurrent stones usually respond poorly to repeated nonsurgical therapy and should be considered for cholecystectomy.

EXTRACORPOREAL SHOCK-WAVE LITHOTRIPSY

The destruction of stones in the gallbladder and bile ducts using shock waves generated outside the body was first introduced in humans in 1985, although today it still remains investigational in the United States. The goal of this therapy is to break stones into pieces smaller than 3 mm, which can then pass through the ducts and be eliminated through the feces. It can also be used in conjunction with oral ursodeoxycholic acid therapy by reducing the surface and volume ratio of stones and making them more amenable to dissolution. The shock waves used are high-pressure waves that are focused to create a limited area of high pressure at the location of the stones while keeping the pressure in the surrounding tissue relatively low to minimize damage. Various strategies with regard to the energy levels used, surface areas exposed, and number of sessions are being investigated. Those using high energy levels usually require an intravenous analgesic.

As with oral dissolution therapy, patients should have typical biliary pain and documented cholelithiasis, but should not have complications such as acute cholecystitis, biliary pancreatitis, or bile duct stones. Patients with coagulopathy or who are anticoagulated must be excluded due to the risk of hematoma. Pregnancy is also an absolute contraindication to lithotripsy.

The major determinants of the success of therapy are degree of fragmentation, which depends on stone characteristics, and gallbladder motility. Patients with a single radiolucent stone less than 20 mm in size are the best candidates for treatment with shock-wave lithotripsy. Since the stones must be eliminated by the gallbladder after treatment, adequate motility (ejection fraction >60 percent of the fasting volume) should be documented prior to the procedure. The efficacy of the procedure varies widely with patient selection. With adjuvant oral dissolution therapy, 76 to 84 percent of patients are stone-free at 12 months. With lithotripsy alone, approximately 80 percent of patients are stone-free at 12 months.

Extracorporeal shock-wave lithotripsy of bile duct stones has been investigated for use in patients in whom endoscopic measures and mechanical lithotripsy have failed. The procedure involves fluoroscopic location of the stone and requires general anesthesia or conscious sedation. Prophylaxis with antibiotics is also recommended.

One-third of patients require more than one lithotripsy session. Endoscopic extraction of the stone fragments is required in 70 to 90 percent of the reported cases. With proper patient selection, the stones can be cleared in 70 to 90 percent of cases. The recurrence rate of stones after shock-wave lithotripsy is approximately 7 percent after 1 year and 31 percent after 5 years.

ENDOSCOPIC RETROGRADE CHOLANGIOPANCREATOGRAPHY

Since the early 1980s, ERCP combined with endoscopic sphincterotomy has been used to treat choledocholithiasis, cholangitis, and acute biliary pancreatitis. In gallstone pancreatitis, ERCP represented a marked improvement over early surgery, which carried a mortality rate of approximately 50 percent in patients with severe pancreatitis.

Indications for early ERCP (within 72 h of hospital admission) include cholangitis with biliary duct obstruction, as evidenced by jaundice and/or ductal dilation on sonography. With early intervention, the complication rate of patients with severe pancreatitis is significantly reduced although improvement in overall mortality remains unproven. One study showed that patients with acute biliary pancreatitis but no evidence of obstruction did not benefit from early intervention. Ideally, patients with gallstone pancreatitis should undergo laparoscopic cholecystectomy at some point even if ERCP is successful. However, in elderly patients who are poor surgical candidates, ERCP with endoscopic sphincterotomy alone can be used to treat gallstone pancreatitis. Over 80 percent of these patients will do well with no further complications of gallstone disease.

In patients undergoing laparoscopic cholecystectomy for complications of gallstone disease, there is always the potential that stones may have migrated into the biliary ducts. Therefore, ERCP is used as an adjuvant to surgery. When patients are at high risk for choledocholithiasis (see Table 17-1), preoperative ERCP with stone extraction is a safe, cost-effective alternative to an intraoperative procedure. Patients with an intermediate risk of having a bile duct stone may benefit from having

an imaging procedure such as endoscopic ultrasound or MRCP with preoperative clearance of the CBD with ERCP when stones are found. Patients at low risk may benefit from either postoperative observation or an intraoperative cholangiogram depending on the surgeon's preferences. If there is evidence of stones remaining in the ducts after surgery, ERCP and stone extraction can be done at that time.

With proper patient selection, ERCP has a success rate of approximately 90 percent. However, ERCP is a technically challenging procedure that is extremely operator-dependent and has failure rates of 3 to 10 percent. In patients with congenital anomalies or surgical alterations of the upper gastrointestinal tract, the failure rate is even higher. Relative contraindications include age, infirmity, allergy to contrast material, and coagulopathy. Serious complications directly related to the procedure include acute pancreatitis, infection, hemorrhage, perforation, and reaction to the medications. These are rare, however, ranging from 0.3 to about 5 percent. This rate is approximately doubled if a sphincterotomy is also done.

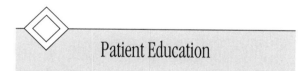

Patient Education

Reassurance is one of the key education points for patients. Often the first attack of biliary colic is distressing, and the fear of another attack may prompt patients to seek unnecessary surgery. It is important to educate patients that recurrent episodes do not occur in many patients and, if they do recur, are infrequent. Patients with asymptomatic stones must also be educated about the likelihood of remaining asymptomatic.

One of the most difficult situations occurs when patients with vague abdominal complaints that may be unrelated to the gallbladder are found to have incidental stones. These patients should not necessarily be denied cholecystectomy, especially if they have some laboratory abnormalities to support a biliary etiology of their symptoms. However, they should be informed that surgery may provide no relief or only partial relief and the risk versus benefit of surgery must be carefully weighed.

Certain groups should be counseled that they might benefit from early gallbladder removal, even if asymptomatic. Patient populations with a high incidence of gallbladder cancer, such as Pima Indians, Mexican-Americans, and Northern American Indian women are likely to benefit from preventative surgery. Individuals with calcification of the gallbladder ("porcelain" gallbladder) also have an increased risk of gallbladder cancer. Children with hemolytic disorders are predisposed to the formation of recurrent pigment stones, and complications may be prevented by early intervention once stones are documented. Individuals with sickle cell anemia prone to sickling crisis may also have a more serious course if they develop complications of cholelithiasis. Patients with short-bowel syndrome tend to develop stones at a more rapid rate than normal, and patients who are undergoing resection of large portions of their small bowel may have a prophylactic cholecystectomy to avoid the need for reoperation. Also, patients undergoing gastric bypass surgery may be given the option of having a cholecystectomy at the same time versus taking ursodeoxycolic acid (Actigall) for several months prior to the procedure.

While it is generally accepted that patients who have diabetes with asymptomatic stones do not develop complications at a rate higher than that of the general population, when complications do arise, they can be more serious. Therefore, surgery should be recommended early when gallstones become symptomatic in patients with diabetes.

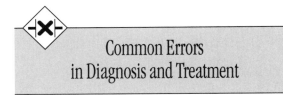

Common Errors in Diagnosis and Treatment

Unneeded Cholecystectomy

It is the nature of a physician to want to act on positive test results. It is therefore easy to see how a clinician could recommend treatment for asymptomatic gallstones. However, the majority of patients will remain asymptomatic and the 30 percent that do become symptomatic will only have a single episode or infrequent episodes of uncomplicated biliary colic. As such, cholecystectomy should be reserved for patients with frequent pain episodes or complications of gallstones.

Cholecystectomy for Vague Symptoms

The clinician, as well as patients, may hold the expectation that cholecystectomy will provide relief for vague complaints, such as dyspepsia, bloating, flatulence, and atypical pain. As previously mentioned, this is only true in about one-half of the patients.

Other gastrointestinal disorders may also produce right upper quadrant pain. Stretching or inflammation of the liver capsule, which can be seen in hepatitis or hepatoma, may produce pain in this area. This pain is constant as opposed to episodic and can usually be correctly diagnosed by blood studies. Burning pain accompanied by a history of relief with food, antacids, and/or antisecretory medications indicates acid peptic disease. Crampy pain suggests an intestinal disorder. A relation to bowel abnormalities, stress, flatulence, and bloating may indicate irritable bowel syndrome.

Errors in Diagnosis

Errors in diagnosis include the confusion of biliary pain with other nongastrointestinal causes of right upper quadrant pain. A right lower lobe pneumonic process can produce pain in the area, although this pain should be more constant in nature and exacerbated by deep inspiration. Fluid and/or consolidation should be visible on a chest radiograph. Renal stones produce intermittent pain but usually have characteristic findings on urinalysis and can be seen on intravenous pyelogram. Cardiac ischemia can be referred to the right upper quadrant but would characteristically be exercise induced. However, this life-threatening process should be ruled out early on if it is suspected in high-risk patients.

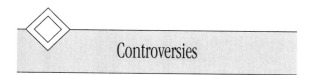

Controversies

Disease Associations with Gallstones

COLON CANCER

Over the last 20 years, a controversy has existed over the possible link between gallstone disease and colon cancer. One theory is that high concentrations of deoxycholate in bile may act as an endogenous carcinogen. Some have noted a higher incidence in right-sided colon cancer in women who have had cholecystectomy, but other large studies have failed to support this finding. In general, the link between gallbladder disease and colon cancer is weak and the presence of stones should not necessarily prompt the physician to recommend studies beyond routine colon cancer screening.

THE ROLE OF *HELICOBACTER PYLORI* IN GALLSTONE DISEASE

Since its discovery in the early 1980s, *Helicobacter pylori* has clearly been linked to peptic ulcer disease, gastritis, gastric adenocarcinoma, and gastric lymphoma. However, its role in gallstone disease is less clear. Studies have detected deoxyribonucleic acid (DNA) from various *Helicobacter* species in the gallbladder mucosa of patients with chronic cholecystitis. These organisms would have the potential to act as a nidus for cholesterol nucleation and thus be a risk factor for gallstone formation.

Other supporting evidence of *Helicobacter's* potential role in gallstone disease is that the incidence of both *H. pylori* infection and gallbladder disease increased with age at similar rates until recent years and is now decreasing at similar rates. Additionally, autopsy studies have shown that patients with peptic ulcer disease also had a higher incidence of gallstone disease.

Decreasing Indications for Cholecystectomy in Asymptomatic Patients

It was not long ago when it was common practice to perform cholecystectomies on patients who have diabetes with asymptomatic cholelithiasis. The reasoning was that patients with diabetes often initially have complications of gallstone disease and have more frequent perioperative complications. It is now generally accepted that patients with diabetes do have complications of gallstones, as opposed to uncomplicated biliary colic, but not at a rate higher than does the general population. It is therefore not cost-effective to do prophylactic cholecystectomies. In a similar situation, patients with large gallstones (>2.0 to 2.5 cm) have a high risk of developing acute cholecystitis, but again, surgery is usually reserved for symptomatic patients.

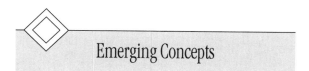

Emerging Concepts

Endoscopic Ultrasonography

Endoscopic ultrasonography has proved its usefulness in diagnosing diseases of the pancreas and its role is rapidly expanding as endoscopists improve their technical skills. Additionally, smaller and more advanced transducers are allowing finer anatomic details to be seen. Endoscopic ultrasonography can visualize the hepatic duct and CBD in 95 to 100 percent of cases. Using very high frequencies, EUS can achieve a resolution of less than 1 mm. In the detection of gallstones including microlithiasis, EUS has a sensitivity of 96 to 100 percent. It has a sensitivity of 91 to 95 percent and a specificity of 96 to 97 percent when compared to ERCP and surgical exploration for the detection of CBD stones.

Because ERCP and endoscopic sphincterotomy may cause morbidity, it is important to select the patients most likely to benefit from this procedure. Endoscopic ultrasonography can be used in this role. In patients with clear evidence of biliary pancreatitis and those at high risk for choledocholithiasis, ERCP is the procedure of choice as therapy can be completed immediately. In patients in whom the diagnosis is less clear and in those at intermediate risk or low risk for ductal stones, EUS can accurately identify patients who would benefit from early ERCP and sphincterotomy.

Convenience, low cost, low complication rate, and relative noninvasiveness are significant advantages to EUS. This study can detect small stones and stones that are present in cases of a small or normal-sized (<8 mm) common bile duct. Another advantage of EUS is that it can be used in obese patients in whom transabdominal ultrasonography may be inadequate.

There are, however, several difficulties with EUS. Imaging of the gallbladder may be difficult when it is in an unusual anatomic location. Patients who have altered gastroduodenal anatomy may also be difficult to study. Many centers lack the necessary technology, but limited availability is becoming less of a problem as EUS use becomes more widespread.

Interventional Magnetic Resonance Scanners and Instruments

While MRCP is useful in detecting CBD stones, surgical or endoscopic techniques must be employed to remove the stones. Currently, intervention-compatible magnetic resonance scanners and instruments are being developed. The hope is that the bile duct could be evaluated noninvasively and treatment rendered immediately if pathology is found. Unnecessary procedures could be avoided if the biliary system is normal. The future of interventional magnetic resonance remains to be determined.

Nonsteroidal Anti-Inflammatory Drug Treatment of Biliary Colic

Similar to dissolution therapy and extrcorporeal shock-wave lithotripsy, nonsteroidal anti-inflammatory drugs (NSAIDs) are a little used therapy in the management of biliary disease. Unlike the other treatments, though, the goal of NSAID use is not to avoid surgery, but to provide patient analgesia and avoid complications of gallstone disease that may make surgery more difficult. When a stone becomes impacted in the cystic duct, it can initiate an intense inflammatory response and lead to acute cholecystitis. Prostaglandins play an important role in this inflammatory process by causing smooth muscle contraction, hyperemia, and edema. One study has suggested that the use of NSAIDs to block this response in patients with uncomplicated biliary colic not only relieves their pain 78 percent of the time, but decreases the occurrence of acute cholecystitis by 64 percent. While more investigation is needed, NSAIDs may be useful as a bridge between an attack of biliary colic and cholecystectomy.

Bibliography

Akriviadis EA, Hatzigavriel M, Kapnias D, et al: Treatment of biliary colic with diclofenac: A randomized, double-blind, placebo-controlled study. *Gastroenterology* 113:225–231, 1997.

Banks PA: Acute and chronic pancreatitis, in Feldman M, Sleissenger MH, Scharschmidt BF (eds): *Sleissenger & Fordtran's Gastrointestinal and Liver Disease,* 6th ed. Philadelphia, W.B. Saunders Company, 1998, p 818.

Barish MA, Yucel EK, Ferrucci JT: Magnetic resonance cholangiopancreatography. *N Engl J Med* 341: 258–264, 1999.

Canfield AJ, Hetz SP, Shriver JP, et al: Biliary dyskinesia: A study of more than 200 patients and review of the literature. *J Gastrointest Surg* 2:443–448, 1998.

Cello JP: Tumors of the gallbladder, bile ducts and ampulla, in Feldman M, Sleissenger MH, Scharschmidt BF (eds): *Sleissenger & Fordtran's Gastrointestinal and Liver Disease,* 6th ed. Philadelphia, W.B. Saunders Company, 1998, p 1026.

Chak A, Hawes RH, Cooper GS, et al: Prospective assessment of the utility of EUS in the evaluation of gallstone pancreatitis. *Gastrointest Endosc* 49: 599–603, 1999.

Coakley FV, Schwartz LH: Magnetic resonance cholangiopancreatography. *J Mag Res Imag* 9:157–162, 1999.

Diehl AK: Symptoms of gallstone disease. *Bailliere's Clin Gastroenterol* 6:635, 1992.

Everhart JE, Khare M, Hill M, et al: Prevalence and ethnic differences in gallbladder disease in the United States. *Gastroenterology* 117:632–644, 1999.

Fenster LF, Lonborg R, Thirlby RC, et al: What symptoms does cholecystectomy cure? Insights from an outcomes measurement project and review of the literature. *Am J Surg* 169:533–539, 1995.

Figura N, Cetta F, Angelico M, et al: Most *Helicobacter pylori*-infected patients have specific antibodies, and some also have *H. pylori* antigens and genomic material in bile. Is it a risk factor for gallstone formation? *Dig Dis Sci* 43:854–861, 1998.

Folsch UR, Nitsche R, Ludke R: Early ERCP and papillotomy compared with conservative management for acute biliary pancreatitis. *N Engl J Med* 336:237–242, 1997.

Fox J, Dewhirst F, Zeli S, et al: Hepatic *Helicobacter* species identified in bile and gallbladder tissue from Chileans with chronic cholecystitis. *Gastroenterology* 114:755–763, 1998.

Gadacz TR: Update on laparoscopic cholecystectomy, including a clinical pathway. *Surg Clin North Am* 80:1127–1149, 2000.

Glasgow RE, Cho M, Hutter MM, et al: The spectrum and cost of complicated gallstone disease in California. *Arch Surg* 135:1021–1027, 2000.

Gracie WA, Ransohoff DF: The natural history of silent gallstones: The innocent gallstone is not a myth. *N Engl J Med* 307:798, 1982.

Huibregtse K: Complications of endoscopic sphincterotomy and their prevention. *N Engl J Med* 335:961–963, 1996.

Jourdan JL, Stubbs RS: Acalculous gallbladder pain: A largely unrecognized entity. *N Z Med J* 112: 152–154, 1999.

Khosla R, Singh A, Miedema BW, et al: Cholecystectomy alleviates acalculous biliary pain in patients with a reduced gallbladder ejection fraction. *South Med J* 90:1087–1090, 1997.

Kratzer W, Mason RA, Kachele V: Prevalence of gallstones in sonographic surveys worldwide. *J Clin Ultrasound* 27:1–5, 1999.

Liu CL, Lo CM: EUS for the detection of occult cholelithiasis in patients with idiopathic pancreatitis. *Gastrointest Endosc* 51:28–32, 2000.

Lyman EB, Horton JD: Gallstone disease and its complications, in Feldman M, Sleissenger MH, Scharschmidt BF (eds): *Sleissenger & Fordtran's Gastrointestinal and Liver Disease,* 6th ed. Philadelphia, W.B. Saunders Company, 1998, pp 948–972.

Mulvihill S: Surgical management of gallstone disease and postoperative complications, in Feldman M, Sleissenger MH, Scharschmidt BF (eds): *Sleissenger & Fordtran's Gastrointestinal and Liver Disease,* 6th ed. Philadelphia, W.B. Saunders Company, 1998, pp 973–984.

NIH Consensus Statement: *Gallstones and Laparoscopic Cholecystomy.* 10:3, 1992.

Opie EL: The etiology of acute hemorrhagic pancreatitis. *Bull Johns Hopkins Hospl* 12:182, 1901.

Palazzo L: Which test for common bile duct stones? Endoscopic and intraductal ultrasonography. *Endoscopy* 29:655–665, 1997.

Patel M, Miedema BW, James MA, et al: Percutaneous cholecystostomy is an effective treatment for high risk patients with acute cholecystitis. *Am Surg* 66: 33–37, 2000.

Patino JF, Quintero GA: Asymptomatic cholelithiasis revisited. *World J Surg* 22:1119–1124, 1998.

Paumgartner G: Nonsurgical management of gallstone disease, in Feldman M, Sleissenger MH, Scharschmidt BF (eds): *Sleissenger & Fordtran's Gastrointestinal and Liver Disease,* 6th ed. Philadelphia, W.B. Saunders Company, 1998, pp 984–993.

Raraty MGT, Finch M, Neoptolemos JP: Acute cholangitis and pancreatitis secondary to common duct stones: Management update. *World J Surg* 22: 1155–1161, 1998.

Shea JA, Berlin JA, Bachwich DR, et al: Indications for and outcomes of cholecystectomy: A comparison of the pre and postlaparoscopic eras. *Ann Surg* 227: 343–350, 1998.

Strausberg, SM: Laparoscopic biliary surgery. *Gastroenterol Clin North Am* 28:117–132, 1999.

Takehara Y: Can MRCP replace ERCP? *J Mag Res Imag* 8:517–534, 1998.

Watanabe Y, Dohke M, Ishimori T, et al: Diagnostic pitfalls of MR cholangiopancreatography in the evaluation of the biliary tract and gallbladder. *Radiographics* 19:415–429, 1999.

Yogesh K. Govil
Minhhuyen T. Nguyen

Chapter

18

Liver Masses

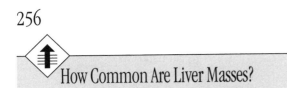

How Common Are Liver Masses?

The frequent use of radiological imaging studies has been associated with the incidental detection of mass lesions in the liver and frequent referral of these patients by primary care physicians to specialists. Benign tumors of the liver were thought to be rare and, by 1944, only 67 histologically proven cases had been reported in the literature. Between 1907 and 1954, only four cases of hepatic adenoma were seen at the Mayo Clinic. Since the 1970s, however, frequent use of radiologic imaging has led to a dramatic increase in the number of cases of liver lesions. In a small series of such incidental liver lesions 81 percent were found to be benign; the remaining were malignant. Hepatic cavernous hemangioma is the most common neoplasm of the liver with a prevalence of up to 20 percent in autopsy series.

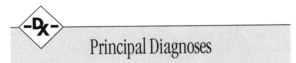

Principal Diagnoses

The hepatic lesions found on imaging studies present spectrums ranging from single to multiple, cystic to solid, benign to malignant, and primary to metastatic. The initial differentiation between cystic and solid can easily be made by ultrasound with a high degree of accuracy. Table 18-1 gives a simple classification of liver lesions encountered by primary care physicians.

Cystic Liver Lesions

Several of the following lesions described are found incidentally. However, many of them may be symptomatic due to their size.

SIMPLE CYSTS

The most common cystic lesions are simple fluid-filled cysts within the liver. They rarely achieve

Table 18-1

Differential Diagnosis of Liver Lesion

CYSTIC	SOLID
Simple cyst	Benign
Amebic abscess	Hemangioma
Echinococcal cyst	Focal nodular hyperplasia
Polycystic liver	Adenoma
Pyogenic abscess	Focal fatty degeneration
Caroli's disease	Regenerating nodule
Cystadenoma	Malignant
Cystadenocarcinoma	Metastatic disease
	Hepatoma
	Cholangiocarcinoma
	Angiosarcoma
	Epithelioid
	hemangioendothelioma

a size of any significance and are usually found incidentally. Cystic lesions less than 2 cm require no further evaluation or treatment. Large cysts or multiple cysts should be further defined by computed tomography (CT) scan.

POLYCYSTIC LIVER DISEASE

Polycystic liver disease may present in childhood, when it has an autosomal-recessive inheritance and is usually rapidly fatal as a result of associated polycystic kidney disease. More commonly, polycystic liver disease presents in adulthood with an autosomal dominant inheritance and a better prognosis, even though it is accompanied by polycystic kidney disease in approximately 50 percent of patients. Polycystic liver disease is usually asymptomatic, but, rarely, extensive replacement of liver parenchyma results in portal hypertension, extrahepatic obstruction, or hepatic failure. Renal disease is usually the predominant clinical manifestation of the cystic process. Therefore, one should continue to observe and clinically evaluate patients. Rarely, surgical intervention, such as cyst unroofing or partial resection, is beneficial.

AMEBIC LIVER ABSCESS

Amebic abscesses are found primarily in patients who live or have traveled in the tropics or subtropics; they have fever and abdominal pain. Computed tomography scanning demonstrates an enhanced rim around a low attenuation center. A positive indirect amebic hemagglutinin will confirm the diagnosis. Initial treatment is with an amebicide, preferably metronidazole. Refractory cases may require percutaneous drainage, when "anchovy-sauce" aspirate without polymorphonuclear leukocytes or organisms on Gram's stain is diagnostic of amebic liver abscess.

ECHINOCOCCAL CYSTS

Echinococcal cysts (hydatid cysts) in the United States are found infrequently in persons travelling from an endemic area (Middle and Far East, Southern Europe, South Australia, New Zealand, Africa, and South America). They are caused by an infestation of the tapeworm *Echinococcus granulosus.* A careful travel history may give a clue into the diagnosis. The indirect hemagglutination test (IHA) is the best serologic test for *Echinococcus,* but this test is available only through the Centers for Disease Control and Prevention and may take 1 to 2 weeks to process. The IHA is sensitive (85 percent) and specific (85 to 95 percent). However, a positive test may merely reflect prior exposure to the organism and is not diagnostic of active ongoing infection. Ultrasound or CT scan is characterized by the finding of classic daughter cysts within the mother cyst. Old inactive lesions may demonstrate calcifications. Treatment consists of therapy with benzimidazole compounds and the cyst may require surgical resection.

PYOGENIC ABSCESS

Pyogenic abscesses often present with fever, chills, and abdominal pain. These patients frequently have had biliary manipulation or surgery or a history of intravenous drug use. The abscesses can be associated with cholecystitis or an obstructing neoplasm. Blood cultures are often positive and imaging may demonstrate multiple abscesses. Computed tomography scanning is beneficial for localization, obtaining a sample for culture, and percutaneous drainage, if the abscess does not respond to culture-directed antibiotics.

OTHER CYSTIC LESIONS

Certain cystic lesions are associated with or contain biliary epithelium. Some have malignant potential. Caroli's disease is a congenital disease of the bile ducts with intrahepatic biliary dilatation and can be confirmed by endoscopic retrograde cholangiopancreatography. The disease causes cholangiocarcinoma.

Biliary cystadenomas and cystadenocarcinomas are rare neoplasms. The great majority (90 percent) occur in women and frequently present with abdominal pain. Any large cyst with lobulations or septations found on ultrasound should be further evaluated with CT or magnetic resonance imaging (MRI) to exclude these conditions. Nodularity is associated with biliary cystadenocarcinoma. The MRI findings will demonstrate a multiloculated septated mass with variable signal intensities due to the consistency of the cystic fluid, which may be serous, biliary, hemorrhagic, or a combination thereof.

Solid Liver Lesions

Solid liver lesions are frequently reported during imaging evaluation of the abdomen. For descriptive purposes, solid lesions can be classified into benign or malignant solid liver lesions.

BENIGN SOLID LIVER LESIONS

Benign solid liver lesions are usually incidentally discovered in patients without a history or clinical or serological evidence of liver disease or malignancy.

Cavernous hemangioma is the most common benign mesenchymal hepatic tumor present in approximately 20 percent of the general population. Most are asymptomatic. Approximately 40 percent of patients experience symptoms of abdominal discomfort if they have lesions >4 cm in diameter, and 90 percent do so if their lesions are >10 cm in diameter.

Ultrasound alone can establish the diagnosis in 80 percent of lesions of <6 cm in diameter. Classically, the lesion is well demarcated, hyperechoic in 67 to 79 percent of the patients, and homogeneous in 58 to 73 percent of the patients.

Larger hemangiomas are more heterogeneous and require further imaging studies. Conventional CT scanning is not very reliable, although dynamic CT scanning with delayed images may be helpful. Radionuclide studies with technetium-99m-pertechnate-labelled red blood cells are considered the method of choice for diagnosing lesions >2 cm, with pooling of the radioactive tracer being pathognomonic. Single-photon emission CT (SPECT) using ^{99m}Tc-red blood cells has been shown to increase the spatial resolution of planar scintigraphy and to have sensitivity and accuracy close to that of MRI. Diagnosis of hepatic cavernous hemangioma could be problematic in patients with known malignancies. The combination of heavily T_2-weighted images with serial dynamic postgadolinium spoiled gradient echo sequences has been found to be a reliable imaging option for hemangiomas and provides much more information about the remainder of the liver and its vasculature than do other modalities.

Focal nodular hyperplasia is the second most common benign solid liver tumor. The incidence in autopsy series has been reported between 0.31 and 0.6 percent and between 2.5 and 8 percent if hemangiomas are excluded. It is a nonneoplastic nodular lesion seen in patients of all ages and both sexes, but more commonly in women between 20 and 50 years of age.

Data suggest that estrogen may have an effect on growth and hemorrhage in focal nodular hyperplasia (FNH). However, its etiologic relation with oral contraceptives is not well established. FNH is believed to occur as a hyperplastic hepatocellular response to either hyperperfusion or vascular injury from a persisting anomalous artery in the location of the lesion. Focal nodular hyperplasia is usually a solitary nodule. Its average size is <5 cm, and its pathognomonic feature is a central scar. Since it is benign and needs not be resected, it is important to differentiate it from lesions that need to be removed. Magnetic resonance imaging is probably the best modality for the diagnosis of FNH, when the central scar is hypointense on T_1-weighted images and hyperintense on T_2-weighted images. The surrounding tumor and liver have the same intensity. The addition of superparamagnetic iron oxide contrast (SPIO), which is phagocytosed by Kuppfer cells, can help establish a highly specific diagnosis in FNH. In instances when a central scar cannot be identified, the lesion should be biopsied to differentiate from more serious lesions.

Hepatocellular adenoma is an uncommon solid liver lesion seen mainly in women of childbearing age. It is caused by proliferation of hepatocytes in an otherwise normal liver. It is associated with the use of oral contraceptives, diabetes mellitus, glycogen storage disease types I and III, and pregnancy.

It is usually asymptomatic, may be solitary or multiple, and may measure more than 20 cm in diameter. Usually, patients have hepatomegaly and abdominal pain. These tumors may undergo malignant transformation, bleeding within the tumor, and rupture of the tumor.

Due to its high sensitivity for fat and hemorrhage, MRI is one of the best methods for hepatocellular adenoma characterization. Lesions are frequently heterogeneous due to varying degrees of necrosis, hemorrhage, and fat within the lesion. Unfortunately, the features of hepatocellular adenoma are nonspecific, and it is difficult to differentiate these tumors from malignant hepatocellular carcinoma.

Adenomas may decrease and even disappear after withdrawal of oral contraceptives. In other instances, tumors continue to grow or rupture. A symptomatic lesion, rising alpha-fetoprotein (AFP), enlarging mass, or one with irregular borders should prompt surgical resection, because malignant transformation may have occurred. If adenomas are not resected, pregnancy should be avoided due to an increased risk for tumor growth, hemorrhage, and fatal complications.

Other benign solid lesions of the liver such as biliary hamartomas, teratomas, hepatic lipomas, angiomyolipomas, and leiomyomas are extremely rare and their description is beyond the scope of this chapter.

MALIGNANT SOLID LIVER LESIONS

Metastatic lesions are commonly encountered liver lesions in clinical practice. Although hepatic metastases may originate from a variety of malignancies, they most frequently arise from tumors of the gastrointestinal tract, lung, and breast. Patient history and tumor markers often help determine the diagnosis.

The natural history and appropriate treatment depend on the site of the primary lesion. Isolated masses to the liver are most often colorectal or neuroendocrine and have a more favorable prognosis. If there is a question of whether the diagnosis is primary hepatic lesion or metastases, a CT- or ultrasound-guided liver biopsy may be necessary. Only few patients benefit from surgical resection. These are individuals with isolated lesions in the absence of extrahepatic metastases. Therefore, optimal imaging evaluation to assess extrahepatic disease, the extent of intrahepatic and perihepatic nodal disease, and laparoscopic examination of the abdomen are essential.

Hepatocellular carcinoma is a leading cause of death from cancer worldwide. It accounts for approximately 80 to 90 percent of all primary malignant hepatic tumors. It occurs two to four times more frequently in males than it does in females. In Western countries, hepatocellular carcinoma (HCC) tends to present at a later age, usually in the 40s through 60s.

Epidemiologic and virologic data support a strong association between hepatitis viruses B and C and HCC. In addition to cirrhosis associated with chronic viral infections, the risk of developing HCC is increased substantially in patients with cirrhosis due to hemochromatosis, alpha$_1$-antitrypsin deficiency, and, to a lesser extent, alcohol-related liver disease.

Diagnosis is relatively simple in patients with a single mass in the liver and elevated AFP. Such patients should be directly evaluated for possible resection if the tumor is confined to the liver. In patients with multiple masses, mildly elevated or normal AFP, or prior history of extrahepatic cancer, needle or laparoscopic biopsy may be indicated.

Imaging (high-resolution helical CT scan and/or contrast-enhanced MRI) is extremely helpful in distinguishing neoplastic nodules from regenerative nodules in cirrhotic livers. Less than 30 percent of patients, however, can be considered for resection because of the large size of the tumor, decompensated liver function secondary to cirrhosis, or tumor spread beyond the liver. Therefore, careful staging is extremely important in the evaluation of HCC. Five-year survival ranges from 10 to 50 percent. Recurrence rate after resection is very high.

Fibrolamellar carcinoma is an uncommon variant of HCC, often occurring in a young population, without the association of cirrhosis or hepatitis virus infection. Often AFP is not elevated. It may be difficult to distinguish from FNH and often has a central scar. Prognosis appears to be better than for HCC.

Angiosarcoma is an extremely aggressive primary hepatic tumor and rarely discovered at a resectable stage. Epithelioid hemangioendothelioma is a rare neoplasm of the liver and other organs with a vascular origin. They are often multifocal, and patients have right upper quadrant pain, anorexia, and weight loss. They can have massive hepatomegaly as well. Treatment is by resection or transplantation.

Cholangiocarcinoma is a tumor arising from biliary epithelium. It may be hilar-type (Klatskin's tumor) or intrahepatic.

The average age at diagnosis is 60 years. It is associated with Caroli's disease, choledochal cysts, large hepatic cysts, congenital hepatic fibrosis, primary sclerosing cholangitis, hepatolithiasis, and infestation with liver flukes. It has also been associated with alpha$_1$-antitrypsin deficiency and exposure to thorium dioxide. Patients may have biliary obstructive symptoms or vague nonspecific symptoms such as weight loss, anorexia, and abdominal distension. Carcinoembryonic antigen and CA 19-9 may be of diagnostic value. Prognosis is extremely poor even with aggressive surgical management, due to extensive disease at the time of diagnosis, but cure is possible in a small percentage. Imaging by ultrasound or CT may show a mass or simply biliary dilatation. Hilar cholangiocarcinoma is more difficult to detect. Endoscopic retrograde cholangiopancreatography or magnetic resonance cholangiography may show a dominant stricture or mass effect.

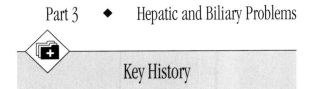

Typical Presentation

In clinical practice, hepatic lesions come to clinical attention when they are incidentally detected on diagnostic radiological studies done for either abdominal or liver symptoms. Occasionally, however, they can be perceived by patients or discovered on physical examination by the physician.

Key History

Patients are frequently alarmed by the diagnosis of "a mass in the liver" and are hoping to be reassured that it can be either "nothing to worry about" or "taken out."

Although it is tempting to order a battery of tests, common sense and thorough history taking will provide the greatest help. Several key points in history taking are illustrated in Table 18-2. Most studies are expensive and may have a small, but definite, risk and should be obtained only if absolutely necessary.

Patients with a liver lesion who are asymptomatic and have normal liver function tests are more likely to have a cyst, hemangioma, adenoma, or FNH. In contrast, patients with a liver

Table 18-2

Key Points in History Taking in Patients with Liver Lesions

KEY POINTS	POSSIBLE DIAGNOSIS
Present history	
Abdominal pain, fever, rigor	Liver abscess
Past history	
Cirrhosis due to hepatitis B/C, alcohol, or	Regenerating nodules or primary hepatocellular
hemochromatosis	carcinoma
Malignancy of gastrointestinal tract, breast, lung	Secondary metastases
Primary sclerosing cholangitis	Cholangiocarcinoma
Abdominal trauma	Hematoma
Diabetes mellitus/glycogen storage	Hepatic adenoma
Disease (I or III)	Polycystic liver disease
Family history	
Polycystic liver/kidney disease	Hepatic adenoma
Drug history	
Oral contraceptives	Primary hepatocellular carcinoma
Social history	Endemic infections, e.g., amebic liver abscess,
Country of origin (Far East)	hydatid cyst, etc.
Travel to endemic areas	Hepatic angiosarcoma
	Cholangiocarcinoma
Occupational history	
Exposure to polyvinylchloride	
Exposure to thorium dioxide	

lesion who are symptomatic and have abnormal liver function tests are much more likely to have a malignant lesion in the liver. However, the clinical context in which a lesion is discovered may help in planning further evaluation. For example, in an otherwise healthy young woman taking oral contraceptives who is found to have an incidental liver lesion, the likeliest diagnosis is hepatocellular adenoma, with FNH or HCC being less likely. Alternatively, HCC is extremely likely in patient with cirrhosis attributable to chronic viral hepatitis or hemochromatosis who have several hepatic lesions accompanied by portal vein occlusion.

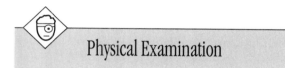

Physical Examination

The physical examination contributes relatively little to the diagnosis of "liver lesions." However, it is useful in identifying patients with liver lesions who have underlying liver disease giving rise to liver lesions. The important physical findings are evidence of systemic infection, stigmata of chronic liver disease, hepatomegaly or presence of a hepatic mass, and evidence of a relevant primary malignancy (particularly of the large bowel, rectum, breast, lung, or melanoma). A bruit or a friction rub may occasionally be heard over hepatomas and metastatic liver nodules. Blood-tinged ascites (hemoperitoneum) occurs in about 20 percent of cases with hepatoma.

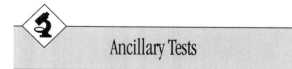

Ancillary Tests

A variety of blood tests and radiologic tests are available for evaluating patients with liver lesions. Although not diagnostic, often these tests may provide important diagnostic clues in evaluation of liver lesions.

Blood Tests

Abnormal liver biochemical tests are infrequent in patients with mass lesions of the liver. An increase in serum alkaline phosphatase may be the only biochemical abnormality. In patients with a history of malignancy, particularly breast and colorectal cancer, the presence of an elevated serum alkaline phosphatase level is of considerable concern and warrants an evaluation for metastasis. The development of HCC in the setting of underlying cirrhosis may also be heralded by a greater than threefold elevation in serum alkaline phosphatase levels.

Hypoalbuminemia, anemia, and, occasionally, mild elevation of aminotransferase levels may be found. A small percentage of patients with HCC may have evidence of *paraneoplastic syndrome;* erythrocytosis may result from erythropoietin-like activity produced by tumor, or hypercalcemia may result from malignant secretion of a "parathyroid-like" hormone. Other manifestations may include hypercholesterolemia, hypoglycemia, acquired porphyria, dysfibrinogenemia, and cryofibrinogenemia.

Serology

Hepatitis serology may help in defining the etiology in patients with liver lesions. Carriers of hepatitis B surface antigen (HBsAg), particularly those infected in infancy or early childhood, and patients infected with hepatitis C virus have an enhanced risk of HCC. In patients with cystic liver lesions and those suspected of abscesses, amebic and ecchinococcal serology should be ordered.

Tumor Markers

Alpha-fetoprotein levels >500 μg/liter are found in about 70 to 80 percent of patients with HCC. Lower levels may be found in patients with large metastases from gastric or colonic tumors. The presence and persistence of high levels of serum

AFP (over 500 to 1000 μg/liter) in an adult with liver disease and without an obvious extrahepatic tumor strongly suggest HCC. Increasing levels over time suggest progression of the tumor or recurrence after hepatic resection. Grossly elevated levels of serum carcinoembryonic antigen are usually found when metastasis is from primary malignancies in the gastrointestinal tract, breast, or lung.

Imaging Studies

A wide variety of imaging modalities is available for evaluating patients with liver lesions. However, one must understand the uses and limitations of each technique before one can make the appropriate choice. In many instances, two or more imaging methods may be needed.

PLAIN ABDOMINAL RADIOGRAPHS

Standard plain films of the abdomen provide little diagnostic information about the liver lesions. They may demonstrate calcified intrahepatic lesions such as echinococcal cysts or, rarely, calcified tumor or vascular lesions.

ULTRASONOGRAPHY

Ultrasonography has the advantages of relatively low cost, portability, and safety, as ionizing radiation is not required. Ultrasonography is a primary screening examination for suspicion of a liver lesion. Hepatic lesions as small as 1 cm may be detected. Ultrasonography can help in distinguishing liver lesions in wide categories of cystic and solid lesions, although it may not identify the nature of a solid liver lesion (adenoma, HCC, metastasis, hemangioma, etc.). Nevertheless, a specific diagnosis may be facilitated by percutaneous "thin"-needle biopsy of hepatic lesion.

Doppler ultrasonography, which may be enhanced by color imaging, allows for the detection of the presence and direction of blood flow based on change in the frequency of back-scattered ultrasound waves caused by the movement of blood. It is useful in detecting vascular tumors such as hemangiomas. Intraoperative ultrasonography involves the application of the ultrasound transducer to the exposed liver at surgery, thereby increasing the sensitivity of detecting occult hepatic metastasis.

COMPUTED TOMOGRAPHY

Computed tomography scanning before and after intravenous administration of a contrast agent is an excellent method of evaluating liver lesions. Cystic lesions are readily identified, and abscesses can usually be distinguished from tumors. Computed tomography scanning can usually identify masses as small as 1 cm, and as with ultrasonography, the lesions can be biopsied under CT-guidance.

Intravenous administration of a contrast agent may result in enhancement of a primary or secondary tumor relative to the surrounding liver, and certain lesions such as cavernous hemangioma, may show a pattern of enhancement that is characteristic enough to confirm the diagnosis. Invasion of blood vessels by tumor may also be demonstrated in this way. Computed tomography portography, in which CT scanning follows injection of contrast into an angiographic catheter placed directly into the superior mesenteric artery, further enhances the sensitivity of detecting mass lesions in the liver.

MAGNETIC RESONANCE IMAGING

Magnetic resonance imaging of mass lesions of the liver appears to have greater sensitivity than does CT scanning; however, like CT scanning, MRI cannot reliably distinguish primary from metastatic lesions. Hepatic abscesses can be detected readily, although on occasion it may be difficult to distinguish abscesses from tumors with necrotic centers.

Magnetic resonance imaging is the technique of choice in the detection of hemangiomas, which have an appearance sufficiently characteristic to permit differentiation from hepatic malignancy. Because rapidly flowing blood is often signal-free on MRI, blood vessels can be distinguished without the need for a contrast agent in most cases; thus MRI may be helpful in assessing the surgical resectability of vascular tumors.

RADIOISOTOPE SCANNING

A variety of radioisotopes can be used to study the anatomy and function of the liver and biliary system. Depending upon the information desired, the study can be performed using radioisotopes that are taken up by hepatic parenchymal cells, Kuppfer cells, or neoplastic and inflammatory cells; or one can use an agent that is rapidly excreted in the bile.

Technetium-99m-labeled sulfur colloid scanning. Reticuloendothelial (Kuppfer) cells in the liver take up ^{99m}Tc-labeled sulfur colloid. Any disease process that results in replacement of Kuppfer cells, including primary and metastatic tumors, cysts, and abscesses, produces a "cold" area in the hepatic scintigram. Lesions >2 to 3 cm in diameter can be readily detected.

Gallium scanning. Gallium-67 citrate accumulates in tissues actively synthesizing protein and is taken up by tumors and abscesses. On scanning, the lesion appears as an area of increased activity, or "hot spot." Imaging with this agent may be helpful in detecting hepatocellular carcinomas and hepatic abscesses.

Tagged blood cell scanning. Intravenous injection of autologous white blood cells labeled with indium increases the specificity of radioisotope scanning for the detection of hepatic (and abdominal) abscesses. Similarly, autologous red blood cells or circulating proteins such as albumin or transferrin labeled with ^{111}In or ^{99m}Tc provide a sensitive method of identifying hemangiomas that are detected as mass lesions by ultrasonography or CT scanning.

Newer scintigraphic techniques designed to improve the sensitivity of liver imaging include SPECT, which permits visualization of the cross-sectional distribution of radioisotope, and positron emission tomography (PET), which utilizes isotopes that decay by positron emission and provides information about regional blood flow and alterations in tissue metabolism. Scintigraphy following the injection of radioactively labeled antibody to tumor antigen has shown promise in distinguishing benign from malignant lesions.

ANGIOGRAPHY

Angiography is required less often now than in the past for evaluating liver lesions. Nevertheless, angiography may be of value in certain situations. Selective cannulation of the hepatic artery or one of its branches may be useful in distinguishing certain vascular lesions of the liver, including hemangiomas, adenomas, FNH, hemangioendotheliomas, and HCC. Angiography may be particularly valuable in assessing the surgical resectability of an isolated hepatic lesion. Therapeutic application of angiography includes embolization of certain highly vascular or inoperable tumors.

LIVER BIOPSY

Percutaneous liver biopsy can be diagnostic, especially if the biopsy is taken in the area of a nodule or mass localized by ultrasound or CT scans. Laparoscopic or open liver biopsy on laparotomy may be required occasionally. This direct approach has the additional advantage of identifying the occasional patient with localized resectable tumor who may be suitable for partial hepatectomy. Percutaneous liver biopsy is contraindicated in patients with hepatic cavernous hemangioma and hepatocellular adenoma because of danger of hemorrhage.

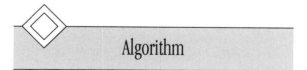

Algorithm

Although no algorithm that describes an approach to liver lesions will satisfy all clinical scenarios, broad guidelines for the sequential use of these tests are given in Table 18-3 and the algorithms in Figure 18-1.

Figure 18-1

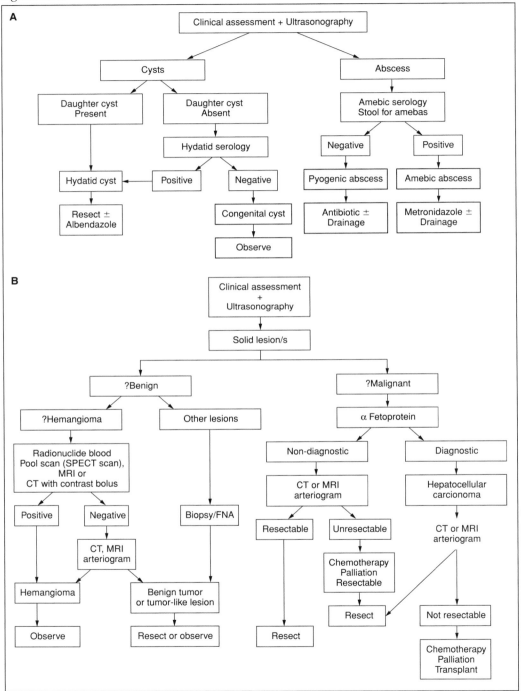

Approach to liver lesions. **A**: Cystic liver lesions. **B**: Solid liver lesions. MRI, magnetic resonance imaging; CT, computed tomography; SPECT, single-photon emission CT; FNA, fine-needle aspiration.

Table 18-3

Problem-Oriented Imaging of Liver Lesions

CLINICAL PROBLEM	INITIAL IMAGING STUDY	SUPPLEMENTAL IMAGING STUDY (IF NEEDED)
1. Known extrahepatic primary carcinoma evaluation for liver metastasis	Dynamic incremental bolus CT (low-attenuation areas within the brighter enhanced liver parenchyma)	
2. Known liver metastasis-follow-up status	CT of liver	
3. Known liver metastasis-evaluation before resection	MRI/CT arterial portography before surgery	Intraoperative ultrasound
4. Suspected primary hepatic or bile duct carcinoma	CT	
5. No known carcinoma-incidental lesion found	Cystic lesion, ultrasound Solid lesion, CT, or ultrasound	Repeat CT scan with dynamic scans in sequential fashion at the level of lesion MRI scanning Radionuclide imaging with ^{99m}Tc tagged RBCs Hepatic arteriography
Symptomatic benign lesion	Ultrasound	

CT, computed tomography; MRI, magnetic resonance imaging; RBCs, red blood cells; ^{99m}Tc, Technetium-99m.

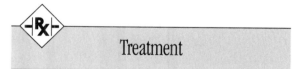

Treatment

With the earlier considerations, the treating clinician should have a reasonable idea about the identity of the liver lesion and, thus, knows which pathway to follow. The treatment of the liver lesions obviously will depend upon their pathology. Following is a brief discussion of the various treatment options that are available to treat liver lesions.

Cystic Lesions

The symptomatic cystic lesions of the liver (fever, leukocytosis, and point tenderness) must be diag-

nosed as quickly and safely as possible. Percutaneous ultrasound- or CT-guided needle aspiration of the lesion under antibiotic coverage (ampicillin, gentamicin, and metronidazole) may be necessary in order to establish the diagnosis. Hydatid disease should be excluded before percutaneous aspiration is attempted, in order to avoid anaphylactic reaction and inadvertent peritoneal seeding. One should describe the gross appearance of the aspirate, use Gram's stain on the material, and obtain both cytologic studies and bacterial culture (anaerobic and aerobic). The gross appearance of anchovy sauce without polymorphonuclear leukocytosis or organisms on Gram's stain is diagnostic of amebic liver abscess. Polymorphonuclear leukocytes with or without organisms on Gram's stain are presumptive evidence of pyogenic liver abscess. In the absence of these findings, one must presume that the cystic lesion represents necrotic tumor and laparoscopy or laparotomy may be needed to confirm this diagnosis.

Metronidazole 750 mg tid for 10 days is adequate therapy for 95 percent of amebic liver abscesses. In cases of relapse, impending rupture of an abscesses, or in situations where patients are unable to take oral medication, therapy with dehydroemetine or emetine should be instituted, and oral chloroquine added as soon as possible. If there is localized swelling over the liver, marked elevation of the diaphragm, severe localized liver tenderness, and failure to respond to systemic amebicide within 72 h, amebic liver abscess should be aspirated. Surgical drainage is rarely necessary.

Although metronidazole and albendazole have been moderately effective in the treatment of hydatid disease, surgery remains the mainstay of therapy for cysts (a) more than 5 cm in diameter, (b) that fail to respond to medical therapy, (c) at risk of imminent rupture, or (d) that compress vital structures. At the time of surgery, instilling hypertonic saline or formaldehyde into the cyst cavity kills any remaining scoleces and prevents intraperitoneal spread of hydatid disease.

Solid Lesions

Hemangiomas should be observed unless severely symptomatic. Most of the remaining solid lesions should be considered for resection, unless the cause is definitely FNH. This may not be possible to determine without tissue diagnosis, and a fine-needle or core biopsy may be necessary with CT or ultrasonographic guidance. If there is clinical suspicion that a mass may be malignant or has malignant potential (adenoma), then resectability needs to be determined. A metastatic work-up should be instituted, including chest CT and bone scan. The tumor should be staged as accurately as possible preoperatively. Laparoscopic exploration may be beneficial to determine resectability

prior to extensive laparotomy. If there is a possibility that it is metastatic to the liver by clinical history or tumor markers, then a biopsy should be considered.

Hepatic Resection

When evaluating patients for possible hepatic resection, several issues need to be addressed. First is to determine if the tumor is anatomically resectable. Preoperative imaging is crucial in order to determine multifocality, vascular invasion, and extrahepatic spread. One must also evaluate if patients are in reasonable general health to withstand major surgery and its subsequent recovery period. With improved understanding of the segmental anatomy of the liver and increasing experience with the techniques learned from liver transplantation, such as total vascular isolation and ex-vivo resection, hepatobiliary surgeons are able to perform extensive resections on very large tumors with low mortality and morbidity in noncirrhotic patients. Several studies have demonstrated a much lower complication rate and shorter hospital stay when hepatic resections are performed at centers with a high volume of liver surgery and experience in liver transplantation.

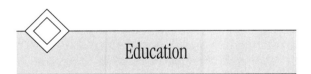

Education

Clinicians should educate patients about the preventable causes of liver lesions. Most importantly, people traveling to regions endemic for amebiasis should be advised about the need to take due precaution to avoid any behavior that will predispose them to infection. People should also be educated about ingestion of safe food and beverages. Avoiding fecally contaminated food and water can best prevent amebic infection. Travelers to endemic areas should follow the general recommendations to avoid drinking local water and to eat only cooked food and peeled fruits.

To prevent infection with *Echinococcus,* contact with infected dogs must be avoided. Infected carcasses should be burned or buried, and infected dogs should be treated with niclosamide or arecoline.

Women taking oral contraceptive pills should be told about the risk of hepatic adenoma. Because these vascular tumors may shrink after withdrawal of oral contraceptive pills, it is usually recommended that these medications be stopped before elective procedures and patients be advised to use alternative methods of contraception.

Hepatocellular carcinoma is one of the few major malignancies in which the cause can usually be determined. Both hepatitis B and C viruses have been definitely implicated in the causation of HCC. At least theoretically, hepatitis-B-virus-related HCC is a preventable malignancy. Although, in practice so far, vaccination programs appear to have made little impact on the prevalence of HCC, even in developed countries, still people at high risk of acquiring hepatitis B virus infection should be encouraged to get vaccinations. Immigrants coming from areas with high prevalence of hepatitis B virus infection should be screened for infection. People with high-risk behavior for hepatitis C virus and history of blood transfusion before 1990 should be screened for hepatitis C infection. Persons infected with hepatitis B and C infections should be offered treatment and kept under surveillance for HCC.

Alcohol and hepatitis C virus are both known to cause cirrhosis. Health care providers should advise patients to abstain from alcohol until they are cured of their viral infection.

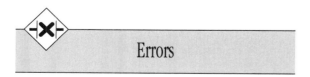

Errors

Clinicians are frequently overwhelmed with choices of diagnostic tests. Not all tests need to be done for each lesion. Clinicians make a variety of errors in the diagnosis and treatment of liver lesions. Two errors are particularly common. One is to order different tests without a definite direction and the other is to order invasive tests without realizing the risks of the procedure.

Recent times have witnessed phenomenal technological growth in radiologic practice, with striking advances in abdominal imaging by nuclear medicine, CT, MRI, ultrasonography, and interventional radiology. It is no wonder that clinicians, confronted with this bewildering array of often unfamiliar procedures, become confused and frustrated over the proper sequencing of tests for a particular problem. Clinicians should aim for an accurate diagnosis with a minimal expenditure of time, money, and risk to the patient.

Finally, it should be stressed that an algorithm is only a guideline and should never be construed as an inviolate strategy. Many factors can influence its application in a given clinical situation including physician expertise, confidence and experience in a given modality, and the general availability of the tests.

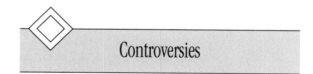

Controversies

Imaging of the liver is complicated. The sporadic appearance of incidental benign lesions and variability in scanning techniques, equipment, and artifacts add difficulties to the evaluation of liver lesions. Therefore, the emphasis should be on the need to define the problem for which patients are being imaged. This information helps in choosing the procedure of choice and the technique needed to give the most expedient and accurate answer with low risk and cost.

A review of the literature shows that there are conflicting statistics about sensitivities of different diagnostic modalities. Some series comparing different methods have shown that CT during arterial portography had the highest sensitivity, but

MRI had the most consistent overall results. In another series comparing single-phase spiral CT and current MRI techniques for liver disease detection and characterization, MRI detected more lesions in 49.4 percent of patients and characterized more lesions in 75.3 percent of patients investigated for focal liver disease. In each of the three series, MRI had a greater effect on patient management than did single-phase spiral CT in more than 67 percent of patients.

Another area of controversy is screening for HCC. Large-scale screening programs have already been established for HCC, particularly in geographic areas with high incidence of the disease, such as in the Republic of China, Taiwan, and Japan. There is some evidence that screening of chronic hepatitis B virus carriers reduces the 1-year case fatality rate associated with the development of HCC, but it has not been confirmed in controlled trials that screening has a beneficial effect on survival. Indeed, a large, well-conducted screening program (employing regular AFP estimations and ultrasonography every 3 to 12 months) concluded that screening did not appreciably increase the rate of detection of potentially curable tumors.

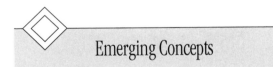

Emerging Concepts

Gains in understanding the biology of liver lesions may permit development of more effective imaging methods and safe treatment. A variety of parenterally administered iron oxides have been developed for contrast-enhanced MRI of the liver. The use of hepatic MRI provides an alternative to the existing multistep diagnosis with CT, CT portography, MRI, and biopsy.

Hepatic metastases are the major cause of morbidity and mortality in patients with gastrointestinal carcinoma and other malignant tumors. For the treatment of patients with unresectable liver metastases, various local ablative interventional

therapeutic modalities (such as laser-induced interventional therapy and microwave, radiofrequency, and ultrasound ablation), cryotherapy, local drug administration (such as alcohol injection), endotumoral chemotherapy, and regional chemoembolization have been developed. The efficacy of these treatment options is still being determined.

Hepatic gene therapy may provide a new approach to treating hepatic malignancies. Genes can be transferred using replication-defective viral vectors either to cultured tumor cells in vitro that can be returned to these patients as a "cancer vaccine" or directly to tumor cells in vivo. Vaccination with deoxyribonucleic acid (DNA) constructs expressing specific tumor antigens characteristic of colorectal neoplasia can trigger immune recognition and destruction of tumor cells. The products of in vivo genes convert prodrugs into cytotoxic derivatives. In the transduced cells the subsequently administered prodrugs are then activated and destroy replicating tumor cells, whereas the infected liver cells are thought to be unaffected because of their minimal proliferative activity. Studies in murine models, combined with human studies, show that such approaches could become an adjunct to current treatments for human colorectal cancer in the near future.

Bibliography

Buetow PC, Midkiff RB: Primary malignant neoplasms in the adult. *Mag Res Imag Clin N Am* 5(2):289, 1997.

Busuttil RW, Farmer DG: The surgical treatment of primary hepatobiliary malignancy. *Liver Trans Surg* 2: 114,1996.

Choti MA, Bulkley GB: Management of hepatic metastases. *Liver Trans Surg* 5(1):65, 1999.

Geoghegan JG, Scheele J: Treatment of colorectal liver metastases. *Br J Surg* 86(2):158, 1999.

Kirchhoff T, Chavan A, Galanski M: Transarterial chemoembolization and percutaneous ethanol injection therapy in patients with hepatocellular carcinoma. *Eur J Gastrenterol Hepatol* 10(11):907, 1998.

Mazzafarro V, Regalia E, Doci R, et al: Liver transplantation for the treatment of small hepatocellular carcinomas in patients with cirrhosis. *N Engl J Med* 334: 693, 1996.

Molmenti EP, Marsh JW, Dvorchik I, et al: Hepatobiliary malignancies. *Surg Clin North Am* 79(1):43, 1999.

Olthoff KM: Surgical options for hepatocellular carcinoma: Resection and transplantation. *Liver Trans Surg* 4(5):S98, 1998.

Reddy KR, Schiff ER: Approach to liver mass. *Semin Liv Dis* 13(4):423, 1993.

Reimer P, Tombach B: Hepatic MRI with SPIO: Detection and characterization of focal liver lesions. *Eur Radiol* 8(7):1198, 1998.

Rubin RA, Mitchell DG: Evaluation of the solid hepatic mass. *Med Clin North Am* 80:907, 1996.

Schiff ER, Sorrell MF, Maddrey WC: *Schiff's Diseases of the Liver*. Philadelphia, Lippincott-Raven Publishers, 1999.

Siegelman ES, Outwater EK: Magnetic resonance imaging of focal and diffuse hepatic disease. *Semin Ultrasound CT MR* 19(1):2, 1998.

Selby R, Kadry Z, Carr B, et al: Liver transplantation for hepatocellular carcinoma. *World J Surg* 19:53, 1995.

Weimann A, Ringe B, Klempnauer J, et al: Benign liver tumors: Differential diagnosis and indications for surgery. *World J Surg* 21(9):983, 1997.

Minhhuyen T. Nguyen

Chapter

19

Abnormal Liver Function Tests

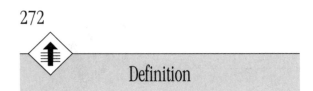

Definition

Laboratory data used to assess liver disease are commonly called liver function tests (LFTs), which include a battery of biochemical tests that lead us to the diagnosis of liver disorders. Since the liver acts as a biochemical powerhouse, carrying out thousands of diverse functions, no single test can serve as a sole reliable indicator of overall liver dysfunction. In fact, the many tests that are available can measure only a limited number of these hepatic activities. Before going further into how to interpret abnormal LFTs, the following points must be kept in mind.

- First, many LFTs such as aminotransferases or alkaline phosphatase do not even measure liver function. Instead, they reflect parenchymal injury or obstructed bile flow.
- Second, LFTs do not identify a specific diagnosis. Instead, they direct us to a certain category of liver disorder.
- Third, LFTs are usually not specific. Many so-called LFTs measure chemicals also produced in other organs. The abnormalities in LFTs may reflect damage to other organs, such as bone, muscles, or heart, instead of the liver.
- Finally, LFTs frequently lack sensitivity and specificity. In many instances, normal LFTs are found in patients with verified liver disease, and vice versa.

Once these limitations are recognized, LFTs are indeed useful clinical tools. They provide a noninvasive sensitive method of screening patients for the presence of liver disease, especially in asymptomatic, anicteric patients with subclinical liver disorders such as chronic viral hepatitis or cirrhosis. When used in composite, the pattern of LFT abnormalities can assist in distinguishing one type of liver dysfunction from another, such as biliary obstruction from viral hepatitis. Liver function tests also allow for the assessment of the severity of the liver disease and, occasionally, prediction of its outcome early on, evaluation of the response to treatment, and adjustment of the therapy accordingly.

This chapter will discuss the most useful LFTs, the common diagnoses associated with their patterns of abnormalities, the approach to arrive at these diagnoses, some common errors in dealing with abnormal LFTs, and when appropriate, treatment recommendations.

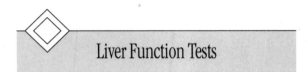

Liver Function Tests

Bilirubin

Bilirubin is a breakdown product of heme, or ferroprotoporphyrin IX. Approximately 80 percent of bilirubin produced daily comes from the breakdown of hemoglobin in old red blood cells. The other 20 percent comes from prematurely destroyed erythroid cells in the bone marrow and other hemoproteins throughout the body, especially from the liver.

Bilirubin, first formed in the reticuloendothelial cells, is lipid soluble and water insoluble due to its molecular configuration. To be transported in blood to the liver, it is reversibly and noncovalently bound to albumin. In the liver, bilirubin, not albumin, is taken up by hepatocytes by a carrier-mediated membrane transport process.

The bilirubin is next solubilized in the liver by conjugation to glucuronic acid, forming bilirubin monoglucuronide and diglucuronide, which are referred to as direct-acting bilirubins. The bilirubin conjugates are then excreted from the hepatocyte into the canalicular system by another carrier-mediated membrane transport, which appears to be the rate-limiting step in hepatic bilirubin excretion.

In the distal ileum and colon, the conjugated bilirubins are hydrolyzed to unconjugated bilirubins, or urobilinogens, by gut flora. The majority of these compounds are excreted in feces. A small fraction is passively absorbed and reexcreted by the liver. A smaller fraction is excreted by the kidney.

CONJUGATED AND UNCONJUGATED BILIRUBIN

Spectrophotometric data measure serum bilirubin in two forms:

1. The water-soluble, conjugated fraction, consisting mainly of bilirubin mono- and diglucuronides and albumin-bound bilirubin, which gives a "direct" reaction to diazo reagent.
2. The lipid-soluble "indirect"-reaction fraction (total minus direct), consisting mainly of unconjugated bilirubin.

Conjugated hyperbilirubinemia indicates some interference with bilirubin excretion into bile or bile flow, and unconjugated hyperbilirubinemia indicates impaired conjugation or uptake, or overproduction of bilirubin. In the majority of hepatobiliary disorders, therefore, one would detect conjugated hyperbilirubinemia. However, fractionation of serum bilirubin does not distinguish cholestasis due to parenchymal disease from that caused by biliary processes. In contrast, unconjugated hyperbilirubinemia has a short list of differential diagnoses, including nonhepatic conditions such as hemolytic anemia, ineffective erythropoiesis, and a few uncommon hepatic disorders such as Gilbert's syndrome, or the rarer Crigler-Najjar or Dubin-Johnson syndromes.

The presence of bilirubin in the urine indicates hepatobiliary disease. Unconjugated bilirubin is tightly bound to albumin and thus not filtered by the renal glomerulus. Only when there is an unusually large amount of conjugated bilirubin in the serum is conjugated bilirubin found in the urine. Rapid assessment of bilirubinuria can be made with commercially available dipsticks and used as a screening test since bilirubinuria can be detected even before clinical jaundice becomes evident.

Serum Enzyme Assays

AMINOTRANSFERASES

Serum aspartate aminotransferase (AST) and alanine aminotransferase (ALT) are the most commonly used enzyme assays to measure hepatocellular injury. Aspartate aminotransferase is found throughout the body, but especially in the liver, heart and skeletal muscle. Alanine aminotransferase is found mainly in the liver and, to a lesser extent, in the kidney and skeletal muscle as well. Although many studies have shown that the magnitude and duration of transaminase elevations often correlate with the extent and degree of hepatocellular damage, precise quantitative correlations cannot be made in most cases.

In cases of acute massive hepatocellular necrosis due to viral hepatitis or drug-induced toxicity, ALT and AST can reach serum levels of 1000 to 3000 U. Less severe necrosis can yield levels of 300 to 1000 U. Serum levels of 300 U or less suggest subclinical hepatitis, chronic liver disease, or alcoholic hepatitis. However, in cases of acute complete, transient or otherwise, biliary obstruction, ALT and AST may reach levels of 1000 to 2000 U with rapid resolution within a few days once the obstruction is removed.

Serial measurements of ALT and AST are helpful in following the course of patients with liver disease. Their persistent elevations, usually of more than 6 months, may point to chronic infection from viral hepatitis. Their relative values over time also allow the clinician to assess whether patients have responded to treatment.

ALKALINE PHOSPHATASE

Alkaline phosphatase hydrolyzes synthetic phosphate esters at pH 9.0. It is found in bone, intestine, liver, and placenta. Most of serum alkaline phosphatase is derived from bone. In the absence of bone disease or pregnancy, the elevation of alkaline phosphatase indicates impaired hepatic excretory function.

In cases of extrahepatic biliary obstruction, intrahepatic cholestasis, or primary biliary cirrhosis, alkaline phosphatase levels are usually 3 to 10 times above normal. In cases of viral hepatitis or other parenchymal diseases, alkaline phosphatase levels are usually one to two times above normal. Elevations of alkaline phosphatase 2 to

10 times above normal occurring on the background of other normal LFTs frequently suggest metastatic disease in the liver or infiltrative disease of the liver from malignancy, such as leukemia or lymphoma, or infections such as fungi or *Cryptosporidium*. In cases of partial biliary obstruction, elevated alkaline phosphatase can occur with normal bilirubin.

The main method to distinguish the source of the elevated alkaline phosphatase is fractionation of the enzyme. The liver fraction is heat-stable, and the bone fraction is heat-labile.

5′-Nucleotidase

5′-Nucleotidase (5′-NUC) is another phosphatase that is found primarily in the liver. It is often used to confirm the presence of liver disease in cases of elevated LFTs.

Gamma-Glutamyl Transpeptidase

Gamma-glutamyl transpeptidase (GGT) is found mainly in the liver and kidney. An isolated elevation of this enzyme assay is usually observed in heavy alcohol drinkers even before other LFTs become abnormal. In comparison, it is a very sensitive assay, and can be abnormal in patients without a significant history of alcohol consumption.

Lactate Dehydrogenase

Lactate dehydrogenase (LDH) is present in all organs and is released into the serum from various tissue injuries; hence it is not a useful test in general. In certain settings, high elevations of LDH are observed in patients with metastatic disease of the liver. Moderate levels are found in acute viral hepatitis. Biliary diseases, in contrast, are associated with minimal elevations of this enzyme assay.

Serum Proteins

Albumin and Globulins

Albumin, prothrombin, fibrinogen and other clotting factors, and alpha- and beta-globulins and many other proteins are produced by hepatocytes. Immunoglobulins, in contrast, are produced by B lymphocytes and plasma cells and do not directly test hepatic function. In cases of liver disease, production is often reduced, while that of the latter group (i.e., immunoglobulins) may vary widely due to the presence of inflammation or sepsis. Other nonhepatic factors such as malnutrition, infections, malignancy, and endocrine disorders can also affect the metabolism of these proteins. In bioassays, albumin and globulins (A/Gs) are measured separately and the A/G fraction is of no clinical significance.

Two conditions associated with clinically significant liver disease are (a) hypoalbuminemia and (b) hyperglobulinemia. Many liver disorders involving massive destruction or replacement of the liver parenchyma, such as cirrhosis, result in hypoalbuminemia. In addition, systemic illnesses such as chronic inflammation, infection, excessive alcohol consumption, or malignancy may inhibit albumin synthesis. Protein-losing disorders, such as nephrotic syndrome and protein-losing enteropathies may also severely affect the serum levels of albumin.

Hyperglobulinemia often reflects chronic inflammation and can present at very high levels in chronic autoimmune hepatitis. Alpha$_2$-globulin levels are usually elevated in neoplastic and inflammatory diseases of the liver. Beta-globulin levels are often high in biliary obstruction. Nonetheless, high levels of globulins do not assist the clinician in arriving at a specific diagnosis of liver disorder.

Clotting Factors

The liver produces multiple clotting factors including fibrinogen (factor I), prothrombin (factor II), and factors V, VII, IX, X, XII, and XIII. The presence of adequate amounts of clotting factors usually reflects good hepatic synthetic function. Factor V level is often measured in cases of fulminant liver failure to assess hepatic biosynthetic capacity.

Normal prothrombin time (PT) tests depend on both normal hepatic synthesis of prothrombin, fibrinogen, factors V, VII, and X, and the presence of adequate vitamin K. Biologically active factors (factors II, VII, IX, and X) require vitamin K in their synthesis (i.e., in their gamma carboxylation). Vitamin K deficiency can occur in the setting of obstructive jaundice and malabsorption of fat-soluble vitamins, destroyed gut flora due to antibiotic use, and dietary deficiency.

It is important to keep in mind that an abnormal PT is not specific for liver disease. Other conditions such as various inborn deficiencies of clotting factors (e.g., hemophilia or Christmas disease), and excessive consumption of coagulation factors (e.g., disseminated intravascular coagulation) can lead to a prolonged PT. Excluding these disorders, to distinguish between hepatic and nonhepatic causes of prolonged PT, vitamin K injection is used. If PT becomes normal, then the likelihood of liver disease is low. If PT remains elevated, the presence of liver disease should be suspected, especially if other LFTs are also abnormal.

Prothrombin time is also a useful prognostic test in cases of acute alcoholic hepatitis and acute hepatocellular necrosis with the potential of fulminant hepatic failure (e.g., viral hepatitis or acetaminophen toxicity), as well as chronic progressive liver disease. A prolonged PT with international normalized ratio (INR) of more than 4 to 6 denotes a poor clinical outcome. In addition, it is a critical test in managing patients with liver disease. An elevated PT not responding to vitamin K administration may point to poor surgical outcome in patients with liver disease. However, if the need for invasive procedures is urgent, fresh frozen plasma can always be used to correct PT value.

The partial thromboplastin time (PTT) test, which mirrors the activities of factors I, II, V, VIII, IX, X, XI, and XII, may also become prolonged in advanced liver disease.

Blood Ammonia Level

In acute hepatocellular damage, the blood ammonia level is usually elevated due to the arrest of the hepatic urea cycle from massive necrosis of liver tissue. In chronic liver disease, especially in the presence of portocaval shunting, ammonia produced by gut bacteria enters the systemic circulation via portal venous flow. This production may increase from excessive protein dietary intake, gastrointestinal bleeding, azotemia, and constipation.

Nonetheless, the correlation between blood ammonia levels and hepatic encephalopathy is not precise since other mechanisms of encephalopathy may be involved. Similar levels can produce lethargy in one patient, but may scarcely affect another. Downward trending of blood ammonia levels may roughly predict neurologic recovery from hepatic encephalopathy.

The best technique to measure ammonia levels is from arterial blood supply. Ammonia levels derived from venous blood are more easily obtained than from arterial blood supply, but they are a less sensitive indicator of hepatic encephalopathy. They should not be obtained on a daily basis; instead, patients with hepatic encephalopathy should be assessed clinically on a frequent basis for signs of neurologic improvement.

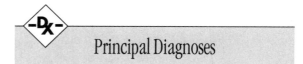

Principal Diagnoses

Liver function tests should be ordered as a battery in patients suspected of liver disease. These include the tests discussed earlier, namely, measurements of total and direct bilirubin, alkaline phosphatase, the aminotransferases, albumin, globulin, and PT. Depending on the patterns of abnormalities, liver diseases can be divided into broad categories that include hepatocellular or parenchymal damage, obstructive liver disease, mixed pattern of injuries, and unconjugated hyperbilirubinemia (Tables 19-1 and 19-2). Once a broad category of liver diseases is focused upon, other diagnostic tests such as viral hepatitis serologies, autoantibodies, percutaneous liver biopsy, endoscopic retrograde cholangiopancreatography,

Table 19-1

Category of Liver Diseases and Associated Liver Function Test Abnormalities

TESTS	HEPATOCELLULAR DAMAGE	OBSTRUCTIVE PATTERN	MIXED PATTERN	UNCONJUGATED HYPERBILIRUBINEMIA
Total bilirubin	N or I	N or I	N or I	I I
Direct bilirubin	N or I	N or I	N or I	N
Indirect bilirubin	N	N	N	I I
ALT/AST	I I I	N or I	I I	N
Alkaline phosphatase	N	I I I	I I	N
Albumin	D D	N	N	N
Prothrombin time	I I	N	N	N

I, mildly increased; II, moderately increased; III, significantly increased; D, decreased; N, normal.

Table 19-2

Some Examples of Hepatobiliary Disorders

Hepatocellular damage	Viral hepatitis
	Autoimmune hepatitis
	Wilson's disease
	Hemochromatosis
	Steatohepatitis (alcoholic and nonalcoholic)
	Budd-Chiaris syndrome
	Ischemic hepatitis
Obstructive pattern	Primary biliary cirrhosis
	Primary sclerosing cholangitis
	Choledocholithiasis
	Mirizzi's syndrome
	Cholangiocarcinoma
	Benign or malignant biliary strictures
	AIDS cholangiopathy
	Caroli's disease
	Oriental cholangiohepatitis
	Granulomatous hepatitis
	Alcoholic hepatitis
	Total parenteral nutrition
Mixed LFT pattern	Drug reactions
Unconjugated hyperbilirubinemia	Gilbert's syndrome
	Dubin-Johnson syndrome
	Crigler-Najjar syndrome
	Rotor syndrome
	Hemolysis
	Ineffective erythropoiesis

LFT, liver function tests.

Figure 19-1

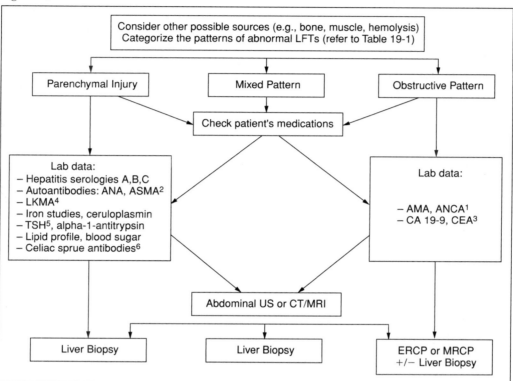

Approach to the patient with abnormal liver function tests. [1]AMA = anti-mitochondrial antibodies; ANCA = anti-neutrophil cytoplasmic antibodies; [2]ANA = antinuclear antibodies; ASMA = anti-smooth muscle antibodies; [3]CA 19-9 = carbohydrate antigen 19-9; CEA = carcinoembryonic antigen; CT, computed tomography; ERCP, endoscopic retrograde cholangiopancreatography; LFTs, liver function tests; [4]LKMA = liver-kidney microsomal antibodies; MRCP, magnetic resonance cholangiopancreatography; MRI, magnetic resonance imaging; [5]TSH = thyroid-stimulating hormone; [6]Celiac sprue antibodies = anti-gliadin antibodies IgA and IgG, anti-reticulin antibodies, anti-endomysial antibodies; US, ultrasound.

abdominal ultrasound, computed tomography, or magnetic resonance imaging can then be chosen to assist in making the final diagnosis (Figure 19-1).

Hepatocellular Damage

The aminotransferases are the most sensitive tests in detecting parenchymal liver injury. Viral, auto-immune, drug-induced, and ischemic hepatitis; hemochromatosis; and Wilson's disease fall into

this category. Liver disease in adults related to alpha₁-antitrypsin deficiency also usually presents with abnormal enzymes; however, in neonates, it may present as jaundice with elevation of the bilirubins. In severe cases of hepatocellular necrosis (i.e., aminotransferase values above 500 IU), bilirubin and alkaline phosphatase levels may also be moderately elevated. The rest of the LFTs are usually mildly affected unless the process is progressive. A rapid steep rise in PT in these cases indicates massive hepatic necrosis and poor prognosis. In alcoholic hepatitis, aminotransferase levels usually do not exceed 300 IU, and the AST/ALT ratio is usually 2 or higher.

In chronic hepatocellular disease, LFT abnormalities may not accurately reflect the extent of liver damage. For example, patients with cirrhosis may have mildly elevated aminotransferase levels and a low or low-normal albumin level may be the only warning to the clinician. In these cases, tests used to measure actual liver function, such as levels of factor V, fibrinogen, PT, albumin, and blood ammonia, may better assist in arriving at the diagnosis of chronic liver disorder.

Obstructive Pattern

The characteristic pattern of the LFTs in obstructive liver disease does not distinguish between intrahepatic and extrahepatic obstruction. Alkaline phosphatase and GGT levels are often highly elevated, out of proportion to other LFTs; alkaline phosphatase level four or more times greater than normal is indicative of some type of cholestasis. In severe cases, the direct fraction of bilirubin is also elevated and bilirubinuria is detected. Examples of extrahepatic obstruction include choledocholithiasis, Mirizzi's syndrome, benign or malignant strictures of the common bile duct and common hepatic duct, and ampullary tumors. Examples of intrahepatic cholestasis include viral hepatitis, alcoholic hepatitis, drug-related cholestasis, primary biliary cirrhosis, benign cholestasis of pregnancy, total parenteral nutrition, postoperative jaundice, and sepsis.

Infiltrative liver diseases such as granulomatous hepatitis (infections, medications, and sarcoidosis) and malignancy may present with elevated alkaline phosphatase levels alone. This clinical picture is almost indistinguishable from that of obstructive liver disease. It may be useful to obtain a fractionation test for alkaline phosphatase (liver versus bone), 5'-NUC, or GGT to confirm the hepatic origin of the abnormality. Careful history taking, physical examination, and imaging studies may also reveal critical data in arriving at the correct diagnosis.

Mixed Pattern of Liver Function Test Abnormalities

Drug reactions are the most common cause of a mixed pattern of LFT abnormalities (i.e., that of partly parenchymal injury and partly cholestatic picture). Some examples are immunosuppressive drugs such as azathioprine, cholesterol-lowering drugs such as mevastatin, anticonvulsants such as phenytoin, and antibiotics such as sulfonamides. Other causes of mixed patterns of LFT abnormalities include the progression of either hepatocellular injury or obstructive jaundice to an advanced stage.

Unconjugated Hyperbilirubinemia

Patients with unconjugated hyperbilirubinemia often do not have significant liver disease. Overproduction of bilirubin (hemolysis and ineffective erythropoiesis), defective hepatic uptake (Gilbert's syndrome), defective conjugation (neonatal jaundice, Crigler-Najjar syndrome, and Gilbert's syndrome), and defective excretion (Dubin-Johnson syndrome, Rotor syndrome, and benign recurrent cholestasis) are the main mechanisms leading to this type of disorder.

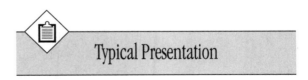

Typical Presentation

Symptoms

Many symptoms related to liver disease are nonspecific, such as fatigue, malaise, nausea, anorexia, and vague abdominal discomfort. Many patients with liver disease are without any symptoms at all. Therefore, it is crucial for primary care clinicians to focus on other aspects of patients' medical history (i.e., history of exposure to viral hepatitis or hepatotoxins; history of blood transfusion; history and extent of illicit drug use, especially intravenous drugs; alcohol consumption; history of medication usage, both prescribed and over-the-counter medications; family history of liver disease; and sexual and travel history).

Key History

HEPATITIS RISK

The diagnosis of viral hepatitis B (HBV) and/or C (HCV) is often associated with a history of blood or blood product transfusion, intravenous drug use with shared needles, sexual promiscuity, needlestick accidents, and tattooing. Although screening for HBV has been a regular procedure at blood banks for more than 30 years, screening for HCV in donated blood became a common practice only in the late 1980s. Hepatitis B is also commonly found in male homosexuals, especially with the advent of the human immunodeficiency virus (HIV) and the AIDS epidemic in the 1980s. It can also be found in immigrants from epidemic areas such as China, Japan, Korea, and Southeast Asia. Hepatitis D should be considered in individuals with active HBV. Hepatitis A should be suspected in patients with a history of recent ingestion of raw seafood, especially raw oysters or clams, history of close contact with day care centers, and history of homosexual contact. Hepatitis E should be suspected in patients immigrating from endemic areas such as India, Southeast Asia, or South America, and especially in pregnant women in whom fulminant liver failure does occur. Further details regarding viral hepatitis can be found in Chapter 16.

HEREDITARY CONDITION

Heredity plays a major role in a host of liver diseases. A careful dissection of family history may reveal hemochromatosis, Wilson's disease,

alpha$_1$-antitrypsin deficiency, all of which are transmitted in an autosomal recessive fashion. Autoimmune hepatitis, primary biliary cirrhosis, and primary sclerosing cholangitis can occur in familial clusters. Other liver disorders with positive family history include benign recurrent intrahepatic cholestasis, arteriohepatic dysplasia or Alagille syndrome, cholelithiasis, and oriental cholangiohepatitis, to name a few.

MEDICATION AND DIET HISTORY

A careful medication and dietary history are always useful in patients presenting with abnormal LFTs of no apparent cause. Medications can cause a wide array of liver disorders ranging from intrahepatic cholestasis, hepatocellular damage, granulomatous infiltration to something in between (Table 19-3). Nonprescription medications should not be overlooked. For instance, hypervitaminosis A (amounts greater than 25,000 IU per day) for prolonged periods can cause transaminitis and possibly cirrhosis. Some herbal medications can also cause liver abnormalities and even hepatic failure. A history of wild mushroom consumption, prolonged total parenteral nutrition, or excessive dieting may lead to liver failure, liver function abnormalities, or the development of cholelithiasis. Occupational exposure to chemicals should also be considered in cases without an obvious cause. Vinyl chloride, carbon tetrachloride, dimethylformamide are some of the organic compounds known to cause liver injury. History of illicit drug use such as cocaine may provide hints of possible vascular events in the liver (ischemic hepatitis).

SEXUAL HISTORY

Sexual history not only provides hints into sexually transmitted viral hepatitis but also directs the clinician to other possible causes of abnormal LFTs. The transmission of HCV is facilitated by the presence of HIV. Contraceptive use is known to be associated with the development of hepatic adenoma, intrahepatic cholestasis, and Budd-Chiari syndrome (hepatic vein thrombosis). Advanced

Table 19-3
Examples of Drug-Related Liver Function Test Abnormalities

PARENCHYMAL INJURY
Anti-inflammatory agents, e.g., ibuprofen (Motrin, Advil), diclofenac (Cataflam, Voltaren), sulindac (Clinoril), and oxaprozin (Daypro)
Acetaminophen (Tylenol)
HMG-CoA reductase inhibitors, e.g., lovastatin (Mevacor), simvastatin (Zocor), and pravastatin (Pravachol)
Antifungals, e.g., ketoconazole (Nizoral), fluconazole (Diflucan), and itraconazole (Sporanox)
Amiodarone
Antibiotics, e.g., penicillins, quinolones, nitrofurantoin, and isoniazid
Beta-blockers, e.g., labetolol and propanolol
Hypoglycemic agents, e.g., glyburide (DiaBeta) and troglitazone (Rezulin)
Immunosuppressives, e.g., methotrexate, azathioprine, and mercaptopurine

OBSTRUCTIVE PATTERN OF INJURY (CHOLESTATIC INJURY AND GRANULOMATOUS CHANGES)
Cholestatic injury
Oral contraceptives
Androgenic anabolic steroids
Antibiotics, e.g., erythromycin, trimethoprim-sulfamethoxazole, and rifampin
Phenothiazines
ACE inhibitors, e.g., captopril, enalapril, and prinivil
Granulomatous changes
Allopurinol
Carbamazepine
Quinidine

MIXED PATTERN OF INJURY
Anticonvulsants, e.g., phenytoin (Dilantin), valproic acid (Depakene/Depakote), and lamotrigine (Lamictal)
Sulfonamides

liver disease may lead to infertility and irregular vaginal bleeding because of anovulation.

SYSTEMIC SYMPTOMS

Liver disease may lead to systemic complications and vice versa. Viral hepatitis can cause polyarthralgias, mixed cryoglobulinemia, immune-complex-mediated glomerulonephritis, and porphyria cutanea tarda. Hemochromatosis can lead to increased skin pigmentation, diabetes mellitus, and cardiac failure in late stages. Wilson's disease may present with neurologic or psychiatric disturbances of unclear etiology and, like primary biliary cirrhosis, can cause osteomalacia and osteoporosis.

In contrast, systemic illness may affect the liver adversely. Sepsis may lead to "shock" liver with subsequent hepatic necrosis. Chronic congestive heart failure may lead to hepatic congestion and abnormal LFTs, especially total and direct hyperbilirubinemia. Hypercoagulable states such as malignancy or myeloproliferative disorders may lead to Budd-Chiari syndrome or portal vein thrombosis. Bone marrow transplantation can lead to venocclusive disease of the liver. Malabsorptive processes such as celiac sprue may cause mild-to-moderate transaminitis. Chronic alcoholic pancreatitis may cause benign common bile duct stricture and extrahepatic cholestasis.

Physical Examination

Findings on physical examination may offer clues to acute versus chronic liver diseases. Presence of splenomegaly, gynecomastia, testicular atrophy, spider angiomata, palmar erythema, and caput medusa point toward the chronicity of the liver disease. In comparison, highly abnormal LFTs in the presence of tender hepatomegaly or ascites, and the absence of the earlier findings suggest acute illnesses such as vascular thrombosis, acute viral hepatitis, medication-related hepatic necrosis, and extrahepatic obstruction from gallstones. Kayser-Fleischer ring and sunflower cataracts are pathognomonic of Wilson's disease. A palpable gallbladder with porcelain appearance on radiographical studies strongly suggests gallbladder malignancy.

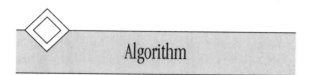

Algorithm

An approach to the patient with abnormal LFTs is depicted in Figure 19-1.

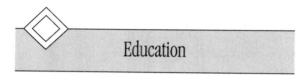

Education

Vaccination for Viral Hepatitis A and B

Viral hepatitis can exact enormous costs on society, so vaccine programs for HBV and hepatitis A have been implemented. The first safe, plasma-derived hepatitis B vaccine (Heptavax B) was first introduced in the early 1980s. However, because its arrival coincided with the beginning of the AIDS epidemic, its plasma origin was poorly received. In the late 1980s, recombinant HBV vaccines (Engerix-B and Recombivax HB) became available. Universal vaccination program for HBV is now widespread in all 50 states. Children are required to have three doses of HBV vaccine by the time they attend elementary school. Adults in high-risk groups such as health care workers, dialysis patients, persons with chronic liver diseases, household and sexual contacts of HBV carriers, those with hemophilia, and prison inmates are strongly recommended to undergo preexposure immunization.

In infants and toddlers, HBV vaccine is given in three doses: birth, 1 to 2 months, and 6 to 18 months. In children older than 2 years of age and adults, HBV vaccine is given in three doses at 0, 1, and 6 months. For postexposure prophylaxis, the vaccine can also be given in combination with hepatitis B immunoglobulins (HBIg) at different sites within 12 h of exposure. Because of some significant, though rare, side effects associated with the vaccine, neurologic and nonneurologic in nature, some concerned parents have mounted legal campaigns against universal vaccination.

The only available hepatitis A vaccine (Havrix) contains inactivated virus. Its use is advocated for travelers to endemic areas, caretakers at mental institutions, childcare workers, military personnel, people with chronic liver diseases, and people exposed to hepatitis A. Adults and children between the ages of 2 through 18 years should receive two intramuscular injections of the vaccine given 6 to 12 months apart. Hepatitis A vaccine can be given concomitantly with immunoglobulins and/or HBV vaccine. The seroconversion rate for HAV vaccine is 100% after the two doses. The duration of the protective immunity provided by the vaccine has not been well-established at this time.

Currently, there is no vaccine for hepatitis C due to the lack of a major neutralizing antibody and the highly mutable and heterogeneous nature of the virus. Researchers, however, have cultured the virus in the laboratory for the first time, which is significant since it is usually the first step in vaccine development.

Testing Pregnant Women for Viral Hepatitis

Vertical transmission of viral hepatitis, especially hepatitis B and C, usually occurs at delivery or soon after and, rarely, in utero. The mode of transmission is considered to be oral contamination of the infant by maternal blood or wastes during the delivery process. The risk of neonatal infection with HBV is the greatest (approximately 90 percent) in newborns, whose mothers have both positive surface and e antigens. The risk is less (approximately 25 percent) in newborns whose mothers are positive for surface antigen alone. It is well known that newborns who are infected at birth usually become chronic carriers, with increased risks of developing cirrhosis and hepatocellular carcinoma. The rate of vertical transmission for hepatitis C is between 10 and 24 percent for newborns whose mothers are infected. This rate may be higher in newborns whose mothers are infected with both HCV and HIV. Hepatitis A is usually not transmitted to the newborn but acute infection during pregnancy can cause premature labor and delivery.

The Centers for Disease Control and Prevention recommend routine hepatitis B surface antigen (HBsAg) screening for all pregnant patients because of the serious risks mentioned earlier and the availability of the highly efficacious combined active-passive vaccination program. Infants at risk are given HBV immunoglobulins and recombinant vaccine concomitantly at birth, and are vaccinated again at 3 and 6 months. Prevention of HBV infection would naturally lead to prevention of hepatitis D infection. If the mother is infected with HCV, close follow-up of the infant is recommended, since there is no effective immunization for the virus at this time. However, routine cesarean section and discouragement against breast-feeding are not advocated in these situations.

Of note, not all pregnant patients with abnormal LFTs have viral hepatitis. Other pregnancy-specific diagnoses that must be entertained include intrahepatic cholestasis of pregnancy, acute fatty liver of pregnancy, preeclampsia and eclampsia, the HELLP (*h*emolytic anemia, *e*levated *l*iver enzymes, and *l*ow *p*latelets) syndrome, and cholelithiasis. Detailed discussion regarding these conditions is beyond the scope of this chapter.

Screening for Hemochromatosis

Hereditary hemochromatosis is a common autosomal recessive disorder of iron metabolism leading to excess iron deposits throughout the body, especially in the liver. In European populations or populations of European ancestry, approximately 1 in 10 persons is a heterozygous carrier, and 0.3 to 0.5 percent are homozygotes. A candi-

date gene (HFE gene) for this condition has been identified on the short-arm of chromosome 6. A single missense mutation (G to A at nucleotide 845) results in the substitution of tyrosine for cysteine at amino acid 282, hence the term *C282Y mutation*. Homozygosity for this mutation is present in 85 to 90 percent of persons who have characteristic symptoms of hemochromatosis. A second missense mutation (C to G at nucleotide 187) results in the substitution of aspartate for histidine at amino acid 63, hence the term *H63D mutation*. This mutation contributes to increased hepatic iron levels, but does not cause the entire syndrome in the absence of C282Y mutation. To complicate the matter, there is other evidence that the hemochromatosis phenotype can occur in the absence of the preceding mutations. Moreover, acquired hemochromatosis can occur in cases of ineffective erythropoiesis such as thalassemia, sideroblastic anemia, and subsequent massive blood or iron transfusions.

Because the disease is treatable with either phlebotomy or chelation if detected early, a high index of suspicion and screening measures for family members of probands have been strongly advocated. Although it is often presumed that women with hereditary hemochromatosis experience mitigated phenotypic disease expression by the effects of menstruation and pregnancy, studies have suggested otherwise. Afflicted women can experience the full spectrum of the illness, including cirrhosis, despite menstrual periods and pregnancy. Women more frequently have fatigue, arthralgia, and pigmentation, while men more frequently have cirrhosis and diabetes. Serum transferrin saturation and serum ferritin levels are both found to be sensitive and complementary screening tests. The sensitivity, specificity, and positive predictive value of serum transferrin saturation alone set at 50 percent or higher would be 94, 96, and 16 percent, respectively. Although the disease has variable degrees of penetrance, biochemical screening identifies virtually all adults with C282Y homozygosity and iron overload. If the disease is detected before the age of 40, and if the serum ferritin level is less than

1000 ng/ml, then it can be managed and treated without a liver biopsy because the likelihood of hepatic fibrosis is low.

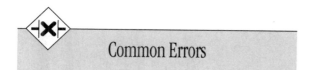

Common Errors

Failure to Consider Other Sources of Abnormal Liver Function Tests

The most common mistake in evaluating patients with abnormal LFTs is not to consider the possibility that these abnormalities may originate from some other organs than the liver itself. For instance, highly elevated values of AST and LDH out of proportion to that of ALT are suggestive of a problem with skeletal or cardiac muscles. They may also point toward possible high rate of cell lysis, or hemolysis, especially in the setting of indirect hyperbilirubinemia. A careful history and physical examination may help the clinician distinguish these problems.

In certain cases, additional liver enzyme tests such as 5'-NUC and GGT may help the clinician distinguish between hepatic and nonhepatic abnormalities. Hodgkin's disease, congestive heart failure, intraabdominal infections, intestinal obstruction, and osteomyelitis, to name a few, are some conditions that can result in abnormal alkaline phosphatase levels without directly involving the liver. In elderly patients, an elevated alkaline phosphatase level may indicate bony disorder, such as Paget's disease. Fractionation of alkaline phosphatase by heat inactivation or electrophoresis may arrive at the correct diagnosis.

Alkaline Phosphatase in Certain Stages of Life

Alkaline phosphatase levels in pregnant women and young children are higher than are the standard adult values. This is a normal finding related to the rapid growth of the placenta and bones,

respectively. In the 15- to 50-year-old age group, mean serum alkaline phosphatase level is higher in men than it is in women. By contrast, above the age of 60, the enzyme activity of women may equal or exceed that of men. Moreover, both sexes in this age group have higher mean alkaline phosphatase values than do young adults. Also notably, in healthy adolescent males, alkaline phosphatase levels that are two to three times above normal adult levels may not indicate hepatobiliary disorder at all. The reasons for these differences are not always clear.

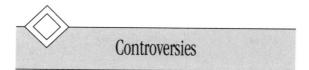

Controversies

Nonalcoholic Steatohepatitis

Nonalcoholic steatohepatitis (NASH) is a liver disease in which the liver pathology is similar to that of alcoholic liver disease, including moderate-to-severe macrovesicular fatty infiltration accompanied by lobular or portal inflammation, with or without Mallory hyaline bodies, fibrosis, or cirrhosis. To distinguish it from alcoholic hepatitis, two other criteria must be met. First, there must be a negligible history of alcohol consumption of less than 40 g of ethanol per week. This calls for a detailed history taken independently by three physicians from the patient and family members and negative random serum alcohol levels. Second, there must be negative viral serology for hepatitis B and C (namely, negative HBsAg and HCV antibody).

Patients with NASH are typically obese, middle-aged women with elevated ALT and AST, and asymptomatic hepatomegaly. Besides morbid obesity, hyperlipidemia, diabetes mellitus, jejunal bypass operation, biliopancreatic diversion, prolonged total parenteral nutrition, and certain medications (e.g., amiodarone, glucocorticoids, synthetic estrogens, and tamoxifen) have been known to contribute to the development of this condition. The pathogenesis of this condition is not well elucidated. Proposed mechanisms for the accumulation of fat in the liver include increased synthesis of fatty acids in the liver, increased delivery of free fatty acids to the liver, decreased beta oxidation of free fatty acids, and decreased secretion of very low density lipoprotein cholesterol. In turn, free fatty acids are highly reactive, leading to the formation of potentially toxic intermediates that can induce an exuberant hepatic inflammatory response and, subsequently, fibrosis.

For many years, clinicians have considered NASH as a stable process without significant risks of developing cirrhosis and, hence, have not found a liver biopsy necessary. This is where the controversy lies. Review of the medical literature on NASH has shown that although this disease usually has an indolent course, and generally good prognosis, nearly half of the patients develop progressive fibrosis and approximately 10 to 15 percent develop cirrhosis. It has also been found that the clinician's ability to diagnose and to predict the course of the disease by following liver function studies alone is inadequate. The predictive value of a diagnosis of NASH before liver biopsy was only 56 percent, compared with 86 percent for alcoholic hepatitis. In addition, an ultrasound finding of diffuse fatty infiltration in the liver is not specific enough and should not be used to diagnose NASH. Therefore, liver biopsy is now generally recommended for the definitive diagnosis of NASH.

To treat or not to treat NASH is the next question. Today, there is no definitive uniform therapy for NASH. In cases of NASH where the liver pathology reveals evidence of fibrosis and active inflammation associated with diffuse fatty infiltration and moderately elevated liver enzymes, treatment is recommended. It includes removal of any offending drug, lowering serum lipid levels, and tight control of diabetic hyperglycemia, which can help in certain cases. Weight loss is often strongly advocated because of the prominent role obesity plays in this condition. However, the effect of weight loss on the liver process is not always predictable. Weight reduction of 10 to 20 percent may result in normalization of the biochemical data. Case reports of treating NASH with ursodeoxycholic acid

for 1 year have shown promising normalization of abnormal LFTs. However, abnormal levels of liver enzymes recurred after the drug was discontinued. Randomized, controlled trials are underway.

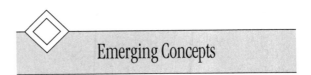

Emerging Concepts

Celiac Sprue as a Cause of Abnormal Liver Function Tests

Studies have suggested that celiac sprue should be considered in the list of differential diagnoses for patients with abnormal LFTs, especially elevated ALT, AST, and alkaline phosphatase levels. In addition, celiac sprue is also common among patients with primary biliary cirrhosis. In patients with celiac disease, the prevalence of primary biliary cirrhosis was approximately 3 percent and in patients with primary biliary cirrhosis, the prevalence of celiac sprue was approximately 6 percent. Screening for primary biliary cirrhosis in patients with celiac sprue using antimitochondrial antibody testing and screening for celiac disease in patients with primary biliary cirrhosis using sprue antibodies (antigliadin, antiendomysial, and antireticulin antibodies) is therefore recommended. A gluten-free diet is the current therapy for celiac disease and ursodeoxycholic acid is that for primary biliary cirrhosis.

Association of Diabetes Mellitus with Hepatitis C

Patients with chronic liver disease are known to have a high prevalence of glucose intolerance. However, several studies have suggested that hepatitis C infection, besides age, is an independent risk factor for the development of diabetes mellitus. Patients with HCV infection of genotype 2a are found to be especially susceptible to developing diabetes. Hepatitis C virus genotype 2a was observed in 29 percent of HCV-positive diabetic patients diagnosed by polymerase chain reaction, compared with 3 to 4 percent of local HCV-positive control population ($p < 0.005$). Prevalence of diabetes was 19 percent in patients with HCV infection, 8 percent in patients with HBV infection, and 1 percent in patients with cholestatic liver disease. The lack of any particular epidemiologic factor for HCV infection in the studied diabetic populations suggests involvement of the virus in the pathogenesis of diabetes. The mechanism for this remains to be discovered. Testing for HCV infection in diabetic patients with abnormal LFTs is mandatory.

Bibliography

American College of Obstetricians and Gynecologists: ACOG educational bulletin No. 248: Viral hepatitis in pregnancy. *Int J Gynaecol Obstet* 63:195–202, 1998.

Bacon BR, Powell LW, Adams PC, et al: Molecular medicine and hemochromatosis: At the crossroads. *Gastroenterology* 116:193–207, 1999.

Bardella MT, Quatrini M, Zuin M, et al: Screening patients with celiac disease for primary biliary cirrhosis and vice versa. *Am J Gastroenterol* 92(9): 1524–1526, 1997.

Burt MJ, George PM, Upton JD, et al: The significance of haemochromatosis gene mutations in the general population: Implications for screening. *Gut* 43: 830–836, 1998.

Dickey W, McMillan SA, Callender ME: High prevalence of celiac sprue among patients with primary biliary cirrhosis. *J Clin Gastroenterol* 25(1):328–329, 1997.

Duff P: Hepatitis in pregnancy. *Semin Perinatol* 22: 277–283, 1998.

Fournier C, Sureau C, Coste J, et al: In vitro infection of adult normal human hepatocytes in primary culture by hepatitis C virus. *J Gen Virol* 79:2367–2374, 1998.

Ito T, Mukaigawa J, Zuo J, et al: Cultivation of hepatitis C virus in primary hepatocyte culture from patients with chronic hepatitis C results in release of high titre infectious virus. *J Gen Virol* 77:1043–1054, 1996.

Kaplan MM: Laboratory tests, in Schiff L, Schiff ER (eds): *Diseases of the Liver,* 7th ed. Philadelphia, JB Lippincott Company, 1993; pp 108–144.

Kingham JG, Parker DR: The association between primary biliary cirrhosis and coeliac disease: A study of relative prevalences. *Gut* 42(1):120–122, 1998.

Mason AL, Lau JY, Hoang N, et al: Association of diabetes mellitus and chronic hepatitis C virus infection. *Hepatology* 29:328–333, 1999.

Moirand R, Adams PC, Bicheler V, et al: Clinical features of genetic hemochromatosis in women compared with men. *Ann Intern Med* 127(2):105–110, 1997.

Moseley RH: Evaluation of abnormal liver function tests. *Med Clin North Am* 80(5):887–906, 1996.

Nguyen MT, Zern MA: An ounce of prevention: The development of viral hepatitis vaccines. *Compr Ther* 21(6):283–289, 1995.

Olynyk JK, Cullen DJ, Aquilia S, et al: A population-based study of the clinical expression of the hemochromatosis gene. *N Engl J Med* 341(10): 718–724, 1999.

Pietrangelo A, Montosi G, Totaro A, et al: Hereditary hemochromatosis in adults without pathogenic mutations in the hemochromatosis gene. *N Engl J Med* 341(10):725–732, 1999.

Sheth SG, Gordon FD, Chopra S: Nonalcoholic steatohepatitis. *Ann Intern Med* 126(2):137–145, 1997.

Simo R, Hernandez C, Genescà J, et al: High prevalence of hepatitis C virus infection in diabetic patients. *Diabetes Care* 19:998–1000, 1996.

Varner MW: General medical and surgical diseases in pregnancy, in Scott JR, DiSaia PJ, Hammond CB, Spellacy WN (eds): *Danforth's Obstetrics and Gynecology,* 7th ed. Philadelphia, JB Lippincott Company, 1994, pp 427–463.

Marc Bernstein

Chapter 20

Biliary Obstruction

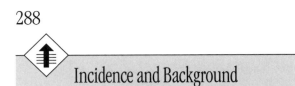

Incidence and Background

Obstruction of the bile ducts is a medical problem that any physician with an active clinical practice will repeatedly encounter. Biliary obstruction from choledocholithiasis (bile duct stones) is present in 5 to 15 percent of patients who undergo cholecystectomy, the most commonly performed abdominal operation in North America. Even among patients whose gallbladder is removed, up to 10 percent may suffer from recurrent choledocholithiasis.

While stones are the most common cause of biliary obstruction, biliary strictures (both benign and malignant) also lead to obstruction. Malignant biliary obstruction from periampullary tumors, such as pancreatic cancer, affects at least 30,000 patients each year. Benign biliary strictures have innumerable underlying etiologies. These etiologies range from the focal iatrogenic injuries that complicate up to 1 percent of all laparoscopic cholecystectomies, to primary sclerosing cholangitis (PSC), which is the fourth leading indication for liver transplantation in the United States.

Therefore, biliary obstruction represents an important and heterogeneous group of clinically related, but pathologically distinct, medical problems. Many principles of diagnosis and care apply to all of the specific entities that embody biliary obstruction. Still, to optimize the care of affected patients, recognition of the specific diseases and an understanding of the advantages and disadvantages of available treatment alternatives are necessary.

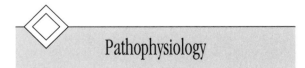

Pathophysiology

The pressure gradient between the biliary tree and the duodenum drives the flow of bile from the liver into the duodenum. This flow serves to flush away tiny crystalline particles that precipitate within bile before they grow and cause obstruction. Without obstruction, this same pressure gradient makes the establishment of bacterial infection within bile virtually impossible. Bacterial decontamination by gastric acid, luminally secreted IgA antibodies, and the barrier effect of the ampulla of Vater may further lower the vulnerability of the biliary tree to bacterial infection. In turn, the sterility of bile prevents the formation of stones since bacterial β-glucuronidases can lead to the precipitation of stone-forming bilirubin-calcium salts. While the functional biliary anatomy is usually protective, there are several inherent weaknesses that can lead to biliary obstruction and secondary infection. Table 20-1 lists the causes of biliary obstruction with the most common causes outlined later.

Cholestasis is the failure of bile to be produced in the liver and then to be delivered into the intestinal lumen. This failure can occur from multiple causes including, but not limited to, biliary obstruction. Any number of acute or chronic liver diseases can also produce cholestasis. The clinical and laboratory manifestations of cholestasis are nonspecific; therefore, distinguishing bile duct obstruction from a primary hepatic disease can be challenging.

Further complicating the diagnosis, the symptoms and laboratory abnormalities of partial or intermittent biliary obstruction may be vague. As a result, biliary obstruction may not be recognized. If allowed to persist or progress, biliary obstruction can acutely result in life-threatening biliary infection and can chronically result in liver failure from biliary cirrhosis. It is essential that the practitioner recognizes even subtle signs and symptoms of cholestasis and maintains a high index of suspicion for biliary obstruction. Once biliary obstruction is diagnosed, vigilance is required for expeditious therapy that maximizes the chance for the best possible clinical outcome.

The causes of biliary obstruction are both common and diverse. Furthermore, obstructions can be focal or diffuse; and the potential locations of obstructions within the biliary tree extend from

Table 20-1

Causes of Biliary Obstruction

AIDS cholangiopathy
Blood clot from hemobilia
Choledochal cysts
Choledocholithiasis
Cholesterol gallstones
Oriental cholangiohepatitis
Pigment gallstones
Chronic pancreatitis
Iatrogenic strictures
Ischemic injury following intraarterial
5-fluorouracil
Liver transplantation
Hepaticojejunostomy
Injury from surgery or trauma
Malignancy
Ampullary neoplasms
Cholangiocarcinoma
Duodenal tumors
Metastatic disease
Pancreatic cancer
Mirizzi's syndrome: extrinsic common duct
compression by gallstone in cystic duct
or gallbladder
Papillary stenosis
Parasites
Ascaris
Clonorchis
Echinococcus
Primary sclerosing cholangitis
Secondary sclerosing cholangitis: bile duct
strictures that result from prior biliary disease
Sphincter of Oddi dysfunction

the smallest intrahepatic ducts through the most distal aspect of the common bile duct to the intestinal lumen. These variables affect clinical presentations and must influence specific management choices. In any case, the essential components of optimal management of patients with biliary obstruction are early recognition, support-ive care, an appropriately limited reliance upon antibiotics, and, most important, efforts to be sure that the obstruction is relieved.

Principal Diagnoses

Choledocholithiasis

Cholesterol and pigment stones are the two principal chemical types of gallstones. *Cholesterol stones* account for 80 percent of the biliary stones in developed Western nations. In an aqueous environment, cholesterol will crystallize. In bile, however, cholesterol associates with bile acids and is kept soluble by the formation of micelles. In at least 50 percent of people, bile will periodically become supersaturated with cholesterol. In most instances, stone formation does not occur because the precipitation of cholesterol crystals is a slow process that may take days. During this period, the supersaturated or crystal-containing bile is periodically flushed from the gallbladder and biliary tree.

Conditions that raise the concentration of cholesterol in bile or lower the bile acid concentration in bile will increase the risk of the formation of gallstones. These conditions include female gender, obesity, Northern European or Native American ancestry, and history of estrogen therapy. Factors that increase bile stasis, such as prolonged bowel rest, weight reduction, or some drugs (such as octreotide), also enhance the risk of gallstone formation.

Pigment stones, though less common than cholesterol stones, are frequently responsible for biliary pathology. Pigment stones are made up of a combination of bilirubin and calcium salts. Pigment stones may be further classified as black or brown. Black pigment stones are noted most commonly among patients with cirrhosis or hemolytic anemia, especially sickle-cell disease.

Brown pigment stones are usually the result of biliary infection and are perhaps more commonly present among patients with relative IgA deficiency, as well as among patients with bacterial colonization of the biliary tree.

Most gallstone formation occurs in the gallbladder, which provides a reservoir for bile stasis and for the precipitation of cholesterol or bilirubin-calcium salts. While most bile duct stones have their origin in the gallbladder, up to 4 percent of patients who undergo surgical bile duct exploration may have primary bile duct stones that have formed outside of the gallbladder. The biliary tree outside of the gallbladder, especially if a large cystic duct remnant, bile duct cysts (choledochocysts), or dilated bile ducts proximal to a stricture are present, can serve as a locus for stasis and the formation of gallstones. Additionally, numerous intrahepatic primary bile duct stones are observed in patients with a rare disorder termed *oriental cholangiohepatitis*. Therefore, it is important not to exclude choledocholithiasis from consideration in evaluating an individual who has had a cholecystectomy. More information about gallstones and their treatment is presented in Chapter 17.

Bile Duct Strictures

Bile is made by hepatocytes and is first deposited into microscopically small ducts within the hepatic parenchyma. These tiny ducts flow into progressively larger ducts within the liver and then into two relatively large ducts within the liver, the right and left hepatic ducts. The hepatic ducts merge to form the common hepatic duct that drains into the extrahepatic portion of the biliary tree. This common duct (called the common hepatic duct above the cystic duct takeoff and common bile duct below that landmark) proceeds past the porta hepatis and through the head of the pancreas. Finally, bile is deposited into the second portion of the duodenum through the ampulla of Vater. The biliary anatomy is susceptible to potential obstruction both from extrinsic mass effect and from intrinsic biliary strictures. Muscular sphincters at the ampulla are, in part, responsible for regulating the flow of biliary (sphincter choledochus) and pancreatic (sphincter pancreaticus) fluids. Focal strictures can occur at isolated or multiple sites along the biliary tree (spanning from the tiny biliary radicals within the liver parenchyma to the duodenal lumen). Aside from bile duct stones, bile duct and ampullary strictures represent the other major category of biliary obstruction. These strictures should be classified, as best as possible, as either malignant or benign; both prognosis and management options are influenced by this determination.

MALIGNANT BILE DUCT STRICTURES

Pancreatic cancers, ampullary neoplasms, cholangiocarcinomas (tumors of the biliary epithelium), and duodenal cancers can be collectively referred to as periampullary tumors. These are the principal malignant processes that cause biliary obstruction. For patients with tumors diagnosed before they have metastasized or locally spread, surgery offers hope for cure. Unfortunately, most of these lesions are advanced before they become clinically evident; thus, curative resection is often an unrealistic goal. In these situations, appropriate recognition and treatment of bile duct obstruction can improve disabling symptoms that accompany cholestasis.

Any other tumor that has locally extended or metastasized to the liver parenchyma or porta hepatis can also lead to biliary obstruction by mass effect. Biliary drainage procedures, similar to those used to treat obstruction from periampullary tumors, may play an important role in treatment. Additionally, chemotherapy or radiation treatment may be used to shrink a tumor, thus resulting in biliary decompression without direct mechanical intervention.

PANCREATIC CANCER   Adenocarcinoma of the head or proximal portion of the pancreas is the most frequent cause of malignant biliary obstruction. Ninety percent of patients with pancreatic cancer have local or distant tumor spread at the time of diagnosis. Also, most patients are elderly (the median age of diagnosis being in the eighth decade of life) and many have comorbid illnesses. These factors, when treating patients with pancreatic cancer, commonly place the emphasis on palliative therapies. Still, an experienced biliary surgeon should evaluate patients before abandoning curative efforts.

CHOLANGIOCARCINOMA Though far less common, like their pancreatic counterparts, about 95 percent of primary malignant tumors of the bile duct are adenocarcinomas. They are usually encountered between the ages of 50 to 70 years, but patients with structural bile duct disease, such as Caroli's disease (congenital cysts of the bile ducts) and PSC, face a markedly increased risk of cholangiocarcinoma and may develop these tumors earlier in life.

Cholangiocarcinomas can occur anywhere within the biliary tree but are usually located in the common bile duct or common hepatic duct (about 70 percent of cases). The eponym, *Klatskin's tumor,* applies to a lesion positioned at the bifurcation of the right and left hepatic ducts (about 20 percent of cases). The remaining small fractions of these tumors are located in the liver, the cystic duct, or diffusely throughout the biliary tree. Unlike pancreatic cancers, about 75 percent of cholangiocarcinomas may be considered "operable" as jaundice and laboratory abnormalities suggestive of bile duct obstruction develop earlier in the course of the disease.

AMPULLARY AND DUODENAL TUMORS Because of their retroperitoneal location and relative isolation from major vascular structures, ampullary and duodenal tumors that cause biliary obstruction are probably the most curable of the periampullary tumors. Ampullary adenomas are dysplastic lesions like adenomatous colon polyps, which may be discovered prior to the development of frankly malignant degeneration. About 40 percent of cancers may not be recognized by endoscopic biopsy of ampullary masses; therefore, it is important that ampullary adenomas be addressed aggressively once they are recognized.

Duodenal cancers, like all small-bowel adenocarcinomas, are unusual lesions that account for less than 4 percent of all gastrointestinal malignancies; duodenal tumors are the least frequently encountered periampullary neoplasm.

BENIGN BILE DUCT STRICTURES

Benign biliary strictures are an especially nonuniform group of conditions. They can result from inherent disorders of the bile duct or from injury, most commonly iatrogenic injury from surgery. Congenital and idiopathic bile duct stricturing diseases present an unusual challenge because the underlying diseases may be benign, yet patients are at increased risk for the development of cholangiocarcinomas that may, by imaging, be indistinguishable from benign bile duct strictures. Thus, separating malignant from benign biliary abnormalities, in this setting, can be problematic.

Iatrogenic biliary obstruction can occur from immediate surgical complication, from late stricturing of a surgical biliary anastomosis, or from scarring or ischemic stricturing of bile ducts following intrahepatic artery chemotherapy or liver transplantation. These complications must always be considered if they are to be recognized and managed expeditiously.

PRIMARY SCLEROSING CHOLANGITIS Primary sclerosing cholangitis is an idiopathic inflammatory disorder of the bile ducts. The inflammation results in strictures that may develop at any location within the intrahepatic and extrahepatic biliary tree. A cholangiographic example of PSC is shown in Figure 20-1.

The disease is present in males more often than it is in females and is usually associated with a history of idiopathic inflammatory bowel disease, especially ulcerative colitis. The natural history of PSC tends to follow a slowly progressive course. It results in cholestatic liver disease, which may span an average period of 9 to 17 years between the time of diagnosis and the development of end-stage disease from secondary biliary

Figure 20-1

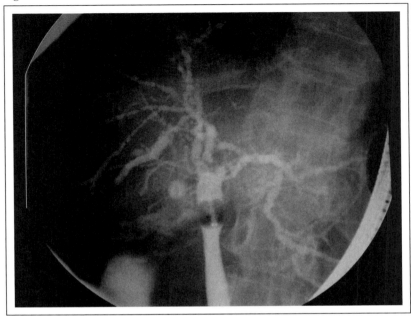

PSC: Cholangiogram showing beading of the intrahepatic ducts.

cirrhosis. During that period, patients' medical course can be punctuated by episodes of cholangitis. Additionally, patients with PSC have a 7 to 15 percent lifetime risk of developing superimposed cholangiocarcinoma.

As a disease, PSC is particularly difficult to characterize and study. The typically slow, but occasionally erratic, progression of the disease limits the ability to prospectively evaluate PSC and available treatments. The study of PSC is also limited by the relatively short history during which physicians have been readily able to establish the diagnosis. In fact, fewer than 100 cases of PSC were reported prior to the early 1970s when endoscopic retrograde cholangiopancreatography (ERCP) became widely available. As a result, PSC management recommendations are based heavily upon anecdotal experience.

CHRONIC PANCREATITIS Stenoses of the intrapancreatic portion of the common bile duct may be present in 10 to 60 percent of adult patients with chronic pancreatitis. These patients are usually asymptomatic; but, over time, symptoms from cholestasis and secondary biliary cirrhosis may occur. Pancreatic pseudocysts located in the head of the pancreas are also a consequence of pancreatitis and can lead to extrinsic compression of the biliary tree. Given the common etiologies of chronic pancreatitis, the possibility of biliary obstruction from pancreatic disease should be entertained in any affected patient with a long history of alcohol abuse or recurrent pancreatitis.

AIDS CHOLANGIOPATHY Cholangiopathy is a recognized complication of advanced HIV infection. It is usually the result of cytomegalovirus and/or *Cryptosporidium* spp. infection of the biliary tree. Though seen less frequently now, as newer antiviral medications have slowed the progression of HIV, AIDS cholangiopathy is still encountered. AIDS cholangiopathy is characterized by strictures of the papilla and extrahepatic biliary tree; the cholangiographic appearance may be similar to that of PSC. Clinically, AIDS cholangiopathy is manifest as abdominal pain and cholestatic clinicopathologic changes.

BILIARY DYSKINESIA Biliary dyskinesia, or sphincter of Oddi dysfunction (SOD), is a disorder of the biliary and pancreatic sphincters. The disorder may be the result of papillary stenosis, perhaps from scarring of the ampulla, or may be a functional disorder of the sphincter mechanism. In any case, SOD may result in biliary dilation and abnormal liver function tests, as well as biliary pain.

IATROGENIC BILIARY STRICTURES Iatrogenic biliary obstructions are encountered for a variety of reasons. While the most common cause of biliary obstruction following cholecystectomy is the presence of a bile duct stone, the possibility of a bile duct injury should not be ignored. Such injuries often result from surgical errors in the setting of congenitally aberrant biliary anatomy. The incidence of such biliary complications rose dramatically with the widespread introduction of laparoscopic cholecystectomy. Fortunately, as surgical experience with this technique has increased, the frequency of these potentially devastating surgical complications has dropped.

Biliary strictures should also be expected as intermittent sequelae after any surgery that alters the typical pattern of biliary drainage. Such situations are not unusual following liver transplantation and can be long-term consequences of healing after hepaticojejunostomy or Roux-en-Y surgery.

Another form of iatrogenic biliary stricturing is the development of an ischemic stricture of the common bile duct. Ordinarily, the extrahepatic biliary tree is protected from ischemic injury by a dual blood supply, with the distal bile duct receiving blood flow from the duodenum and the proximal bile duct receiving blood flow from the hepatic artery. If one of these blood supplies is interrupted, collateral circulation is ordinarily sufficient to meet the oxygen demands of the remaining portion of the bile duct. A few situations may interrupt these

collateral connections. These conditions include liver transplantation with a duct-to-duct anastomosis, radiation therapy to the portal region, or the intraarterial administration (via the hepatic artery) of 5-fluorouracil chemotherapy; the result is ischemic damage to the biliary system.

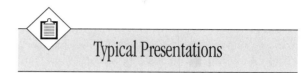

Typical Presentations

While no two patients are the same, most patients with biliary obstruction fit into one of a few clinical presentation patterns. Recognition of these patterns is useful for appropriate triage in arranging medical and procedural intervention.

Aseptic Biliary Obstruction

Aseptic biliary obstruction can result from both complete and partial biliary obstruction. Affected patients may be asymptomatic and only have abnormalities incidentally detected on routine blood testing or imaging studies (obtained for unrelated purposes) that demonstrate dilatation of the biliary tree. It is this presentation for which the medical cliché regarding "painless jaundice" as a sign of malignant biliary obstruction most aptly applies. While many of these patients remain symptom-free for prolonged intervals, progression to more severe disease can occur. Other patients can develop the symptomatic and metabolic consequences that result from cholestasis.

Acute Cholangitis

Acute cholangitis is the development of bacterial infection in the biliary tree proximal to an obstructed bile duct. The most frequent causative organisms are lactose fermenting, gram-negative organisms including *Escherichia coli* and *Klebsiella* spp. Other common offending bacteria include *Streptococcus fecalis*, *Enterococcus*, and *Bacteroides fragilis*.

Cholangitis can range in form from mild to severe and may evolve in a progressive fashion if the biliary obstruction persists or worsens. In its mildest form, *ascending cholangitis* (as some authors refer to it), the clinical presentation of cholangitis resembles that of aseptic biliary obstruction. Only 50 to 60 percent of patients with cholangitis will present with Charcot's triad of fever, jaundice, and right upper quadrant abdominal pain (the classic description of cholangitis). It is imperative to attempt to recognize and promptly treat milder forms of cholangitis to prevent progression to more advanced life-threatening disease, sometimes termed *suppurative cholangitis*.

Only 10 to 15 percent of patients with infected bile present with suppurative cholangitis. Suppurative cholangitis is best characterized by Raynaud's pentad, which adds mental obtundation and septic shock to Charcot's triad. The prognosis faced by patients with suppurative cholangitis is guarded. Suppurative cholangitis represents a life-threatening septic condition, and management requires emergency efforts toward biliary decompression.

Liver Abscess

The predominant cause of pyogenic liver abscesses has changed with the widespread availability of antibiotics and with the improved management of appendicitis and diverticulitis. While colonic diseases remain important etiologies of liver abscesses, biliary tract diseases have supplanted them as the leading cause. Typically, affected patients present acutely in their sixth decade of life or later with symptoms of jaundice, fever, nausea and vomiting, and sometimes pleurisy. Most patients follow a fulminant septic course, so that even with prompt intervention the mortality rate can be as high as 40 percent.

The causative organism of pyogenic liver abscesses is most commonly *E. coli*, but other gram-negative organisms such as *Klebsiella*, *Proteus*, and *Pseudomonas* are also important pathogens that may produce liver abscesses. Gram-positive organisms such as streptococci and staphylococci can also produce liver abscesses.

Biliary Cirrhosis

With long-standing biliary obstruction from any etiology, chronic inflammatory changes will occur around the intrahepatic bile ducts and portal tracts. Initially, the response is the proliferation of bile ducts within the liver. Over time, bile leaks from the biliary system into the liver parenchyma. This is followed by the development of a scarring pattern with fibrous expansion of the portal tracts. Finally, there is obliteration of intrahepatic bile ducts and evolution of irreversible liver failure.

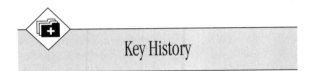

Key History

Patients with early biliary obstruction may be minimally symptomatic; therefore, the absence of symptoms does not exclude milder forms of obstruction. On the opposite end of the spectrum, the clinical presentation of patients with advanced or high-grade biliary obstruction may be virtually identical to patients with severe liver failure. Patients with cholestatic drug reactions, aggressive autoimmune hepatitis, or acute viral hepatitis may have symptoms of fever, abdominal pain, and jaundice that are indistinguishable from symptoms caused by acute cholangitis. Biliary obstruction should be among the differential diagnoses of any patient who has new or worsened cholestasis.

When cholestatic symptoms are identified, a directed review of symptoms, past medical history, and past surgical history should be obtained from patients as well as from available medical records. This should include inquiries for symptoms of biliary colic and risk factors for primary liver diseases. The characteristic pattern of biliary colic is prolonged episodes (lasting 2 to 3 h) of right upper quadrant abdominal pain that may radiate to the shoulder. Most patients who develop complications from gallstones have had prior episodes of biliary colic so this history can be particularly useful. Finally, when biliary obstruction is suspected, the past medical history should be used to evaluate for prior history of liver disease, biliary obstruction, biliary surgery, and biliary instrumentation.

Cholestatic Symptoms

A few symptoms, including jaundice, urine and stool color changes, and pruritus are characteristic of cholestasis from any cause.

JAUNDICE

Jaundice is the most widely recognized of all cholestatic symptoms. In its earliest manifestation, patients may notice only slight yellowing of the sclera. As cholestasis worsens, this is followed by the development of more diffuse mucous membrane and skin discoloration. The development of jaundice may be gradual and go unnoticed by patients, so it is often useful to ask relatives or friends if jaundice is present. Normal serum bilirubin levels are typically less than 1.1 mg/dl, but jaundice is not visibly apparent until the serum bilirubin is at least 2.5 mg/dl. Therefore, jaundice is not a sensitive indicator of either cholestasis or hyperbilirubinemia.

DARK URINE AND ACHOLIC STOOL

With the normal flow of bile, bilirubin (in bile) is metabolized in the digestive tract into stercobilinogen. It is this chemical that is responsible for the typical brown color of stool. If the flow of bile is blocked, stool may become pale with a gray shade.

As bilirubin accumulates in the blood, it is conjugated by the liver and rendered filterable by the kidney. As the serum bilirubin increases, there is typically an increase in urinary bilirubin excretion and this produces brown discoloration of the urine. Simply asking patients if their urine is darker

often leads to misleading answers, with patients simply answering that the urine is "more yellow"; this is very nonspecific. Rather, asking patients if their urine has a brown color similar to iced tea or cola may result in more meaningful answers.

PRURITUS

Patients with cholestasis may experience diffuse pruritus that occurs in the absence of a causative rash. The exact mechanism of this pruritus remains poorly understood and, while this symptom alone is far from diagnostic, in the right clinical context, it does further support consideration of biliary obstruction or cholestatic liver disease.

Fever

Fever is an important symptom to recognize. About 90 percent of patients with cholangitis will have fevers. Fevers coupled with abnormal liver function tests should be an alert to possible cholangitis.

Constitutional Symptoms

While symptoms such as anorexia and weight loss are nonspecific, they can result from cholestasis and are often relieved with decompression of the biliary tract. Chronicity of these symptoms may suggest an underlying malignancy. Abdominal pain also may be a useful but highly nonspecific symptom. Abdominal pain is common with acute biliary obstruction from gallstones, but is less common with slowly evolving obstruction from tumors. The pattern of pain should therefore be noted.

Prior History of Biliary Disease

Patients who have an established history of biliary obstruction should be evaluated and treated promptly. The stents, appliances, and surgical interventions that are utilized to provide biliary drainage are prone to failure. Such failures might result from stricturing of a previous biliary anastomosis, occlusion or displacement of a biliary stent or drain, or stenosis of a biliary sphincterotomy. It is therefore imperative that any patient who has a history of biliary intervention and fever, laboratory abnormalities, or cholestatic symptoms be evaluated promptly for recurrent obstruction or cholangitis.

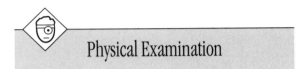

Physical Examination

General Examination

The general examination is perhaps the most important part of any physical exam. In the setting of cholestasis, patients who are febrile, diaphoretic, obtunded, and with unstable vital signs require immediate evaluation and intervention to assess for and treat cholangitis. More stable patients may be able to be resuscitated and treated with antibiotics. Following this, biliary decompression can be pursued in a semielective fashion.

Like clinical history, the physical examination may help to identify patients with biliary obstruction. Further examination can demonstrate cutaneous signs, such as jaundice, or skin excoriation from scratching, which suggest cholestasis. The abdominal exam may be invaluable by revealing the presence of masses, surgical scars, or areas of tenderness. More in-depth examination may provide further clues regarding the etiology of the cholestasis aiding in the distinction of biliary from liver disease.

Cutaneous Signs

JAUNDICE

As described in "Key History," the discovery of overt jaundice may be a relatively late finding. Additionally, jaundice can occur from hyperbilirubinemia caused by hemolysis or inherited disorders of bilirubin glucuronosyltransferase, such as Gilbert's disease. So while jaundice is a clue, its presence is neither sensitive nor specific for cholestasis.

To examine for jaundice, a generalized skin examination for overt yellow discoloration and for skin excoriation that may indicate scratching from severe pruritus is the initial step. If no overt jaundice is seen, the sclera should be inspected along with the interior aspect of the lower eyelid. While examining the eyes, the upper eyelid should be inspected for xantholasmas, a nonspecific sign of disordered cholesterol metabolism that can result from chronic cholestatic liver diseases, such as primary biliary cirrhosis. Finally, icteric changes of the oropharyngeal mucosa, especially on the floor of the mouth, may be the first area where jaundice is clinically evident by examination.

Cutaneous bruising or bleeding may be seen both among patients with liver disease and patients with cholestasis from biliary obstruction that has led to vitamin K deficiency and clotting time abnormalities. Bruising along the anterior abdominal wall (Cullen's sign) or abdominal flank (Grey-Turner's sign) is an indicator of abdominal bleeding and is most associated with hemorrhagic pancreatitis.

Abdominal Examination

The abdominal examination may provide important clues regarding the source of biliary obstruction. The finding of an epigastric mass or palpation of an enlarged gallbladder (Courvoisier's sign) strongly suggests the presence of a periampullary tumor. The presence of lymphadenopathy may indicate metastatic spread of a tumor. Among patients from whom history is limited, the findings of abdominal scars should raise suspicion for prior disease and surgery.

Examining For Chronic Liver Disease

The physical examination of patients with suspected biliary obstruction should include assessments for the presence of ascites, hepatic encephalopathy, and spider angioma. Ascites, though possibly a manifestation of a widely metastatic tumor, is more commonly seen with liver disease. Metabolic encephalopathy and spider angioma are nonspecific findings, but when present, suggest that liver disease (rather than biliary obstruction) is responsible for cholestasis.

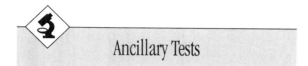

Ancillary Tests

Like clinical history and clinical examination, laboratory assessment is a useful aid for the identification of patients with potential biliary obstruction. Such tests can be especially helpful in distinguishing patients who have liver disease as a cause of jaundice from patients with bile duct obstruction. Table 20-2 lists several patterns of liver test abnormalities.

Transaminases

Serum aspartate aminotransferase (ALT) and serum alanine aminotransferase (AST) levels are sensitive, but nonspecific, markers of hepatocellular injury. They are often increased in all varieties of liver injuries. Biliary obstruction must be considered as a possible cause of relatively modest elevation of the transaminases. In contrast, marked elevations of the ALT or AST (higher that 500 IU/dl) are unusual with bile duct obstruction alone. While markedly elevated serum transaminases do not exclude biliary obstruction, they should prompt a search for other causes of liver injury as well.

Alkaline Phosphatase

The serum alkaline phosphatase is the most widely available blood test that, when compared to the transaminases, is relatively specific for cholestasis as opposed to other forms of liver injury. The protein itself is localized to the luminal side of the bile duct epithelium. Most assays for alkaline phosphatase measure the enzymatic activity not only from the biliary tree, but also from the enzymatic activity of alkaline phosphatases that are present in bone and intestine. Therefore, an elevated serum alkaline phosphatase is not specific for biliary injury. Other blood tests including heat fractionation of alkaline phosphatase, mea-

Table 20-2

Characteristic Patterns of Liver Test Abnormalities*

Test	Biliary Obstruction	Acute Hepatitis	Cirrhosis	Hemolysis or Gilbert's Syndrome
Albumin	Normal	Normal, low	Low, very low	Normal
ALT and AST	Mild, modest elevation	Modest, marked elevation	Normal, modest elevation	Normal
Bilirubin direct	High total and direct	Normal, high total and direct	Normal, high total and direct	High total, normal and direct
Alkaline phosphatase	Modest to severe elevation	Mild, modest elevation	Mild, modest elevation	Normal
Prothrombin time	Normal, elevated if chronic	Normal to marked prolongation	Mild to marked prolongation	Normal
Platelet count	Normal	Normal	Low	Normal

*While helpful, overlap of patterns prevents laboratory tests alone from being diagnostic.

surement of 5′-nucleotidase, or assay of γ-glutamyl transpeptidase (γ-GT) may further delineate the source of an elevated serum alkaline phosphatase, as γ-GT is more specific for biliary obstruction.

Bilirubin

The serum bilirubin is frequently, but not invariably, elevated with bile duct obstruction or cholestatic liver injury. Care must be taken to assess that an elevated serum bilirubin represents a true hepatic or biliary abnormality. Most laboratories routinely report the serum bilirubin as a total value that includes both conjugated and unconjugated bilirubin. In typical bilirubin metabolism, serum bilirubin is conjugated by the liver and is thus rendered soluble and filterable by the renal glomerula. This type of conjugated bilirubin is reported as direct bilirubin.

Several disorders, such as hemolysis and inherited deficiencies of glucuronyltransferase activity, can produce elevation in total bilirubin, but with the unconjugated bilirubin accounting for the major portion of the elevation. In these situations, an extensive evaluation for liver or biliary disease may not be required. It is therefore important to recognize the possibility of unconjugated hyperbilirubinemia. To evaluate patients with an elevated serum bilirubin but no other clinical, laboratory, or radiographic evidence of biliary obstruction (or liver disease), fractionation of direct and indirect bilirubin is the first step.

Prothrombin Time

Prothrombin time (PT) should be measured in all patients with biliary obstruction. Patients who have had prolonged biliary obstruction may become deficient in fat-soluble vitamins; the deficiency of vitamin K can lead to prolongation of the PT and a consequent bleeding tendency. For these patients without other liver failure, the parenteral administration of vitamin K can produce overnight correction of coagulopathy. The PT can also be elevated

because of primary hepatic insufficiency, disseminated intravascular coagulation, and pharmacologic anticoagulation. Assessment of the PT and platelet count may both help in understanding the underlying disease from which a patient is suffering and aid in realizing and minimizing the bleeding risks involved with invasive interventions.

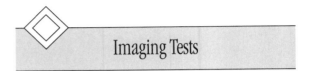

Imaging Tests

Multiple imaging modalities of the biliary tree are available. These imaging techniques represent the backbone for the diagnosis of biliary obstruction. The tests can be segregated into two fundamental categories: (a) noninvasive, and (b) invasive studies. Noninvasive tests include ultrasound, computer tomography (CT) scan, and magnetic resonance cholangiopancreatography (MRCP). The invasive studies include ERCP and percutaneous transhepatic cholangiography (PTC). As a general rule, the noninvasive tests are utilized for initial evaluation, with the invasive tests being reserved for situations when intervention to relieve obstruction is anticipated. Furthermore, the invasive tests are applied when suspicion for biliary obstruction persists, even if not demonstrated by the noninvasive methods. Table 20-3 lists the imaging tests, their advantages, and their limitations.

Noninvasive Biliary Imaging

The noninvasive tests have the advantages of ease of performance, minimal risk to patients, and low cost. Additionally, CT scanning, magnetic resonance imaging, and ultrasound offer the ability to evaluate not just the biliary tree but also the adjacent anatomy, including lymph nodes, liver, gallbladder, pancreas, kidneys, and, sometimes, intestines. This allows for evaluation for abscesses, metastases, and other structural or inflammatory problems. The drawbacks of the noninvasive tests

Table 20-3

Imaging of the Biliary Tree for Suspected Obstruction

TEST	STRENGTHS	WEAKNESSES
Ultrasound	• Noninvasive • High sensitivity for gallstones • Allows assessment of liver echotexture	• Study limited by bowel gas • Limited view of bile duct
Computed tomography	• Noninvasive • Sensitive for biliary dilation • Good visualization of surrounding anatomy	• Optimal study requires intravenous contrast • Fair detection of gallbladder stones
MRCP	• Noninvasive • Sensitive indicator of cholangitis	• Requires alert patient to follow breath holding instructions • Variable experience with the technique may limit quality of the study. Operator- and interpreter-dependent • Poorly tolerated by claustrophobic patients
ERCP	• Sensitive test for biliary pathology • Allows direct visualization of the papilla • Provides images of biliary and pancreatic ducts • Provides avenue for biliary drainage	• Invasive, typically requires sedation • Risks include pancreatitis, cholangitis, duodenal perforation, bleeding • Technical challenges can result in failed biliary cannulation and failed drainage
PTC	• Sensitive test for biliary pathology • Provides avenue for biliary drainage	• Invasive, typically requires sedation • Risks include bleeding, trauma to adjacent organs, bile peritonitis, biliary fistula • Internal-external drainage often required prior to internalization of drains. • Especially difficult in chronically strictured biliary tracts that can result from sclerosing cholangitis

MRCP, magnetic resonance cholangiopancreatography; ERCP, endoscopic retrograde cholangiopancreatography; PTC, percutaneous transhepatic cholangiography.

are their limited sensitivity for biliary obstruction, and their performance may delay invasive tests that are both more sensitive for biliary obstruction and allow an avenue for intervention.

ULTRASOUND

Ultrasound affords excellent visualization of the gallbladder and is the preferred imaging test for patients with right upper quadrant pain suggestive of biliary colic. In experienced hands, US has a better than a 95 percent sensitivity for the detection of cholelithiasis, though much less for choledocholithiasis. Additionally, US allows some evaluation of the intra- and extrahepatic bile ducts with a good sensitivity for detecting dilatation of these ducts. However, the distal common bile duct and part of the pancreas are often not visualized by ultrasound because of their retroperitoneal locations and the potential presence of overlying bowel gas. Ultrasound is also limited in the identification of choledocholithiasis with about a 50 to 75 percent sensitivity for the detection of common duct stones, and a much lower sensitivity for the detection of stones in the intrahepatic bile ducts.

COMPUTED TOMOGRAPHY

CT scan is evolving into the preferred noninvasive method for evaluation of the biliary tree. While less sensitive than US for the detection of gallbladder stones, it seems equally effective for the detection of biliary dilatation and bile duct stones. Because it is not adversely affected by the presence of air, CT scans afford some evaluation of the duodenum, pancreas, and retroperitoneal lymph nodes that may not be assessed with US.

To be maximally effective for detecting the presence of tumors, CT scans should be performed with administration of oral and intraveneous contrast. If endoscopic procedures are anticipated shortly after the performance of a CT, aqueous oral contrast (as opposed to thin barium) should be the oral contrast of choice. Clinicians should keep in mind that intravenous contrast agents are nephro-

toxic and should be avoided or used cautiously in patients at risk for renal injury.

MAGNETIC RESONANCE CHOLANGIOPANCREATOGRAPHY

Magnetic resonance cholangiopancreatography is a relatively new technique developed for imaging the biliary tree. This imaging modality when used to maximal effectiveness may be 95-percent sensitive for the detection of bile duct stones, which is similar to the sensitivity provided by invasive studies. However, MRCP remains a new technology. Therefore, the experience and equipment required for optimization of this study are not universally available. Cooperation with breath-holding is needed so this test may not be possible if patients are suffering from respiratory failure or if patients are obtunded. In summary, while MRCP holds great promise, it has yet to become universally established as a tool for assessing biliary obstruction.

Invasive Biliary Imaging and Nonsurgical Approaches to Biliary Drainage

The invasive tests have the advantages of being the most sensitive and specific tests for biliary obstruction. Furthermore, they offer the opportunity for simultaneous mechanical therapy to relieve biliary obstruction. Endoscopic retrograde cholangiopancreatography and PTC evolved virtually concurrently in the early 1970s. Since then the ability to diagnose biliary disease and to intervene on patients' behalf has grown tremendously. Still, the techniques are relatively new ones and this imposes some limitations. Other drawbacks are more obvious. Invasive tests can be uncomfortable and pose risks related both to the procedure itself in addition to the sedation that may be necessary. There is also the possibility for introduction of infection into a previously sterile biliary tree. Last, many biliary strictures are not technically amenable to therapy; this is especially true

Figure 20-2

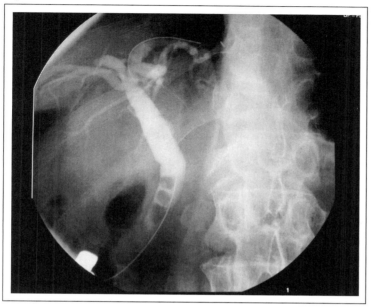

CBD stone: Cholangiogram reveals three stones in the distal common bile duct.

for multiple strictures and strictures of smaller (more proximal) bile ducts.

ENDOSCOPIC RETROGRADE CHOLANGIOPANCREATOGRAPHY

Endoscopic retrograde cholangiopancreatography is a combined endoscopic and radiographic procedure. The study is typically performed with sedated patients lying prone on a fluoroscopy table. A specialized endoscope designed for visualization and manipulation of the ampulla of Vater is advanced through the oropharynx and into the second portion of the duodenum. Once the papilla is localized, small cannulae are used to selectively gain access to the common bile duct or, if desired, the pancreatic duct. Though technically challenging, skilled endoscopists can achieve selective cannulation of the bile duct in 95 percent of patients.

Once cannulation of the desired duct is achieved, water-soluble contrast is injected under fluoroscopic observation. This technique allows identification of filling defects, such as stones (see Figure 20-2), and ductal irregularities, such as strictures (Figure 20-3). Specially designed electrocautery instruments that allow for incising and releasing the muscular portion of the biliary or pancreatic sphincters are utilized to perform sphincterotomy. Biliary sphincterotomy enhances the flow of bile through the papilla and improves access to the bile ducts. Additional endoscopic tools are available to aid in the extraction of bile duct stones and the dilation of biliary strictures.

At ERCP, the physician can aspirate bile for examination and obtain tissue samples from biliary strictures for histolopathology or cytology. Although useful, the sensitivity of these sampling techniques for diagnosing tumors is limited to about 60 percent. Finally, endoprostheses such as temporary plastic stents or permanent self-expanding metal stents can be positioned to provide biliary drainage. *Plastic stents* are relatively easy to place, exchange, and remove should they no longer be necessary. Unfortunately, they are prone to clogging from bacterial infection and the accumulation of bile duct sludge and mucus. *Metal stents* (while markedly more costly) typically have a longer patency than do their plastic counterparts. Tumor ingrowth can still lead to stent failure and, unlike plastic stents, metal stents cannot be routinely removed endoscopically.

In most cases, ERCP should be the first choice of the invasive diagnostic and therapeutic biliary imaging. However, ERCP has a few specific limitations. As previously mentioned, access to the bile duct can be difficult, especially when intestinal or biliary anatomy has been altered by mass effect or by previous foregut surgery. Endoscopic retrograde cholangiopancreatography is associated with a risk of procedure-related pancreatitis. The risk of pancreatitis varies from 2 to 20 percent, with the most important determinants of the risk being the indication for which the ERCP is performed and the presence or absence of biliary dilatation. The risk of procedure-related pancre-

atitis is lowest among patients with biliary dilatation and among those who undergo ERCP for pancreatic cancer or choledocholithiasis; the risk is highest for those with suspected sphincter of Oddi dysfunction. Typically, post-ERCP pancreatitis is mild and resolves within 2 to 3 days of bowel rest. However, on occasion post-ERCP pancreatitis can be severe with potential complications, including pancreatic necrosis and pseudocyst development. Common risks from sphincterotomy include duodenal perforation and bleeding that may complicate up to 1 percent of sphincterotomies.

PERCUTANEOUS TRANSHEPATIC CHOLANGIOGRAPHY

Percutaneous transhepatic cholangiography is performed by interventional radiologists with consciously sedated patients lying supine on a fluoroscopy table. A right-side approach is preferred, but an anterior approach can also be used if primary access to the left biliary tree is required.

Figure 20-3

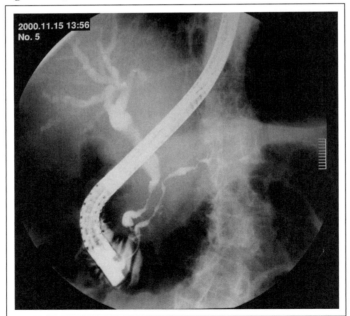

Stricture: Pancreatic mass causing a stricture in the pancreatic duct and intrapancreatic portion of the bile duct.

After local anesthesia, a flexible needle is advanced into the liver and access into the biliary tree is confirmed by the aspiration of bile. Once into the biliary tree, cholangiography and intervention can be performed.

Percutaneous transhepatic cholangiography is an important invasive biliary imaging tool. Like ERCP, PTC combines detailed imaging of the biliary tree and an opportunity for intervention. Unlike ERCP, PTC (by the nature of its percutaneous approach) may be considered to be somewhat more invasive and does not allow visualization of the papilla or imaging of the pancreatic duct. However, PTC does have a few advantages over ERCP. It is frequently successful when surgically altered intestinal anatomy places the papilla out of the reach of the ERCP scope. PTC drainage may also be preferred for the management of strictures proximal to the common hepatic duct, where endoscopic decompression is less successful.

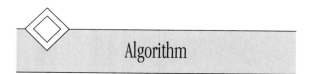

Algorithm

Much of the foundation of the management of biliary obstruction has been alluded to in the pre-vious sections of this chapter. There are a few principles that should be followed religiously. A clinician should consider the possibility of biliary obstruction in any patient with liver function test abnormalities. If these abnormalities are not easily explained by other pathology, testing for biliary obstruction needs to be pursued. An algorithm for the evaluation of such patients is shown in Figure 20-4.

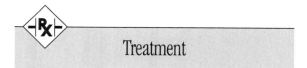

Treatment

Patients who have biliary obstruction or cholangitis might need to be resuscitated to treat dehydration, coagulopathy, and possible sepsis.

Antibiotics are a useful adjunct to therapy but, except in rare cases (where biliary drainage is technically unfeasible), they should never be considered as primary therapy without accompanying efforts to relieve any persistent biliary obstruction. In some instances, biliary obstruction can be self-limited, such as when a bile duct stone passes into the duodenum without intervention; still, in this situation, efforts should be pursued to assess for recurrent obstruction.

Resuscitation

The resuscitation of patients with suspected biliary obstruction follows general guidelines. Since these patients are frequently volume-depleted, efforts at intravenous rehydration may be invaluable. Also patients who are hypotensive from sepsis should be treated promptly with fluids, vasoconstricting agents, if needed, and antibiotics (see next section). Patients who are coagulopathic should receive parenterally administered vitamin K; however, if bleeding is present or if urgent procedures for decompression are necessary, fresh frozen plasma offers the advantage of more prompt correction of coagulopathy.

Antibiotics

There have been few studies to scientifically compare the utilities of different antibiotics to treat biliary tract infections. As a general rule, a broad-spectrum regimen with activity against gram-negative organisms and anaerobes is appropriate. Additional factors to consider include the secretion of various antibiotics into the bile. The few randomized studies suggest that the ureidopenicillins, including mezlocillin and piperacillin, might be good choices for the first-line management of bacterial biliary tract infections. Data (uncontrolled) support the utility of other antibiotics that may be equally or more effective. These include cephalosporins with activity against anaerobes, such as cefotetan or cefoperazone; monobactams, such as imipinem; and the quinolones.

Figure 20-4

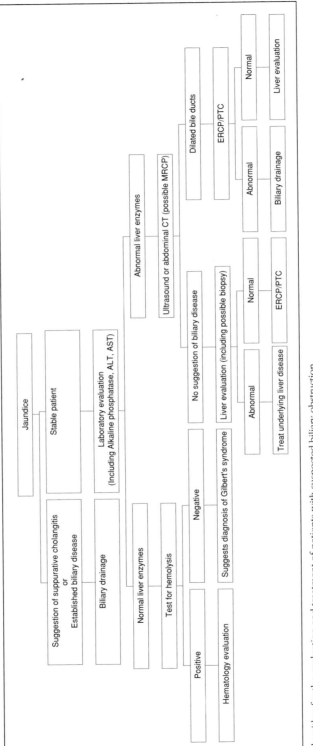

Algorithm for the evaluation and treatment of patients with suspected biliary obstruction.

Orally available antibiotics such as ciprofloxacin and amoxicillin or clavulanate may be useful in the outpatient management of patients who are recovering from biliary tract infections. Oral antibiotics may also be used to suppress cholangitis for patients among whom biliary drainage is not feasible. In this setting, however, recurrent episodes of cholangitis in an otherwise appropriate candidate become an indication for liver transplantation.

Biliary Drainage

A number of techniques, endoscopic, radiological, and surgical, are available to treat biliary obstruction. The unifying feature in all of these groups is that intensive and specialized training is required. The selection of the drainage approach should be based upon the advantages of the specific procedures as well as the available expertise.

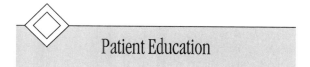

Patient Education

The role of patient education in the prevention of biliary obstruction is limited. At-risk patients, especially those with indwelling stents or biliary stricturing diseases, should be taught to recognize the signs and symptoms of biliary obstruction (stent failure) and early cholangitis. If symptoms occur, patients should seek medical attention immediately

In truth, there is little patients can do to prevent or self-manage biliary obstruction. Prompt recognition and expeditious intervention are essential. When patients with indwelling stents, biliary malignancy, or PSC experience fevers (even low grade), cholangitis should be presumed until testing excludes the diagnosis. The physician should consider the possibility of biliary obstruction in almost all patients as a part of the differential of liver test abnormalities.

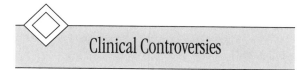

Common Clinical Errors

The most frequent errors in management are the failure to recognize and to treat biliary obstruction. Biliary obstruction must be considered in the differential diagnosis of almost any patient with even mildly abnormal liver enzymes. A high index of suspicion should be maintained for biliary obstruction and, when present, obstruction should be promptly treated. It is important that consultants appropriately experienced in the treatment of biliary obstruction be involved early in the management.

Clinical Controversies

As ERCP and PTC are new and rapidly evolving therapeutic modalities, their appropriate role in the management of patients is an expanding one. Controversy is prone to develop in any such situation.

One area of controversy in the diagnosis and management of biliary obstruction is the timing of ERCP in relation to cholecystectomy when common bile duct stones might be present. In some centers, routine preoperative ERCP is still used. In others, MRCP may become a more widely used tool. A third approach is the use of intraoperative cholangiography and, if stones are present, ERCP is performed following the operation.

The role of biliary drainage prior to surgery for malignant bile duct strictures is also controversial. Cholestasis has systemic implications and may worsen surgical outcomes. Therefore, some surgeons prefer the biliary drainage be achieved by ERCP or PTC prior to surgical treatment of either benign or malignant biliary obstruction. However, several studies that evaluated PTC suggest that the risks of preoperative biliary drainage do not justify the modest improvement in surgical outcomes. Other studies implied an increased risk of postoperative cholangitis among patients with bile duct strictures located in the proximal biliary tree, where endoscopic drainage is least possible. Whether preoperative endoscopic drainage in patients with malignant biliary obstruction more distal in the bile ducts is appropriate remains unresolved.

One final area of controversy that may deserve mentioning here is the application of permanent metal stents for benign biliary strictures. Typically, metal stents are reserved for the palliative treatment of patients with limited life expectancy because of unresectable tumors. With metal stents, obstruction is often the result of tumor ingrowth into the stent. As this ingrowth does not occur in benign strictures, the applicability of metal stents in this situation might evolve.

Bibliography

Choudari CP, Fodel E, Gottlieb K, et al: Therapeutic biliary endoscopy. *Endoscopy* 30:163, 1998.

Cvetkovski B, Gerdes H, Kurtz RC: Outpatient therapeutic ERCP with endobiliary stent placement for malignant common bile duct obstruction. *Gastrointest Endosc* 50:63, 1999.

England RE, Martin DF: Endoscopic and percutaneous intervention in malignant obstructive jaundice. *Cardiovasc Intervent Radiol* 19:381, 1996.

Freeman ML, Nelson DB, Sherman S: Complications of endoscopic biliary sphincterotomy. *N Engl J Med* 335:909, 1996.

Hochwald SN, Burke EC, Jarnagin WR: Association of preoperative biliary stenting with increased postoperative infectious complications in proximal cholangiocarcinoma. *Arch Surg* 134:261, 1999.

Johnston DE, Kaplan MM: Pathogenesis and treatment of gallstones. *N Engl J Med* 328:412-421, 1993.

Kadakia SC: Biliary tract emergencies: Acute cholecystitis, acute cholangitis and acute pancreatitis. *Med Clin North Am* 77:1015, 1993.

Kamath PS: Clinical approach to the patient with abnormal liver test results. *Mayo Clin Proc* 71:1089, 1996.

Lee YM, Kaplan MK: Primary sclerosing cholangitis. *N Engl J Med* 332:924, 1995.

Lehman GA, Sherman S: Sphincter of Oddi dysfunction. *Int J Pancreatol* 20:11, 1996.

Men S, Hekimogly, Pinar A, et al: Palliation of malignant obstructive jaundice: Use of self-expandable metal stents. *Acta Radiol* 37:259, 1996.

Mosely RH: Evaluation of abnormal liver function tests. *Med Clin North Am* 80:887, 1996.

Rosenthal RJ, Rossi RL, Martin RF: Options and strategies for the management of choledocholithiasis. *World J Surg* 22:1125, 1998.

Saini S: Imaging the hepatobiliary tract. *N Engl J Med* 336:1889, 1997.

Schoeman MN, Huibregtse K: Pancreatic and ampullary carcinoma. *Gastrointest Endosc Clin N Am* 5:217, 1995.

Shimizu S, Kutsumi H, Fujimoto S, et al: Diagnostic endoscopic retrograde cholangiopancreatography. *Endoscopy* 30:158, 1998.

Sinanan MN: Acute cholangitis. *Infect Dis Clin North Am* 6: 571, 1992.

Soehendra N, Binmoeller KF, Seifert H, et al: *Therapeutic Endoscopy: Color Atlas of Operative Techniques for the Gastrointestinal Tract*. Stuttgart, Thieme, 1998.

Srivastava ED, Mayberry JF: Pyogenic liver abscesses: A review of etiology, diagnosis, and intervention. *Dig Dis* 8:287, 1990.

Strasberg SM, Hertl M, Soper NJ: An analysis of the problem of biliary injury during laparoscopic cholecystectomy. *J Am Coll Surg* 180:101, 1995.

Van Thiel DH, Fagiuoli S, Wright HI, et al: Biliary complications of liver transplantation. *Gastrointest Endosc* 39:455, 1993.

Vitale GC, George M, McIntyre K, et al: Endoscopic management of benign and malignant biliary strictures. *Am J Surg* 171:553, 1996.

Voegeli DR, Crummy AB, Weese JL: Percutaneous transhepatic cholangiography, drainage, and biopsy in patient with malignant biliary obstruction. *Am J Surg* 150:243, 1985.

Westphal JF, Brogard JM: Biliary tract infections: A guide to drug treatment. *Drugs* 57:81, 1999.

Yeo CJ, Pitt HA, Cameron JL: Cholangiocarcinoma. *Surg Clin North Am* 70:1429, 1990.

Yu JL, Ljungh A: Infections associated with biliary drains. *Scand J Gastroenterol* 31:625, 1996.

Index

Page numbers followed by *t* indicate tables; page numbers followed by *f* indicate figures.